A HISTORY

OF

EPIDEMICS IN BRITAIN.

BY

CHARLES CREIGHTON, M.A., M.D.,

FORMERLY DEMONSTRATOR OF ANATOMY IN THE UNIVERSITY OF CAMBRIDGE.

VOLUME II.

From the Extinction of Plague to the present time.

CAMBRIDGE:

AT THE UNIVERSITY PRESS.

1894

 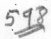

A HISTORY

OF

EPIDEMICS IN BRITAIN.

𝕷onðon: C. J. CLAY AND SONS,
CAMBRIDGE UNIVERSITY PRESS WAREHOUSE,
AVE MARIA LANE.

AND

H. K. LEWIS,
136, GOWER STREET, W.C.

𝕮ambriðge: DEIGHTON, BELL AND CO.
𝕷eipჳig: F. A. BROCKHAUS.
𝕹ew 𝕪ork: MACMILLAN AND CO.

Cambridge:

PRINTED BY C. J. CLAY, M.A. AND SONS,

AT THE UNIVERSITY PRESS.

PREFACE.

THIS volume is the continuation of 'A History of Epidemics in Britain from A.D. 664 to the Extinction of Plague' (which was published three years ago), and is the completion of the history to the present time. The two volumes may be referred to conveniently as the first and second of a 'History of Epidemics in Britain.' In adhering to the plan of a systematic history instead of annals I have encountered more difficulties in the second volume than in the first. In the earlier period the predominant infection was Plague, which was not only of so uniform a type as to give no trouble, in the nosological sense, but was often so dramatic in its occasions and so enormous in its effects as to make a fitting historical theme. With its disappearance after 1666, the field is seen after a time to be occupied by a numerous brood of fevers, anginas and other infections, which are not always easy to identify according to modern definitions, and were recorded by writers of the time, for example Wintringham, in so dry or abstract a manner and with so little of human interest as to make but tedious reading in an almost obsolete phraseology. Descriptions of the fevers of those times, under the various names of synochus, synocha, nervous, putrid, miliary, remittent, comatose, and the like, have been introduced into the chapter on Continued Fevers so as to show their generic as well as their differential character; but a not less important purpose of the chapter has been to illustrate the condition of the working classes, the unwholesomeness of towns, London in particular, the state of the gaols and of the navy, the seasons of dearth, the

times of war-prices or of depressed trade, and all other vicissitudes of well-being, of which the amount of Typhus and Relapsing Fever has always been a curiously correct index. It is in this chapter that the epidemiology comes into closest contact with social and economic history. In the special chapter for Ireland the association is so close, and so uniform over a long period, that the history may seem at times to lose its distinctively medical character.

As the two first chapters are pervaded by social and economic history, so each of the others will be found to have one or more points of distinctive interest besides the strictly professional. Smallpox is perhaps the most suitable of all the subjects in this volume to be exhibited in a continuous view, from the epidemics of it in London in the first Stuart reigns to the statistics of last year. While it shares with Plague the merit, from a historical point of view, of being always the same definite item in the bills of mortality, it can be shown to have experienced, in the course of two centuries and a half, changes in its incidence upon the classes in the community, upon the several age-periods and upon town and country, as well as a very marked change relatively to measles and scarlatina among the infective scourges of infancy and childhood. For certain reasons Smallpox has been the most favoured infectious disease, having claimed an altogether disproportionate share of interest at one time with Inoculation, at another time with Vaccination. The history of the former practice, which is the precedent for, or source of, a whole new ambitious scheme of prophylaxis in the infectious diseases of men and brutes, has been given minutely. The latter practice, which is a radical innovation inasmuch as it affects to prevent one disease by the inoculation of another, has been assigned as much space in the chapter on Smallpox as it seems to me to deserve. Measles and Whooping-cough are historically interesting, in that they seem to have become relatively more prominent among the infantile causes of death in proportion as the public health has improved. Whooping-cough is now left to head the list of its class by the shrinkage of the others. It is in the statistics of Measles and

Whooping-cough that the principle of population comes most into view. The scientific interest of Scarlatina and Diphtheria is mainly that of new, or at least very intermittent, species. Towards the middle of the 18th century there emerges an epidemic sickness new to that age, in which were probably contained the two modern types of Scarlet Fever and Diphtheria more or less clearly differentiated. The subsequent history of each has been remarkable: for a whole generation Scarlatina could prove itself a mild infection causing relatively few deaths, to become in the generation next following the greatest scourge of childhood; for two whole generations Diphtheria had disappeared from the observation of all but a few medical men, to emerge suddenly in its modern form about the years 1856–59.

The history of Dysentery, as told by the younger Heberden, has been a favourite instance of the steady decrease of a disease in London during the 18th century. I have shown the error in this, and at the same time have proved from the London bills of mortality of the 17th and 18th centuries that Infantile Diarrhoea, which is now one of the most important causes of death in some of the great manufacturing and shipping towns, was formerly still more deadly to the infancy of the capital in a hot summer or autumn. Asiatic Cholera brings us back, at the end of the history, to the same great problem which the Black Death of the 14th century raised near the beginning of it, namely, the importation of the seeds of pestilence from some remote country, and their dependence for vitality or effectiveness in the new soil upon certain favouring conditions, which sanitary science has now happily in its power to withhold. I have left Influenza to be mentioned last. Its place is indeed unique among epidemic diseases; it is the oldest and most obdurate of all the problems in epidemiology. The only piece of speculation in this volume will be found in the five-and-twenty pages which follow the narrative of the various historical Influenzas; it is purely tentative, exhibiting rather the *disjecta membra* of a theory than a compact and finished hypothesis. If there is any new light thrown upon the subject, or new point of view opened, it is in

bringing forward in the same context the strangely neglected history of Epidemic Agues.

Other subjects than those which occupy the nine chapters of this volume might have been brought into a history of epidemics, such as Mumps, Chickenpox and German Measles, Sibbens and Button Scurvy, together with certain ordinary maladies which become epidemical at times, such as Pneumonia, Erysipelas, Quinsy, Jaundice, Boils and some skin-diseases. While none of these are without pathological interest, they do not lend themselves readily to the plan of this book ; they could hardly have been included except in an appendix of *miscellanea curiosa*, and I have preferred to leave them out altogether. It has been found necessary, also, to discontinue the history of Yellow Fever in the West Indian and North American colonies, which was begun in the former volume.

I have, unfortunately for my own labour, very few acknowledgements to make of help from the writings of earlier workers in the same field. My chief obligation is to the late Dr Murchison's historical introduction to his 'Continued Fevers of Great Britain.' I ought also to mention Dr Robert Willan's summary of the throat-distempers of the 18th century, in his 'Cutaneous Diseases' of 1808, and the miscellaneous extracts relating to Irish epidemics which are appended in a chronological table to Sir W. R. Wilde's report as Census Commissioner for Ireland. For the more recent history, much use has naturally been made of the medical reports compiled for the public service, especially the statistical.

September, 1894.

CONTENTS.

CHAPTER I.

TYPHUS AND OTHER CONTINUED FEVERS.

CHAPTER II.

FEVER AND DYSENTERY IN IRELAND.

CHAPTER III.

INFLUENZAS AND EPIDEMIC AGUES.

CHAPTER IV.

SMALLPOX.

CHAPTER V.

MEASLES.

CHAPTER VI.

WHOOPING-COUGH.

CHAPTER VII.

SCARLATINA AND DIPHTHERIA.

CHAPTER VIII.

INFANTILE DIARRHOEA, CHOLERA NOSTRAS, AND DYSENTERY.

CHAPTER IX.

ASIATIC CHOLERA.

CHAPTER I.

TYPHUS AND OTHER CONTINUED FEVERS.

IT was remarked by Dr James Lind, in 1761, that a judicious synopsis of the writings on fevers, in a chronological sense, would be a valuable book: it would bring to light, he was fain to expect, treasures of knowledge; "and perhaps the influence of a favourite opinion, or of a preconceived fancy, on the writings of some even of our best instructors, such as Sydenham and Morton, would more clearly be perceived[1]." Lind himself was the person to have delivered such a history and criticism. He was near enough to the 17th century writers on fevers to have entered correctly into their points of view; while so far as concerned the detection of theoretical bias or preconceived fancies, he had shown himself a master of the art in his famous satire upon the "scorbutic constitution," a verbal or mythical construction which had been in great vogue for a century and a half, and was still current, at the moment when Lind destroyed it, in the writings of Boerhaave and Haller. A judicious historical view of the English writings on fevers, such as this 18th century critic desired to see, may now be thought superfluous. The theories, the indications for treatment, the medical terms, have passed away and become the mere objects of a learned curiosity. But the actual history of the old fevers, of their kinds, their epidemic prevalence, their incidence upon rich or poor, upon children or adults, their fatality, their contagiousness, their connexion with the seasons and other vicissitudes of the people—all this is something more than curious.

[1] James Lind, M.D., *Two Papers on Fevers and Infection*. Lond. 1763, p. 79.

C. II.

I

Unfortunately for the historian of diseases, he has to look for the realities amidst the " favourite opinions " or the " preconceived fancies " of contemporary medical writers. Statements which at first sight appear to be observations of matters of fact are found to be merely the necessary truths or verbal constructions of some doctrine. One great doctrine of the 17th and 18th centuries was that of obstructions : in this doctrine, as applied to fevers, obstructions of the mesentery were made of central importance ; the obstructions of the mesentery extended to its lymphatic glands ; so that we come at length, in a mere theoretical inference, to something not unlike the real morbid anatomy of enteric fever. Another great doctrine of the time, specially applied by Willis to fevers, was that of fermentations and acrimonies. " This ferment," says a Lyons disciple of Willis in 1682, " has its seat in the glandules of the velvet coat of the stomach and intestines described by Monsieur Payer[1]." But the Lyons physician is writing all the while of the fevers that have always been common in the Dombes and Bresse, namely intermittents ; the tertian, double tertian, quotidian, quartan, or double quartan paroxysm arises, he says, from the coagulation of the humours by the ferment which has its seat in the glandules described by M. Payer, even as acids cause a coagulation in milk, the paroxysm of ague continuing, " until this sharp chyle be dissipated and driven out by the sweat or insensible perspiration." The lymphatic follicles of the intestine known by the name of Payer, or Peyer, were then the latest anatomical and physiological novelty, and were chosen, on theoretical grounds, as the seat of fermentation or febrile action in agues. On the ground of actual observation they were found about a century and a half after to be the seat of morbid action in typhoid fever.

While there are such pitfalls for the historian in identifying the several species of fevers in former times, there are other difficulties of interpretation which concern the varieties of a continued fever, or its changes of type from generation to generation. Is change of type a reality or a fiction ? And, if a reality, did it depend at all upon the use or abuse of a certain regimen or treatment, such as blooding and lowering, or heating and corroborating ? A pupil of Cullen, who wrote his thesis in

[1] *Observations on Fevers and Febrifuges.* Made English from the French of M. Spon. London, 1682.

1782 upon the interesting topic of the change in fevers since the time of Sydenham[1], inferred that the great physician of the Restoration could not have had to treat the low, putrid or nervous fevers of the middle and latter part of the 18th century, otherwise he would not have resorted so regularly to blood-letting, a practice which was out of vogue in continued fevers at the time when the thesis was written, as well as for a good many years before and after. Fevers, it was argued, had undergone a radical change since the time of Sydenham, in correspondence with many changes in diet, beverages and creature comforts, such as the greatly increased use of tea, coffee and tobacco, and of potatoes or other vegetables in the diet, changes also in the proportion of urban to rural population, in the use of carriages, and in many other things incident to the progressive softening of manners. In due time the low, putrid, nervous type of typhus fever, which is so much in evidence in the second half of the 18th century, ceased to be recorded, an inflammatory type, or a fever of strong reaction, taking its place; so that Bateman, of London, writing in 1818, said: "The putrid pestilential fevers of the preceding age have been succeeded by the milder forms of infectious fever which we now witness"; while Armstrong, Clutterbuck, and others, who had revived the practice of blood-letting in fevers shortly before the epidemic of 1817–18, claimed the comparatively slight fatality and short duration of the common fever of the time as an effect of the treatment. After 1831, typhus again became low, depressed, spotted, not admitting of the lancet; on which occasion the doctrine of "change of type" was debated in the form that the older generation of practitioners still remember.

Thus the task of the historian, whose first duty is to ascertain, if he can, the actual matters of fact, or the realities, in their sequence or chronological order, is made especially difficult, in the chapter on continued fevers, by the contemporary in-fluence of theoretical pathology or "a preconceived fancy," by the ascription of modifying effects to treatment, whether cooling or heating, lowering or supporting, and, most of all, by the absence of that more exact method which distinguishes the records of fever in our own time. Nor can it be said that the work of historical research has been made easier in all respects, by the

[1] James Hutchinson, M.D., *De Mutatione Febrium e tempore Sydenhami, etc.* Edin. 1782. Thesis.

exact discrimination and perfected diagnosis to which we are accustomed in present-day fevers. In the years between 1840 and 1850, the three grand types of fever then existing in Britain, namely, spotted typhus, enteric, and relapsing fever, were at length so clearly distinguished, defined and described that no one remained in doubt or confusion. Thereupon arose the presumption that these had always been the forms of continued fever in Britain, and that the same fevers, presumably in the same relative proportions to each other, might have been left on record by the physicians of former generations, if they had used the modern exactness and minuteness in observing both clinical history and anatomical state, which were seen at their best in Sir William Jenner. It would simplify history, indeed it would make history superfluous, if that were really the case. There are many reasons for believing that it was not the case. As Sydenham looked forward to his successors having experiences that he never had, so we may credit Sydenham with having really seen things which we never see, not even those of us who saw the last epidemics of relapsing fever and typhus. It is due to him, and to his contemporaries and nearest successors, to reciprocate the spirit in which he concludes the general chapter on epidemics prefatory to his annual constitutions from 1661 to 1676:

> "I am far from taking upon myself the credit of exhausting my subject in the present observations. It is highly probable that I may fail even in the full enumeration of the epidemics. Still less do I warrant that the diseases which during the years in question have succeeded each other in the sequence about to be exhibited shall remain the same in all future years. One thing most especially do I aim at. It is my wish to state how things have gone lately; how they have been in this country, and how they have been in this the city which we live in. The observations of some years form my ground-work. It is thus that I would add my mite, such as it is, towards the foundation of a work that, in my humble judgment, shall be beneficial to the human race. Posterity will complete it, since to them it shall be given to take the full view of the whole cycle of epidemics in their mutual sequences for years yet to come[1]."

The epidemic fever of 1661, according to Willis.

On the very threshold of the period at which the history is resumed in this volume, we find a minute account by Willis of an epidemic in the year 1661, which at once raises the question whether a certain species of infectious fever did really exist at

---

[1] *Observationes Medicae*, 3rd ed. 1676, I. 2. § 23. English by R. G. Latham, M.D.

that time which exists no longer, or whether Willis described as "a fever of the brain and nervous stock" what we now call enteric fever. Willis's fever corresponds in every respect to the worm fever, the comatose fever, the remittent fever of children, the acute fever with dumbness, the convulsive fever, which was often recorded by the medical annalists and other systematic observers as late as the beginning of the 19th century[1]. It ceased at length to be recorded or described, and it has been supposed that it was really the infantile or children's part of enteric fever, which had occurred in former times as now[2]. The epidemic fever which Willis saw in the summer of 1661, after a clear interval of two years from the great epidemics of agues, with influenzas, in 1657–59, is called by him "a certain irregular and unaccustomed fever[3]." It was not, however, new to him altogether; for he had seen the same type, and kept notes of the cases, in a particular household at Oxford in 1655, as well as on other occasions. It was an epidemical fever "chiefly infestous to the brain and nervous stock." It raged mostly among children and youths, and was wont to affect them with a long and, as it were, a chronical sickness. When it attacked the old or middle-aged, which was more rarely, it did sooner and more certainly kill. It ran through whole families, not only in Oxford and the neighbouring parts, "but in the countries at a great distance, as I heard from physicians dwelling in other places." Among those other witnesses, we shall call Sydenham; but meanwhile let us hear Willis, whose account is the fullest and least warped by theory.

Its approach was insidious and scarce perceived, with no immoderate heat or sharp thirst, but producing at length great debility and languishing, loss of appetite and loathing. Within eight days there were brain symptoms— heavy vertigo, tingling of the ears, often great tumult and perturbation of the brain. Instead of phrensy, there might be deep stupidity or insensibility; children lay sometimes a whole month without taking any notice of the bystanders, and with an involuntary flux of their excrements; or there might be frequent delirium, and constantly absurd and incongruous chimaeras in their sleep. But in men a fury, and often-times deadly phrensy, did succeed. If, however, neither stupidity nor great distraction did fall upon them, swimmings in the head, convulsive movements, with convulsions of the

[1] Reports of Whitehaven Dispensary (Dixon) and of Nottingham General Hospital (Clarke), cited in the sequel.

[2] Rilliet, *De la Fièvre Typhoïde chez les Enfants*, Thèse, Paris, 2 *Janv.* 1840, based on 61 cases; West, *Diseases of Infancy and Childhood*, 3rd ed. Lond. 1854.

[3] "Febris epidemicae cerebro et nervoso generi potissimum infestae, anno 1661 increbescentis descriptio," in *Pathologia Cerebri*, Cap. VIII, "De Spasmis universalibus qui in febribus malignis" etc., Eng. transl. p. 51.

members and leaping up of the tendons did grievously infest them. In almost all, there were loose and stinking motions, now yellow, now thin and serous ; vomiting was unusual ; the urine deep red. The sufferers in this prolonged sickness wasted to a skeleton, with no great heat or evacuations to account for the wasting. Some, at the end of the disease, had a severe catarrh. In others, with little infection of the head, soon after the beginning of the fever a cruel cough and a stinking spittle, with a consumptive disposition, grew upon them, and seemed to throw them suddenly into a phthisis, from which, however, they recovered often beyond hope. In some there were swellings of the glands near the hinder part of the neck, which ripened and broke, and gave out a thin stinking ictor for a long time. "I have also seen watery pustules excited in other parts of the body, which passed into hollow ulcers, and hardly curable. Sometimes little spots and *petechiales* appeared here and there." But none of the spots were broad and livid, nor were there many malignant spots.

Willis then gives several cases clinically, in his usual manner. The first is of a strong and lively young man, who was sick above two months and seemed near death, but began to mend and took six weeks to recover, sweating every night or every other night of his convalescent period. The second case, aged twelve, was restored to health in a month. Numbers three and four were children of a nobleman, who both died, the convulsive type being strongly marked ; one of the two was examined after death, and found to have several sections of the small intestine telescoped, but all the abdominal viscera free from disease[1], the lungs engorged, the vessels of the brain full, much water in the sub-arachnoid space, and more than half a pint in the lateral ventricles.

In farther illustration of this type of fever, epidemic in 1661, Willis goes back to his notes of a sporadic outbreak of what he thinks was the same disease in a certain family at Oxford in the winter of 1653-4[2] : "yea I remember that sometime past very many laboured with such a fever." In the family in question, five children took the fever one after another during a space of four months, two of the cases proving fatal ; the domestics also took it, and some strangers who came in to help them, "the evil being propagated by contagion." The cases in the children are fully recorded[3], the following being some of the symptoms :

In case 1, aged seven, the illness began at the end of December, 1653 (or 1655): there were contractions of the wrist tendons, red spots like flea-bites on his neck and other parts, drowsiness, and involuntary passage of the excrements. At the end of a fortnight, a flux set in and lasted for four days ; next, after that, a whitish crust or scurf, as it were chalky, began to spread over the whole cavity of his mouth and throat, which being often in a day wiped away, presently broke forth anew. He mended a little, but had paralysis of his throat and pharynx, was reduced to a living skeleton, but at length got well.

Case 2, a brother, aged nine, had frequent loose and highly putrid motions on the eleventh day ; and next day, the flux having ceased, the most severe colic, so that he lay crying out day and night, his belly swollen and hard as a drum, until, on the 24th day, he died in an agony of convulsions.

Case 3, a brother, aged 11, was taken with similar symptoms on the 13th February, and died on the 13th day.

---

[1] "Itaque ventrem inferiorem primo aperiens, viscera omnia in eo contenta satis sana et sarte tecta inveni"—the small intestine being telescoped in several places.

[2] Elsewhere he says the first case of the series was "circa solstitium hyemale anno 1655."

[3] *De Febribus*, chapter "De febribus pestilentibus."

Case 4, a sister, was taken ill in March, with less marked symptoms, and recovered slowly, having had no manifest crisis.

Case 5, a boy of the same family, and the youngest, fell ill about the same time as No. 4, and after the like manner, "who yet, a looseness arising naturally of itself, for many days voiding choleric and greenish stuff, was easily cured."

Then comes a general reference to the domestics and visitors, who fell sick of the same and all recovered.

The prolonged series of cases in the household of this "venerable man" appears to have made a great impression upon Willis, as something new in his experience, as well as in the experience of several other physicians who gave their services. That it was malignant he considers proved "ex contagio, pernicie, macularum pulicularum apparentia, multisque aliis indiciis." He adds that he had seen the same disease sporadically at other times; and again "I remember that formerly several laboured under such a fever." Those cases were all previous to the general prevalence of the fever which he identifies with them in the summer of 1661, under the name of a "fever of the brain and spinal cord."

The signs given by Willis are as nearly as may be the signs of infantile remittent fever, or worm fever, or febris synochus puerorum, or hectica infantilis, or febris lenta infantum, or an acute fever with dumbness, of which perhaps the first systematic account in this country was given by Dr William Butter of Lower Grosvenor Street, in 1782[1]. It is, he says, both a sporadical and an epidemical disease, "and when epidemical it is also contagious." The age for it is from birth up to puberty; but "similar symptoms are often observed in the disorders of adults." Morton, writing in 1692–94, clearly points to the same fever under the name of worm fever (febris verminosa). He adds it at the very end of his scheme of fevers, as if in an appendix, having been unable to find a place for it in any of his categories owing to its varying forms—hectic, acute, intermittent, continued, συνεχής, inflammatory, but for the most part colliquative or σύνοχος, "and malignant according to the varying degrees of the venomous miasm causing it[2]." Butter also recognizes its varying types: it has many symptoms, but they seldom all occur in the same case; there are three main varieties—the acute, lasting from eight to ten days up to two or three weeks;

---

[1] *Treatise on the Infantile Remittent Fever.* London, 1782.
[2] *Pyretologia*, 2 vols. Lond. 1692—94, i. 68, at the end of "Synopsis Febrium":— "Febris verminosa, quae nulli e specibus memoratis praecisé determinari potest."

the slow, lasting two or three months; and the low, lasting a month or six weeks. The slow form, he says, is only sporadic; the low is only epidemic, and is never seen but when the acute is also epidemical; it is rare in comparison with the latter, and not observed at all except in certain of the epidemical seasons. Waiving the question whether the remittent fever of children, thus systematically described, was not a composite group of maladies, of which enteric fever of children was one, we can hardly doubt that Willis found a distinctive uniform type in the epidemic of 1661, in Oxford as he saw it himself, in other parts of England by report. It had symptoms which were not quite clearly those of enteric fever: spots, like fleabites, on the neck and other parts, swelling and suppuration of the glands in the hinder part of the neck, effusion of fluid on the brain and in the lateral ventricles, and the intestine free from disease[1].

Confirming Willis's account for Oxford, is the case of Roger North, when a boy at Bury St Edmunds Free School in 1661, as related by himself in his 'Autobiography[2].' Being then "very young and small," after a year at school he had "an acute fever, which endangered a consumption." Elsewhere he attributes his bad memory with "confusion and disorder of thought," to that "cruel fit of sickness I had when young, wherein, I am told, life was despaired of, and it was thought part of me was dead; and I can recollect that warm cloths were applied, which could be for no other reason, because I had not gripes which commonly calls for that application." That "great violence of nature," while it had impaired his mental faculties, had sapped his bodily vigour somewhat also, of which he gives a singular illustration.

This special prevalence of epidemic fevers in the summer and autumn of 1661 is noticed also by the London diarists.

Evelyn says that the autumn of 1661 was exceedingly sickly and wet[3]. Pepys has several entries of fever[4]. On 2 July, 1661: "Mr Saml. Crewe died of the spotted fever." On 16 August: "At the [Navy] Office all the morning, though little to do;

[1] Häser gives a reference to an essay in which Willis's fever of 1661 is compared to enteric fever: C. M. W. Rietschel, *Epidemia anni* 1661 *a Willisio et febris nervosa lenta ab Huxhamio descriptae, etc. cum typho abdominali nostro tempore obvio comparantur.* Lips. 1861. Not having found this essay, I cannot say on what grounds the comparison is made.
[2] *Lives of the Norths.* New ed. by Jessopp. 3 vols. 1890, iii. 8, 21.
[3] *Diary of John Evelyn, Esq., F.R.S.,* 1641—1706, under the date of 18 Sept.
[4] *Diary of Samuel Pepys, Esq., F.R.S.,* 1659—69.

because all our clerks are gone to the burial of Tom Whitton, one of our Controller's clerks, a very ingenious and a likely young man to live as any in the office. But it is such a sickly time both in the city and country everywhere (of a sort of fever) that never was heard of almost, unless it was in a plague-time. Among others the famous Tom Fuller [of the 'Worthies of England'] is dead of it; and Dr Nichols [Nicholas], Dean of St Paul's; and my Lord General Monk is very dangerously ill." On 31 August: "The season very sickly everywhere of strange and fatal fevers." On 15 January, 1662: "Hitherto summer weather, both as to warmth and every other thing, just as if it were the middle of May or June, which do threaten a plague (as all men think) to follow; for so it was almost the last winter, and the whole year after hath been a very sickly time to this day."

The great medical authority of the time is Sydenham. His accounts of the seasons and reigning diseases of London extend from 1661 to 1686, so that they begin with the year for which Willis described the epidemic fever "chiefly infestous to the brain and nervous stock," popularly called the new disease. But Sydenham did not describe the epidemic in the same objective way that Willis did. He records a series of "epidemic constitutions of the air," the particular constitution of each year being named from the epidemic malady that seemed to him to dominate it most. It was, perhaps, because it had to conform to Sydenham's "preconceived fancy," as Lind said, that his account of the dominant type of fever in 1661 differs somewhat from that given by Willis.

Sydenham's epidemic Constitutions.

Sydenham adopted the epidemic constitutions from Hippocrates, as he did much else in his method and practice. In the first and third books of the 'Epidemics,' Hippocrates describes three successive seasons and their reigning diseases in the island of Thasos, as well as a fourth plague-constitution which agrees exactly with the facts of the plague of Athens as described by Thucydides. The Greek term translated "constitution" is κατάστασις, which means literally a settling, appointing, ordaining, and in the epidemiological sense means the type of reigning disease as settled by the season. The method of Hippocrates is first to give an account of the weather—the winds,

the rains, the temperature and the like,—and then to describe the diseases of the seasons[1]. Sydenham followed his model with remarkable closeness. The great plague of London has almost the same place in his series of years that the plague-constitution, the fourth in order, has in that of Hippocrates. It looks, indeed, as if Sydenham had begun with the year 1661, more for the purpose of having several constitutions preceding that of the plague than because he had any full observations of his own to record previous to 1665. He is also much influenced by the example of Hippocrates in giving prominence to the intermittent type of fevers. It was remarked by one of our best 18th century epidemiologists, Rogers of Cork, and with special reference to Sydenham's " intermittent constitutions," that fevers proper to the climate of Thasos were not likely to be identified in or near London excepted by a forced construction.

Sydenham's Constitutions.

	Constitutions	Total deaths in London	Plague	Fever and Spotted Fever	Small-pox	Measles	Griping in the Guts
1661	"Intermittent" con-	16,665	20	3,490	1,246	188	1,061
1662	stitution: with a con-	13,664	12	2,601	768	20	835
1663	tinued fever through-	12,741	9	2,107	411	42	866
1664	out.	15,453	5	2,258	1,233	311	1,146
1665	Constitution of plague	97,306	68,596	5,257	655	7	1,288
1666	and pestilential fever.	12,738	1,998	741	38	3	676
1667	Constitution of small-	15,842	35	916	1,196	83	2,108
1668	pox, with a continued	17,278	14	1,247	1,987	200	2,415
1669	" variolous " fever.	} 19,432	3	1,499	951	15	4,385
1669	Constitution of dysen-						
1670	tery and cholera nostras,	20,198	0	1,729	1,465	295	3,690
1671	with a continued fever.	15,729	5	1,343	696	17	2,537
1672	Measles in 1670.	18,230	5	1,615	1,116	118	2,645
1673	Constitution of " co-	17,504	5	1,804	853	15	2,624
1674	matose" fevers.	21,201	3	2,164	2,507	795	1,777
1675	Influenza in 1675.	17,244	1	2,154	997	1	3,321
1676		18,732	2	2,112	359	83	2,083
1677	Not recorded.	19,067	2	1,749	1,678	87	2,602
1678	Return of the "inter-	20,678	5	2,376	1,798	93	3,150
1679	mittent" constitution,	21,730	2	2,763	1,967	117	2,996
1680	absent since 1661-64.	21,053	0	3,324	689	49	3,271
1681	"Depuratory" fevers,	23,951	0	3,174	2,982	121	2,827
1682	or dregs of the inter-	20,691	0	2,696	1,408	50	2,631
1683	mittents.	20,587	0	2,250	2,096	39	2,438
1684		23,202	0	2,836	1,560	6	2,981
1685	Constitution of a	23,222	0	3,832	2,496	197	2,203
1686	"new" continued fever.	22,609	0	4,185	1,062	25	2,605

[1] An analysis of the four Hippocratic constitutions, with modern illustrative cases, is given by Alfred Haviland, *Climate, Weather, and Disease.* London, 1855.

The foregoing is a Table of Sydenham's epidemic constitutions from 1661 to 1686, compiled from his various writings, with the corresponding statistics from the London Bills of Mortality.

I give this Table both as a convenient outline and in deference to the great name of Sydenham. But we should be much at fault in interpreting the figures of the London Bills, or the history of epidemic diseases in the country at large, if we had no other sources of information than his writings. Only some of the figures in the Table concern us in this chapter; plague has been finished in the previous volume, smallpox, measles and "griping in the guts" are reserved each for a separate chapter, as well as the influenzas and epidemic agues which formed the chief part of the "strange" or "new" fevers. If this work had been the Annals of Epidemics in Britain, it would have been at once proper and easy to follow Sydenham's constitutions exactly, and to group under each year the information collected from all sources about all epidemic maladies. But as the work is a history, it proceeds, as other histories do, in sections, observing the chronological order and the mutual relations of epidemic types as far as possible; and in this section of it we have to cull out and reduce to order the facts relating to fevers, beginning with those of 1661.

Cases of fever, says Sydenham, began to be epidemic about the beginning of July 1661, being mostly tertians of a bad type, and became so frequent day by day that in August they were raging everywhere, and in many places made a great slaughter of people, whole families being seized. This was not an ordinary tertian intermittent; indeed no one but Sydenham calls it an intermittent at all, and he qualifies the intermittence as follows:

"Autumnal intermittents do not at once assume the genuine type, but in all respects so imitate continued fevers that unless you examine the two respectively with the closest scrutiny, they cannot be distinguished. But, when by degrees the impetus of the 'constitution' is repelled and its strength reined in, the fevers change into a regular type; and as autumn goes out, they openly confess themselves, by casting their slough (*larva abjecta*) to be the intermittents that they really were from the first, whether quartans or tertians. If we do not attend to this diligently" etc. And again, in a paragraph which does not occur in the earlier editions, he writes as follows in the context of the "Intermittent Fevers of the years 1661–1664:"

"It is also to be noted that in the beginning of intermittent fevers, especially those that are epidemic in autumn, it is not altogether easy to distinguish the type correctly within the first few days of their accession, since they arise at first with continued fever superadded. Nor is it always

easy, unless you are intent upon it, to detect anything else than a slight remission of the disease, which, however, declines by degrees into a perfect intermission, with its type (third-day or fourth-day) corresponding fitly to the season of the year."

The intermittent character of these fevers seems to have struck Sydenham himself in a later work as forced and unreal. Writing in 1680, when the same kind of fevers were prevalent, after the epidemic agues of 1678 and 1679, he calls them "depuratory," and says that "doubtless those depuratory fevers which reigned in 1661–64 were as if the dregs of the intermittents which raged sometime before during a series of years," i.e. the agues of 1657–59[1].

Theory or names apart, Sydenham's account of the fatal epidemic fever of the summer and autumn of 1661, comes to nearly the same as Willis's. Without saying expressly, as Willis does, that the victims were mostly children or young people, he speaks in one place of those of more mature years lying much longer in the fever, even to three months, and he specially mentions the same sequelae of the fever in children that Willis mentions, and that Roger North remembered in his own case—namely that they sometimes became hectic, with bellies distended and hard, and often acquired a cough and other consumptive symptoms, "which clearly put one in mind of rickets." He refers also to pain and swelling of the tonsils and to difficulty of swallowing, which, if followed by hoarseness, hollow eyes, and the *facies Hippocratica*, portended speedy death. Among the numerous other *accidentia* of the fever, was a certain kind of mania. Among the symptoms were phrensy, and coma-vigil; diarrhœa occurred in some owing, as he thought, to the omission of an emetic at the outset; hiccup and bleeding at the nose were occasional.

But, although Sydenham must have had the same phenomena of fever before him that Willis had, the epidemic being general, according to the statements of both, one would hardly guess from his way of presenting the facts, that the fever was what Willis took it to be—a slow nervous fever, with convulsive and ataxic symptoms, specially affecting children and the young. Both Willis and Sydenham recognised something new in it; the common people called it, once more, the "new disease," and Pepys calls it a "sort of fever," and "strange and fatal fevers."

[1] *Epist. I. Respons.* § 57.   Greenhill's ed. p. 298.

As Sydenham maintains that the same epidemic constitution continued until 1664 (although the fever-deaths in London are much fewer in 1662–3–4 than in the year 1661, which was the first of it), we may take in the same connexion Pepys's account of the Queen's attack of fever in 1663. The young princess Katharine of Portugal, married to Charles II. in 1662, had the beginning of a fever at Whitehall about the middle of October, 1663; Pepys enters on the 19th that her pulse beat twenty to eleven of the king's, that her head was shaved, and pigeons put to her feet, that extreme unction was given her (the priests so long about it that the doctors were angry). On the 20th he hears that the queen's sickness is a spotted fever, that she was as full of the spots as a leopard : "which is very strange that it should be no more known, but perhaps it is not so." On the 22nd the queen is worse, 23rd she slept, 24th she is in a good way to recovery, Sir Francis Prujean's cordial having given her rest; on the 26th "the delirium in her head continues still; she talks idle, not by fits, but always, which in some lasts a week after so high a fever, in some more, and in some for ever." On the 27th she still raves and talks, especially about her imagined children; on the 30th she continues "light-headed, but in hopes to recover." On 7th December, she is pretty well, and goes out of her chamber to her little chapel in the house; on the 31st "the queen after a long and sore sickness is become well again."

Typhus fever perennial in London.

Sydenham says that a continued fever, the symptoms of which so far as he gives them suggest typhus, was mixed with the masked intermittent, (or the convulsive fever of children, as in Willis's account), in every one of the years 1661–4; and that statement raises a question which may be dealt with here once for all. Fever in the London bills is a steady item from year to year, seldom falling below a thousand deaths and in the year 1741, during a general epidemic of typhus, rising to 7500. The fevers were a composite group, as we have seen, and shall see more clearly. But the bulk of them perennially appears to have been typhus fever. Where the name of "spotted fever" is given there can be little doubt. Every year the bills have a small number of deaths from "spotted fever," and the number of them

always rises in the weekly bills in proportion to the increase of "fever" in general, sometimes reaching twenty in the week when the other fevers reach a hundred. It would be a mistake to suppose that only the fevers called spotted were typhus, the other and larger part being something else. The more reasonable supposition is that the name of spotted was given by the searchers in cases where the spots, or vibices or petechiae of typhus were especially notable. If a score, or a dozen or half-a-dozen deaths in a week are set down to spotted fever, it probably means that a large part of the remaining hundred, or seventy, or fifty cases of "fever" not called spotted were really of the same kind, namely typhus. In the plague itself, the "tokens," which were of the same haemorrhagic nature as the larger or more defined spots of typhus, were exceedingly variable[1]. One of the synonyms of typhus (the common name in Germany) is spotted typhus; but the spots were of at least two kinds, a dusky mottling of the skin and more definite spots, sometimes large, sometimes like fleabites.

Assuming that the cases specially called "spotted" in the London Bills were only a part of all that might have been called by the same name in the wider acceptation of the term (as in Germany), it is a significant fact that there are few of the weekly bills for a long series of years in the 17th and 18th centuries without some of the former. Such a case as that of Mr Samuel Crewe, brother of Lord Crewe, who died of the "spotted fever" on 2 July, 1661, probably means that there were more cases of the same kind in the poorer parts of the town, from which no account of the reigning sicknesses ever came unless it were the number of deaths in the bills. The conditions of endemic typhus were there long before we have authentic accounts, towards the end of the 18th century, of that disease being ever present in the homes of the lower classes. In the time of Sydenham, and even in the time of Huxham two generations after, there was no thought of the unwholesome domestic life graphically described by Willan and others, as a cause of typhus—the overcrowding, the want of ventilation, the foul bedding and the excremental effluvia.

If there had been any reason to suppose that the London of the Restoration, or of the time of Queen Anne, or of the first

[1] Tillison to Sancroft, 14 Sept. 1665. Cited in former volume, p. 677: "One week full of spots and tokens, and perhaps the succeeding bill none at all."

Georges had enjoyed better public health in its crowded liberties and out-parishes than we know it to have done from the time when the authentic accounts of Lettsom and other dispensary physicians begin, then one might err in assuming the perennial existence of typhus fever and in assigning to that cause the bulk of the deaths under the heading of "fevers" in the Parish Clerks' bills. But the public health was undoubtedly worse in the earlier period. A writer as late as the year 1819, who is calling for that reform of the dwellings of the working classes in London which was soon after carried out, namely the construction of regular streets instead of mazes of courts and alleys, speaks of the "silent mortality" that went on in the latter[1]. It was still more silent in earlier times, when the west end of London knew nothing of what was passing in the east end[2].

In all matters of public health, after the somewhat romantic interest in plague had ceased, the poorer parts of London were for long an unexplored territory. Dr John Hunter, who had been an army physician and was afterwards in practice in Mayfair, began about the year 1780 to visit the homes of the poor in St Giles's or other parishes near him, and was surprised to find in them a fever not unlike the hospital typhus of his military experience. I quote at this stage only a sentence or two[3].

"It may be observed, that though the fever in the confined habitations of the poor does not rise to the same degree of violence as in jails and hospitals, yet the destruction of the human species occasioned by it must be much greater, from its being so widely spread among a class of people whose number bears a large proportion to that of the whole inhabitants. There are but few of the sick, so far as I have been able to learn, that find their way into the great hospitals in London." I shall defer the subject of the dwellings of the working class in London until a later stage.

The "constitution" in Sydenham's series which succeeded the febrile one of 1661–64 was "pestilential fever." It began in the end of 1664, lasted into the spring of 1665, and passed by an easy transition into the plague proper. The bills for those months have very large weekly totals of deaths from "fever," as well as a good many deaths from "spotted fever," before they begin to have more than an occasional death from plague. It is

---

[1] H. Clutterbuck, M.D., *Obs. on the Epidemic Fevers prevailing in the Metropolis.* Lond. 1819, pp. 58—60.

[2] Horace Walpole's *Letters* give two instances: he himself had never set foot in Southwark; a small tradesman in the City had never heard of Sir Robert Walpole.

[3] *Transactions of the College of Physicians,* iii. 366.

this particular form of typhus fever that Bateman had in mind when he wrote, in 1818, "We never see the pestilential fever of Sydenham and Huxham"; although Willan, who preceded him at the Carey Street dispensary, described in 1799 a fever of so fatal a type that it gave rise to the rumour that the plague was back in London. The term "pestilential" was technically applied to a kind of fever a degree worse than the "malignant."

Willis, the earliest of the Restoration authorities on fevers, had three names in an ascending scale of severity—putrid, malignant and pestilential. The putrid fevers were what we might call idiopathic, engendered within the body in some way personal to the individual from "putrefaction" or fermentation of the humours; all the intermittents were included in that class, and the theory of their cure by bark was that the drug corrected putridity. In the malignant and pestilential, an altogether new element came in—the τὸ θεῖον of Hippocrates, the mysterious something which we call infection; and of these two infectious fevers, the malignant was milder than the pestilential[1].

Morton drew out the scale of fevers in an elaborate classification, of which only the last section of continued contagious fevers concerns us at present[2]:

Synochus	Simple Malignant Fever	Fever mostly with sweats and other signs of malignity, but without buboes, carbuncles, petechiae or miliary rash.
	Pestilential Fever	Fever with petechiae, purple spots, miliaria, morbillous rash on the chest.
	Plague	With buboes, carbuncles and black spots.

The order in this Table was also the order in time: the fever of 1661, which Willis calls malignant, remained as the constitu-

---

[1] Willis, Op. ed. 1682, Amstelod. p. 110. "De febribus pestilentibus": "Etenim vulgo notum est febres interdum populariter regnare, quae pro symptomatum vehementia, summa aegrorum strage, et magna vi contagii, pestilentiae vix cedant; quae tamen, quia putridarum typos innotantur, nec adeo certo affectos interemunt aut alios inficiunt haud *pestis* sed diminutiori appellatione *febris pestilens* nomen merentur. Praeter has dantur alterius generis febres, quarum et pernicies et contagium se remissius habent, quia tamen supra putridarum vires infestae sunt, et in se aliquatenus τὸ θεῖον Hippocratis continere videntur, tenuiori adhuc vocabulo *febres malignae* appellantur."

The war-typhus of 1643, which was sometimes bubonic, and was succeeded by plague in 1644, is given as an example of *febris pestilens*; the epidemic of 1661 as an example of *maligna*.

[2] *Pyretologia*, i. 68.

tion of the years following until the end of 1664; then began the pestilential, which passed definitely in the spring of 1665 into the plague proper. Willis, Sydenham and Morton, differing as they did on many points of theory and treatment, all alike taught the scale of malignity in fevers and plague, and all used the language of "constitutions." The Great Plague of 1665 was, in their view, the climax of a succession of febrile constitutions of the air, being attended by much pestilential fever and followed by a fever which Morton places in the milder class of συνεχής.

The epidemic Constitutions following the Great Plague.

During the ten or twelve years following the Great Plague of London, the epidemic maladies which Sydenham dwelt most upon as the reigning types will appear on close scrutiny to have been on the whole proper to the earlier years of life. This cannot be shown in the simple way of figures; for the ages at death from the several maladies, although they were in the books of the Parish Clerks, were not published.

There was some continued fever every year, which we may take to have been chiefly the endemic typhus of a great city, and there were also deaths among adults due to those reigning epidemics which fell most on the young. In 1667 and 1668 the leading epidemic was smallpox, with a continued fever towards the end of the period which Sydenham called "variolous," for no other reason, apparently, than that it was part of a variolous constitution. In the autumn of 1669, and in the three years following, the epidemic mortality was peculiarly infantile, in the form of diarrhoea or "griping in the guts," with some dysentery of adults, and some measles in 1670. From 1673 to 1676, the constitution was a comatose fever, which chiefly affected children, with a sharp epidemic of measles in the first half of 1674, attended by a very high mortality from all causes, and a severe smallpox in the second half of 1674, attended by a much lower mortality from all causes. There was also an influenza for a few weeks in 1675. In 1678 the "intermittent" constitution returned, having been absent for thirteen years, and continued through 1779–80, until its "strength was broken." In 1681 smallpox was unusually mortal, the deaths being more than in any previous year. Most of these constitutions fall to be dealt with fully in

C. II.

other chapters: but as we are here specially concerned with the succession to the plague, it is to be noted how largely the epidemic mortality in London fell upon the age of childhood for a number of years after the Great Plague of 1665. It was observed both by English and foreign writers that the next epidemic following the Black Death of 1348–49, namely, that of 1361 in England and of 1359–60 in some other parts of Europe, fell mostly upon children and upon the upper classes of adults. There is doubtless some particular application of the population principle in the earlier instance as in the later, but not the same application in both. The conditions at the beginning of the three hundred years' reign of plague in Britain were different from those at the end of it. The increased prevalence of smallpox in the generation before the last great outburst of plague, and the infantile or puerile character of the epidemic fever of 1661, as described by Willis, show that the incidence of infectious mortality had already begun to shift towards the age of childhood. It looks as if the conditions of population, intricate and obscure as they must be confessed to be, were somehow determining what the reigning infectious maladies, with their special age-incidence, should be. Such a gradual change is the more probable for the reason that infectious mortality came in due time to be mostly an affair of childhood. The plague, which was the great infection of the later medieval and earlier modern period, was peculiarly fatal to adult lives; on the other hand, the mortality from infectious diseases in our own time falls in much the larger ratio upon infants and children. It looks as if this change, now so obvious, had begun before the end of plague in Britain, having become more marked in the generation following its extinction. The direct successor of plague, so far as concerns age-incidence and nosological affinity, was the pestilential or malignant typhus, which came into great prominence in 1685–86, in circumstances that seemed to contemporaries to forebode a return of the plague. But before we come to that, there remains a little to be said of some other fevers, especially of the comatose fever of 1673–76, which was largely an affair of childhood.

Pepys says that he went on 3 May, 1668, to Old Street (St Luke's) to see Admiral Sir Thomas Teddiman, "who is very ill in bed of a fever," and, in a later entry, that he "did die by a thrush in his mouth" on the 12th of May. Next year, 1669,

Pepys and his wife went on tour through several parts of Europe, and had hardly returned to their house in Seething Lane when the lady fell ill of a fever; on 2nd November, it was "so severe as to render her recovery desperate," and on 10th November she died in her 29th year,—a surprising sequel, as her husband felt, to a "voyage so full of health and content." These two years, for which we have a sample of the London fevers, were marked in the Netherlands by epidemics of fevers which are among the most extraordinary in the whole history. At Leyden in 1669 the fever reached such a height as to cut off 7000—a mortality which would not have been surprising if the disease had been plague; but it was not plague, it wanted the buboes, carbuncles &c., was longer in its course, and, strangest of all, affected the upper classes far more severely than the poor, so much so "that of seventy men administering the public affairs, scarcely two were left[1]," while, according to Fanois, who was the Leyden poor's doctor, the lower classes, "protected as it were by having survived the simpler forms of fever," suffered from this malignant epidemic far less than the rich[2]. The mortality is said to have risen as high as three-fourths of the attacks. At Haarlem the burials in a week rose to three or four hundred (which was a fair week's average for London itself in an ordinary season), the epidemic lasting four months and leaving hardly one family untouched. Among the symptoms were extreme praecordial anxiety, weight at the pit of the stomach, constant nausea and loathing, vomiting, in part bilious but chiefly "pituitous," thirst and restless tossing. It was attended by an affection of the throat and mouth—an angina with aphthae or thrush of the palate. The pools and other sources of water for domestic use were unusually stagnant that summer in Holland, and were commonly blamed for the epidemic; but Fanois points out that at Haarlem and Emden, where similar fevers raged, "salubriores non desunt aquae[3]."

---

[1] C. L. Morley, *De morbo epidemico, in 1678—9, narratio.* Lond. 1680.

[2] Guido Fanois, *De morbo epidemico hactenus inaudito, praeterita aestate anni 1669 Lugduni Batavorum vicinisque locis grassante.* Lugd. Bat. 1671.

[3] Brownrigg cites the Leyden epidemic of 1669, which he calls an intermitting fever, as an instance of the effects of changes in the ground water; it was "powerfully aggravated by the mixture of salt water with the stagnant water of the canals and ditches. This fever happened in the month of August, 1669, and continued to the end of January, 1670." "Observations on the Means of Preventing Epidemic Fevers." Printed in the *Literary Life of W. Brownrigg, M.D., F.R.S.* By Joshua Dixon, Whitehaven. 1801.

After such an instance as the Leyden fever of 1669, nothing is incredible in the records of fever subsequent to the extinction of plague. Turning to Sydenham's account of the continued fever which occurred in London during the same season, the latter half of 1669, as well as in the three years following, we find that it was characterized rarely by diarrhoea or sweats, commonly by pain in the head, by a moist white tongue which afterwards became covered by a dense skin, and by a greater tendency than Sydenham had ever seen to aphthae (the "thrush in the mouth" of Admiral Teddiman in 1668) when death threatened—the same being a "deposition from the blood of foul and acrid matter upon the mouth and throat." But London in 1668 and 1669 suffered little from fevers in comparison to Leyden, Haarlem and other Dutch towns, its high mortality in the summer and autumn of 1669 being from infantile diarrhoea, cholera nostras and dysentery.

Sydenham's continued fever from 1673 to 1676 (he was absent from his practice in 1677 owing to ill health) was a malady which affected adults as well as children, but, it would appear, the latter especially. The only characteristic case given is of a boy of nine who did not begin to mend until the thirtieth day. Many recovered in a fortnight, while others were not clear of the fever in a month. On account of the remarkable stupor which almost always attended it, Sydenham called the fever of this constitution a comatose fever. It began with sharp pains in the head and back, pains in the limbs, heats and chills, etc. His account of the comatose state is exactly like that given by Willis for the fever of children in 1661—profound stupor, sometimes for a week long, so profound in some as to pass into absolute aphonia (the "acute fever with dumbness" of later writers), while others would talk a few words in their sleep, or would seem to be angry or perturbed by something (the chimaeras mentioned by Willis) and would then become tranquil again; when roused to take physic or to drink they would open the eyes for a moment and then fall back into stupor. When they began to mend, they would crave for absurd things to eat or drink. During convalescence the head, through weakness, could not be kept straight but would incline first to one side and then to the other[1].

---

[1] *Obs. Med.* 3rd ed., v. 2.

The years 1678–1680 witnessed remarkable epidemics of ague, such as had occurred on several occasions before, the last in the years 1657–59. They engross so much of Sydenham's writing, especially in connexion with the Peruvian-bark controversy, that we hear little of any other fever until the great epidemic of continued fever, or typhus, in 1685–6. But he does mention briefly that the interval between the decline of the agues in 1680 and the beginning of the "new fever" of 1685, was occupied by "continued depuratory" fevers—depuratory of the dregs of the preceding intermittent constitution, and comparable in that respect to the fevers of 1661–64 which followed the agues of 1657–59[1].

Sydenham's term "depuratory" does not help us much; but we learn something from Morton as to what fevers were prevalent, besides the epidemical intermittents, in the years preceding the epidemic of 1685–86. Morton classes them as continued συνεχής (*Synocha*), by which he means something less malignant than *Synochus*. A fever which began in the milder form would often degenerate into the more malignant, the cause assigned, in the usual recriminatory manner of the time between rival schools, being mistaken treatment. But sometimes the fever was malignant from the outset, with purple spots, petechiae, morbillous efflorescence, watery vesicles on the neck and breast, buboes, and anthraceous boils. All these fevers, says Morton, whether they were spurious forms of synocha, or malignant from the outset, were sporadic, "neque contagione, ut in pestilentiali constitutione, sese propagabant[2]." This points to their having been part of that strange aguish epidemic of which an account is given in another chapter. In Short's abstracts of parish registers, the year 1680 seems to have been the most unhealthy of the series in country parishes, and that is borne out by one Lamport, or Lampard, an empiric who practised in Hampshire: "I will tell you somewhat concerning a malignant fever. In the year '80 or '81 there were great numbers of people died of such fevers, many whereby were taken with vomitings, etc., yet I had the good fortune to cure eighteen in the parish of Aldingbourn, not one dying, in that great compass, of that disease[3]." The moral is that the empiric recovered his

---

[1] *Epist. I. Respons.* §§ 56, 57.
[2] *Pyretologie,* i. 429.
[3] John Lamport *alias* Lampard, *A direct Method of ordering and curing People of that loathsome disease the Smallpox.* Lond. 1685, p. 28.

cases, whereas the regular faculty lost theirs; which means that the fevers were of various degrees, some aguish, some typhus, as in the exactly similar circumstances a century after, 1780–85.

In the London Bills from 1681 to 1684, the deaths from fever were many, with some from "spotted fever" nearly every week, while the annual mortalities from all causes were high. It is the more remarkable, therefore, that Sydenham should have discovered, in the beginning of 1685, the outbreak of a new fever, different from any that had prevailed for seven years before. The explanation seems to be that a malignant typhus fever, such as might have been discovered in any year in the crowded parishes where the working classes lived, broke out at the Court end of the town, where Sydenham's practice lay.

The epidemic fever of 1685–86.

A letter of 12 March, 1685, says: "Sir R. Mason died this morning in his lodging at Whitehall. A fever rages that proves very mortal, and gives great apprehensions of a plague[1]." Sydenham also was reminded of the circumstances preceding the Great Plague of London in 1665. In his first account of the epidemic of fever in 1685[2], which began with a thaw in February, he points out that the thaw in March, 1665, had been followed by pestilential fever and thereafter by the plague proper. In a later reference, when the epidemic of fever was in its second year (1686) he says: "How long it may last I shall not guess; nor do I quite know whether it may not be a certain more spirituous, subtle beginning, and as if *primordium*, of the former depuratory fever [1661–64] which was followed by the most terrible plague. There are some phenomena which so far incline me to that belief[3]." However, no plague followed the malignant, if not pestilential, fever of 1685–86. The reign of plague, as the event showed, was over; the fever which had been on former occasions its portent and satellite, came into the place of reigning disease. It is true that Sydenham does not identify the fever of 1685–86 by name as pestilential fever; on

---

[1] *Hist. MSS. Com.* v. 186. Duke of Sutherland's historical papers.
[2] *Schedula Monitoria I.* "De novae febris ingressu." §§ 2, 3.
[3] *Ibid.* § 46.

the contrary, he entitles his essay "De Novae Febris Ingressu." But the novelty of type was partly in contrast to the fevers immediately preceding, which admitted treatment by bark, and its principal difference from the pestilential fever of former occasions seems to have been that it was not followed by plague[1]. Its antecedents and circumstances were very much those of plague itself. Its mortality was greatest in the old plague-seasons of summer and autumn, it had slight relation to famine or scarcity, or to other obvious cause of domestic typhus. Sydenham can find no explanation of the new constitution but "some secret and recondite change in the bowels of the earth pervading the whole atmosphere, or some influence of the celestial bodies." He enlarges, however, on the character of the seasons preceding, which would have affected the surface, if not the bowels, of the earth, and the levels of the ground-water.

The winter of 1683–84 was one of intense frost; an ice-carnival was held on the Thames during the whole of January. The long dry frost of winter was followed by an excessively hot and dry summer, the drought being such as Evelyn did not remember, and as "no man in England had known." For eight or nine months there had not been above one or two considerable showers, which came in storms. The winter of 1684–85 set in early, and became "a long and cruel frost," more interrupted, however, than that of the year before. The spring was again dry, and it was not until the end of May 1685 that "we had plentiful rain after two years' excessive drought and severe winters[2]."

The two years of excessive drought, with severe winters, had their effect upon the public health, as will appear from Short's abstracts of parish registers in town and country[3]; the years 1683–85 being conspicuous for the excess of burials over baptisms:

[1] In the Belvoir Letters (*Hist. MSS. Com. Calendar*) Charles Bertie writes from London to the Countess of Rutland, 26 January, 1685, that "many are sick of pestilential fevers." Evelyn says that the winter of 1685–6 was extraordinarily wet and mild, but does not mention sickness until June, 1686, when the weather was hot and the camp at Hounslow Heath was broken up owing to sickness.

[2] Evelyn's *Diary*, which gives other particulars, including a description of the ice-carnival on the Thames.

[3] Thomas Short, M.D. of Sheffield, *New Observations on City, Town and Country Bills of Mortality*. London, 1750.

Country Parishes.

Year	Registers examined	Registers with excess of death	Deaths in them	Births in them
1683	140	37	923	685
1684	140	31.	900	629
1685	140	19	574	478
1686	140	16	419	301
1687	143	19	522	427
1688	143	11	327	267

Towns.

Year	Registers examined	Registers with excess of death	Deaths in them	Births in them
1683	25	8	1398	1169
1684	25	8	1243	865
1685	25	4	1191	741
1686	25	2	555	418
1687	25	1	313	269
1688	25	2	191	146

There is no clue to the forms of sickness that caused the excessive mortality· in country parishes and provincial towns. But in London it appears from the Bills that the one great cause of the unusual excess of deaths in 1684 was an enormous mortality from infantile diarrhoea, from the end of July to the middle of September, during the weather which Evelyn describes as excessively hot and dry with occasional storms of rain.

It was in the second year of the long drought, February, 1685, that Sydenham dated the beginning of his new febrile constitutions. The mortality of 1685 was just twenty deaths more than in 1684 (23,222); but fever (with spotted fever) and smallpox had each a thousand more out of the total than in the year before. Sydenham says that the fever did not spare children, which might be alleged of typhus at all times; but a fever of the kind, even if it ran through the children of a household, seldom cut off the very young, the mortality being in greatest part of adults and adolescents. Excepting smallpox for the year 1685, infantile and children's maladies were not prominent during the constitution of the "new fever;" the usual items of high infantile mortality, such as convulsions and "griping in the guts" or infantile diarrhoea, were moderate and even low. Hence, although the weekly fever-deaths in the following Table may not appear sufficient for the professional and other interest that they excited, it is to be kept in mind that they had been ·mostly of adult lives. It is probable also that a good many of them had been among the well-to-do, and perhaps at first in the

West End; for there is nothing in the height of the weekly bills for all London to bear out the remark of the letter of 12 March, already quoted, "A fever rages that proves very mortal and gives apprehensions of a plague."

Weekly Mortalities in London.

1685.

Week ending	Dead	Of fever	Of spotted fever	Of small-pox	Of griping in the guts
March 3	376	49	0	11	35
10	458	73	2	30	3:
17	367	53	1	25	17
24	441	63	3	33	27
31	366	53	5	24	36
April 7	421	47	10	28	30
14	433	64	8	32	27
21	473	66	6	47	45
28	470	68	3	49	45
May 5	385	50	6	35	39
12	447	75	3	59	41
19	437	79	4	58	43
26	452	61	2	74	39
June 2	469	65	8	65	36
9	521	88	14	62	41
16	499	91	9	66	34
23	478	76	12	71	53
30	526	82	13	84	45
July 7	497	81	8	87	53
14	478	82	11	78	51
21	464	79	11	87	47
28	488	62	6	68	54
Aug. 4	493	82	5	86	51
11	529	109	13	89	47
18	580	74	13	99	71
25	536	91	7	67	85
Sept. 1	556	94	13	53	104
8	539	82	10	81	77
15	485	90	7	63	70
22	459	90	10	37	51
29	502	114	3	58	53
Oct. 6	444	108	11	40	54
13	445	89	13	61	38
20	369	86	5	40	28
27	379	73	7	29	45
Nov. 3	443	96	8	55	43
10	410	84	7	26	35
17	432	103	8	35	39
24	471	107	6	56	31
Dec. 1	384	87	4	36	24
8	452	98	8	49	24
15	403	69	3	29	47
22	438	99	2	34	27
29	432	80	9	28	28

Weekly Mortalities in London.

1686.

Week ending	Dead	Of fever	Of spotted fever	Of small-pox	Of griping in the guts
Jan. 5	394	80	5	28	29
12	400	80	3	27	48
19	396	67	5	36	32
26	366	76	2	21	30
Feb. 2	452	87	8	16	30
9	416	78	5	37	30
16	405	94	9	20	25
23	419	74	7	16	40
March 2	417	84	1	20	37
9	455	95	6	18	30
16	415	71	10	31	21
23	453	78	11	22	46
30	372	58	8	17	35
April 6	392	80	11	13	27
13	393	72	7	21	29
20	420	61	10	26	37
27	471	99	9	27	22
May 4	429	78	21	28	46
11	374	71	6	16	22
18	395	69	5	17	3 (sic)
25	395	66	11	24	36
June 1	383	63	4	15	49
8	404	66	6	26	38
15	523	88	9	43	64
22	503	99	9	25	73
29	473	90	10	31	62
July 6	430	71	6	18	62
13	401	76	2	19	56
20	464	87	14	24	74
27	508	99	3	23	76
Aug. 3	506	86	9	14	90
10	493	74	7	14	104
17	522	99	7	26	101
24	536	115	5	18	104
31	520	90	8	22	93
Sept. 7	531	94	4	21	104
14	498	84	6	18	110
21	540	100	3	17	101
28	443	90	5	13	67
Oct. 5	425	81	4	13	60
12	432	96	2	9	56
19	391	73	1	9	33
26	402	79	3	11	43
Nov. 2	373	64	1	23	39
9	456	85	1	19	31
16	401	73	2	9	23
23	359	61	4	10	54
30	397	68	1	7	34
Dec. 7	359	76	0	9	21
14	438	60	0	8	46
21	354	49	1	8	39
28	356	53	2	9	32

Sydenham says that he regarded the new fever at first as nothing more than the "bastard peripneumony" which he had described for previous seasons; but he had soon cause to see that it wanted the violent cough, the racking pain in the head during coughing, the giddiness caused by the slightest movement, and the excessive dyspnoea of the latter (Huxham likewise distinguished typhus from "bastard peripneumony"). The early symptoms of the "new fever" were alternating chills and flushings, pain in the head and limbs, a cough, which might go off soon, with pain in the neck and throat. The fever was a continued one, with exacerbation towards evening; it was apt to change into a phrensy, with tranquil or muttering delirium; petechiae and livid blotches were brought out in some cases (Sydenham thought they were caused by cordials and a heating regimen), and there were occasional eruptions of miliary vesicles. The tongue might be moist and white at the edges for a time, latterly brown and dry. Clammy sweats were apt to break out, especially from the head. If the brain became the organ most touched, the fever-heat declined, the pulse became irregular, and jerking of the limbs came on before death.

Later writers, for example those who described the great epidemic fever of 1741, have identified the fever of 1685–86 with the contagious malignant fever afterwards called typhus, and Murchison, in his brief retrospect of typhus in Britain, has included it under that name. Sydenham mentions petechiae and livid blotches in some cases, and the Bills give a good many of the deaths in the worst weeks of the epidemic under the head of "spotted fever." It is not at first easy to understand why Sydenham should have written an essay specially upon it, in September, 1686, to claim it as a new fever[1] and not rather as the old pestilential fever—" populares meos admonens de subingressu novae cujusdam Constitutionis, a qua pendet Febris nova species, a nuper grassantibus multum abludens." It should be kept in mind that his motive was correct treatment,

[1] Freind (*Nine Commentaries upon Fever, &c.*, engl. by Dale, Lond. 1730, p. 4) has the following general criticism upon Sydenham's varying constitutions of fevers: " I believe also I may truly affirm that those very fevers which Sydenham explains as distinct species, according to the various temperature of the seasons, do not differ much from one another. For, if perhaps you should except the *Petechiae*, they differ rather in degree than in kind. There hardly ever appeared a fever in any season where the signs so constantly answered one another, that those which you found collected in one person should unite after the same manner in another; however upon this account you would not deny their labouring under the same distemper."

and that the fashionable treatment of the day by Peruvian bark was, in his judgment, unsuited to this fever, however much it may have suited the epidemical intermittents of 1678–79 and the "depuratory" dregs of them for several years after. Physicians, he says, had learned to drive off by bark the fevers of the former constitution, from 1677 to the beginning of 1685, even when the fever intermitted little and sometimes when it intermitted not at all; and they saw an indication for bark in the nocturnal exacerbations of the new fever. Sydenham found that even large doses of bark did not free the patient from fever, and that restoration to health under treatment with the bark was due "magis fortunato alicui morbi eventu quam corticis viribus." He seeks to establish the indications for another treatment by setting forth the symptoms minutely; and as the question of bark in fevers was the great medical question of the time, this may well have been Sydenham's motive for discovering in the epidemic of 1685–6 a "new fever" although he does not say so in as many words. We have a good instance of how the bark-craze was at this time influencing the very highest circles of practice in the case of Lord Keeper Guildford, in July, 1685, as related in another chapter.

It will be seen from the table of weekly deaths that the second of the two hard winters was over before the fever began to attract notice. Sydenham compares its beginning after the thaw in February, 1685, to the beginning of the plague when the frost broke in March, 1665.

If it had been merely the typhus of a hard winter, of overcrowding indoors, of work and wages stopped by the frost, and of want of fuel (which things Evelyn mentions as matters of fact), it would have come sooner than the spring of 1685. The Bills for years before have regularly a good many deaths from fever, and always some from spotted fever; but these may have come from parishes wholly beyond the range of Sydenham's practice. The fever began definitely for him in February, 1685, and was at its worst in the old plague-seasons of summer and autumn. If the seasons had any relation at all to it, the epidemic was a late effect of the long drought, an effect which was manifested most when the rain came, in the summer of 1685 and throughout the mild winter and normal summer of 1685–86. It must have been for that reason that Sydenham traced the source of it to "some secret and recondite change in the bowels

of the earth," rather than to a change in the sensible qualities of the air. One must ever bear in mind that the physicians of the Restoration gave no thought to insanitary conditions of living; in that respect the later Stuart period seems to have been behind the Elizabethan or even the medieval; we cannot err in assuming, behind all Sydenham's speculative causes, a great deal of unwholesomeness indoors. Sydenham's fullest reference to the subterranean sources of poisonous miasmata occurs in his tractate on Gout:

"Whether it be that the bowels of the earth, if one may so speak, undergo various changes, so that by the accession of vapours exhaled therefrom the air is disturbed, or that the whole atmosphere is infected by a change which some peculiar conjunction of certain of the heavenly bodies induces in it;—the matter so falls out that at this or that time the air is furnished with particles that are adverse to the economy of the human body, just as at another time it is impregnated with particles of a like kind that agree ill with the bodies of some species of brute animals. At these times, as often as by inspiration we draw into the naked blood miasmata of this kind, noxious and inimical to nature, and we fall into those epidemical diseases which they are apt to produce, Nature raises a fever,—her accustomed means of vindicating the blood from some hostile matter. And such diseases are commonly called *epidemical;* and they are short and sharp because they have thus a quick and violent movement[1]."

It was Sydenham's intimate friend Robert Boyle who worked out the hypothesis of subterraneous miasmata as a cause of epidemic (and endemic) diseases. An account of his theory will be found in the chapter on Influenzas and Epidemic Agues. It may be said here that it needs only a few changes, especially the substitution of organic for inorganic matters in the soil, to bring it into line with the modern doctrine of miasmatic infective disease as expounded by the Munich school.

It has not been usual to think of spotted fever, (or of influenzas), in that connexion; but a telluric source of the epidemic constitution of 1685–86 was clearly Sydenham's view; and as the fever came in circumstances like those of the last great plague, and was thought at the time to be the forerunner of another great plague, its connexion with recondite decompositions in the soil, dependent on the phenomenal drought of two whole years before, cannot be set aside as a possibility, the less so that the fever, although of the type of typhus, was not a fever of cold, hunger, and domestic distress, but mainly of the warm, or mild, or soft weather following the long drought, and of many well-to-do-people, as in the great Netherlands fever of 1669.

[1] *Tractatus de Podagra,* § 35. Greenhill's edition, p. 428.

My view of it is that it was the modified successor of plague, the *pestis mitior*, which used to precede and accompany the plague, now become the dominant constitution. The authentic figures of its mortality come from London; but Sydenham says that its "effects were felt far more in other places"; although Short's abstracts of parish registers, given above, do not indicate excessive mortality throughout England.

Retrospect of the great Fever of 1623–25.

The most instructive instance of *pestis mitior* in Britain is not the pestilential fever which led up to the last plague (1665–6), but the great epidemic of fever all over England and Scotland which reigned for two or three years before the great outburst of plague in 1625. I go back to this because it was not wholly or even mainly a famine fever (although it was as general as one of the medieval famine-fevers), and because in that respect it furnishes a close parallel to the fever of 1685–86, which I regard as the successor of the plague. After this interlude in the history, we shall proceed to consider the question of the final extinction of plague.

In Scotland the fever of 1622-23 was directly connected with famine, but in England it was not obviously so according to the records that remain. The dearth in Scotland began as early as the autumn of 1621: "Great skarsitie of cornes throw all the kingdome," the harvest having been spoiled by wet weather and unheard-of river floods; however, abundance of foreign victual came in, and the scarcity was got over[1]. In England the same harvest of oats was abundant, and probably yielded the "foreign victual" which relieved the Scots; but the price of wheat rose greatly[2]. It was the year following, 1622, that really brought famine and famine-sickness to Scotland, as the second of two bad harvests had always done. On 21 July, 1622, a fast was proclaimed at Aberdeen for "the present plague of dearth and famine, and the continuance thereof threatened by tempests, inundations and weets likely to rot the fruit on the ground[3]."

In an entry of the Chronicle of Perth, subsequent to July, 1622, it is said: "In this yeir about the harvest and efter, thair wes suche ane universall seiknes in all the countrie as the ellyke hes not bene hard of. But speciallie in this burgh, that no familie in all the citie was frie of this visitation. Thair was also great mortalitie amonge the poore." From which it appears that the autumnal fever of 1622 was among all classes in Scotland. The famine in Scotland became more acute in the spring and summer of 1623; the country swarmed with beggars, and in July, says Calderwood, the famine increased daily until "many, both in burgh and land, died of hunger." At Perth ten or twelve died every day from Mid-

[1] *Chronicle of Perth* (Maitland Club) under date 14 Oct. 1621.
[2] Thorold Rogers, *Hist. of Agric. and Prices*, sub anno.
[3] *Extracts from Kirk Session Records.* Spalding Club, 1846.

summer to Michaelmas ; the disease was not the plague, but a fever[1]. At Dumfries 492 died during the first ten months of 1623, perhaps a ninth part of the inhabitants, about one hundred of the deaths being specially marked as of "poor[2]." The "malignant spotted fever" which caused numerous deaths in 1623 in Wigton, Penrith and Kendal is clearly part of the famine-fever of Scotland extending to the Borders and crossing them. This is a famine-fever of the old medieval type; like that of 1196 which, according to William of Newburgh "crept about everywhere," always the same acute fever, putting an end to the miseries of the starving, but attacking also those who had food.

The same spotted fever was all over England in 1623, but it did not, as in Scotland, come in the wake of famine. It is true that the English harvest of 1622 was a good deal spoiled ; a letter of 25 September says[3]: "Though the latter part of this summer proved so far seasonable, yet the harvest is scant, and corn at a great price by reason of the mildews and blasting generally over the whole realm," rye being quoted a few weeks later at 7/- the bushel and wheat at 10/-, although the average of wheat for the year, in Rogers's tables, is not more than 51/1d. per quarter, while the average of next year falls to 37/8d. These were not famine-prices in England, and there is no evidence of general sickness directly after the harvest of 1622, when corn was dearest. Also, although the autumn of 1623 was a time of "continual wet" in England[4], the price of wheat remained moderate, and even low as compared with the rather stiff price of the winter of 1622-23. But it was not until the summer and autumn of 1623 that the spotted fever became epidemic in England. Short's abstracts of the registers of market towns show how sickly that year was :

Year.	No. of registers examined.	No. with excess of burials.	Buried in the same.	Baptised in the same.
1622	25	4	442	345
1623	25	16	2254	439 (sic)
1624	25	9	978	714
1625	25	9	666	563

In September, 1623, the corporation of Stamford made a collection "in this dangerous time of visitation," and sent £10 of it to Grantham, the rest to go "to London or some other town, as occasion offered." A London letter of 6 December, 1623, from Chamberlain to Carleton says[5]:—

"Here is a contagious spotted or purple fever that reigns much, which, together with the smallpox, hath taken away many of good sort, as well as meaner people." He then gives the names of notables dead of it, and adds: "Yet many escape, as the dean of St Paul's [Dr Donne, who used the occasion to compile a manual of devotion] is like to do, though he were in great danger." One of the Coke family writes early in January, 1624, from London[6]: "Having two sons at Cambridge, we sent for them to keep Christmas with us, and not many days after their coming my eldest son Joseph fell suddenly into the sickness of the time which they call the spotted fever, and which after two days' extremity took away his life." From another letter it appears that one of his symptoms was "not being able to sleep," the unmistakable vigil of typhus. Although there is no word of the epidemic continuing in Scotland in 1624, it was undoubtedly as prevalent in England in that year as the year before, and prevalent in country houses as

[1] *Chronicle of Perth.*
[2] *History of the Burgh of Dumfries.* By W. MacDowall. 2nd ed. Edin. 1873, p. 381.
[3] *Court and Times of James I.,* ii. 331.
[4] *Ibid.,* under date 25 Oct. 1423.
[5] *Ibid.* ii. 439.   [6] *Cal. Coke MSS.* (Hist. MSS. Com.) i. 158.

well as in towns and cities. Thus, on 7 August, 1624, Chamberlain writes: "The [king's] progress is now so far off that we hear little thence, but only that there be many sick of the spotted ague, which took away the Duke of Lennox in a few days. He died at Kirby," a country house in Northampton- shire[1]. On 21 August he writes again : "This spotted fever is cousin- german to it [the plague] at least, and makes as quick riddance almost. The Lady Hatton hath two or three of her children sick of it at her brother Fanshaw's in Essex, and hath lost her younger daughter, that was buried at Westminster on Wednesday night by her father ; a pretty gentlewoman, much lamented." A letter of 4 September says there was excessive mortality in London, in great part among children (doubtless from the usual infantile trouble of a hot autumn, diarrhoea), while "most of the rest are carried away by this spotted fever, which reigns almost everywhere, in the country as ill as here." Sir Theodore Mayerne, the king's physician, confirms this, under date 20 August, 1624 : the purple fever, he says, was "not so much contagious as common through a universal disposing cause," seizing upon many in the same house, and destroying numbers, being most full of malignity[2]. It was clearly an inexplicable visitation. The summer was hot and dry, from which character of the season, says Chamberlain, "some have found out a far-fetched speculation, which yet runs current, and would ascribe it [the spotted fever] to the extraordinary quantity of cucumbers this year, which the gardeners, to hasten and bring forward, used to water out of the next ditches, which this dry time growing low, noisome and stinking, poisoned the fruit. But," adds Chamberlain, "that reason will reach no farther than this [London] town, whereas the mortality is spread far and near, and takes hold of whole households in many places." He then gives the names of several eminent persons dead of it, and speaks of others who were "still in the balance[3]." On 9 October, "the town continues sickly still," and Parliament had been put off, "in consideration of the danger," from 2 November, 1624, to 15 February, 1625. On Ash Wednesday, 1625, the Marquis of Hamilton died of the pestilent fever at Moor Park, Rickmansworth. Thus far there had been no plague ; and if the spotted fever were cousin-german to the plague, as Chamberlain said, it was remark- able in this that it prevailed in the mansions of the rich in town and country and took off more victims among the upper classes than the plague itself even in its most terrific outbursts. However, a plague of the first rank followed in London and elsewhere in the summer and autumn of 1625.

The cucumber-theory, above mentioned, shows how puzzled people must have been to account for the spotted fever, or "spotted ague" as it was also called, in 1624. Sir Theodore Mayerne did not think contagion from person to person could explain it, but referred it to "some universal disposing cause." It is conceivable that the famine-fever of 1622 and 1623 in Scotland and the Marches may have spread by contagion into England in the latter year ; but in 1624 there is nothing said of fever in Scotland or of scarcity as a primary cause in England.

Besides the famine-fever of Scotland in 1622–23, there was another associated thing which should not be left out of account. Before the famine and fever had begun in that country, the notorious Hungarian fever was raging in the Palatinate, and continued to rage for four years. "Hungarian fever" had become the dreaded name for war-typhus of a peculiar malignity and diffusive power. It had been so often engendered since the 16th century in campaigns upon Hungarian soil as to have become known everywhere under the name of that country. Its infection spread, also, everywhere through Europe ; thus it is said to have even reached England

[1] *C. and T. James I.*, ii. 469.
[2] Mayerne, *Opera Medica*, Lond. 1700.   [3] *Ibid.* ii. 473.

in 1566, and again in 1589, although it is not easy to find English evidence of it for either year. It was this type of fever which broke out in the Upper Palatinate, occupied by troops of the Catholic powers, in 1620, and continued through the years 1621, 1622 and 1623; as the title of one of the essays upon this outbreak somewhat fantastically declares, it spread "ex castris ad rastra, ex rastris ad rostra, ab his ad aras et focos[1]." Was the epidemic constitution of "spotted ague" in England in 1623 and 1624 derived from the centre of famine-fever in Scotland, or from the centre of camp-fever in the Palatinate? In the last years of James I. communications were frequent with the latter country, and there was of course much intercourse with Scotland.

The spotted fever or spotted ague of 1623–24, the plague of 1625, and the country agues of the same autumn make really a more instructive series of epidemic constitutions than any that fell under Sydenham's observation, so instructive, indeed, that it has seemed worth while to revert to it for the sake of illustrating the doctrine of epidemics then in vogue. That doctrine made little of contagion from person to person; yet the idea of contagion was familiar, and had been so since medieval times. If we might assume contagion to explain such cases as those that occurred in the houses of squires and nobles, we might find a source of it either in the famine-fever of Scotland or in the war-fever of the Palatinate. But the teaching of the time was that it was in the air; and if the infective principle had been generated either in Scotland or on the upper Rhine it had diffused itself in some inscrutable way. The doctrine of epidemic constitutions seems strange to us; but some of the facts that it was meant to embrace are also strange to us. Were it not for an occasional reminder from influenza, we should hardly believe that any fevers could have travelled as the Hungarian fevers, the spotted fevers or "spotted agues" of former times are said to have done.

On the other hand, we have now a scientific doctrine of the effects of great fluctuations of the ground-water upon the production of telluric miasmata, which may be used to rationalize the theory of emanations adopted by Sydenham and Boyle. From this modern point of view the remarkable droughts preceding the pestilential fevers and plagues of 1624–25 and 1665, and preceding the fever of 1685–86, which is the one that immediately concerns us, may be not without significance.

The London fever of 1685–86 having been suspected at the time to be the forerunner of a plague, as other such fevers in

[1] Janus Chunradus Rhumelius, *Historia morbi, qui etc.* Norimb. 1625.

the earlier part of the century had been, and no plague havi[ng]
ensued, the question arises most naturally at this stage, why t[he]
plague should have never come back in London or elsewhere [in]
Britain after the great outbreak of 1665–66.

The extinction of Plague in Britain.

Plague had been the grand infective disease of Britain fro[m]
the year of the Black Death, 1348–9, for more than thre[e]
centuries, down to 1666. The last of plague in Scotland wa[s]
in 1647–8, in the west and north-west of England about 165[0]
(in Wales probably in 1636–8), in Ireland in 1650, and in al[l]
other parts of the kingdom including London in 1666, the
absolute last of its provincial prevalence having been at Peterborough in the first months of 1667[1], while two or three occasional
deaths continued to occur annually in London down to 1679.
False reports of plague, contradicted by public advertisement,
were circulated for Bath in 1675[2], and for Newcastle in 1710[3];
while in London as late as 1799, during a bad time of typhus
fever, the occurrence of plague was alleged[4].

It is not easy to say why the plague should have died out.
It had been continuous in England from 1348, at first in general
epidemics, all over the country in certain years, thereafter mostly
in the towns, either in great explosions at long intervals or at a
moderate level for years together. The final outburst in 1665,
which was one of the most severe in its whole history, had
followed an unusually long period of freedom from plague in
London, and was followed, as it were, by a still longer period
of freedom until at last it could be said that the plague was
extinct. In some large towns it had been extinct, as the event
showed, at a much earlier date; thus at York the last known
epidemic was in 1604, and it can hardly be doubted that many

---

[1] W. D. Cooper, *Archæologia*, XXXVII. (1857) p. 1. I had overlooked this
important paper on English plagues in my former volume. The chief additional facts
that it contains are the very severe plague at Cambridge in the summer of 1666,
the deaths of 417 by plague at Peterborough in 1666, and of 8 more in the first
quarter of 1667, and the slightness of the Nottingham outbreak, which was in
August, 1666 (p. 22).

[2] *London Gazette*, 17–21 June, 1675, repeated in the number for 28 June–1 July.

[3] Brand, *Hist. of Newcastle*, II. 509. Report contradicted on 18 Dec.

[4] "The habitations of the poor within or adjoining to the City," says Willan,
"have suffered greatly; and some, I am informed, have been almost depopulated, the
infection having extended to every inmate. The rumour of a plague was totally devoid
of foundation."

other towns in England, Scotland and Ireland would have closed their records of plague earlier than they did had not the sieges and military occupations of the Civil Wars given especial occasion for the seeds of the infection to spring into life. Plague seemed to be dying out all over England and Scotland (in Ireland it is little heard of except in connexion with the Elizabethan and Cromwellian conquests) for some time before its final grand explosion in London in 1665.

In seeking for the causes of its decline and extinction we must keep prominently in view the fact that the virus was brought into the country from abroad as the Black Death of 1348-9. But for that importation it is conceivable that there would have been no signal history of plague in Britain. Its original prevalence was on a great scale, and there were several other widespread epidemics throughout the rest of the 14th century. In the first volume of this history I have collected evidence that plague was endemic or steady for long periods of the 15th and 16th centuries in London, with greater outbursts at intervals, and that in the 17th century it came chiefly in great explosions. Something must have served to keep the virus in the country, and more especially in the towns, until at length it was exhausted. An exotic infection, or one that had not arisen from indigenous conditions, and would probably never have so arisen, does not remain indefinitely in the country to which it is imported. Thus Asiatic cholera, imported into Europe on six, or perhaps five, occasions in the 19th century, has never become domesticated; and yellow fever had a career in the southern provinces of Spain during some twenty years only. Plague did become domesticated for about three centuries in England, and for longer in some other countries of Europe; but it died out at length, and it would almost certainly have died out sooner had it not found in all European countries some conditions not altogether unsuited to it. What were the favouring conditions?

If, as I believe, the virus of plague had its habitat in the soil, from which it rose in emanations, and if it depended therein, both remotely for its origin in some distant country, as well as immediately for its continuance in all countries, upon the decomposition of human bodies, then it is easy to understand that the immense mortalities caused by each epidemic would preserve the seeds of the disease, or the crude matters of the disease, in the soil. Buried plague-bodies would be the most obvious

sources of future plagues.   But if the theory given of the Black
Death be correct, bodies dead of famine or famine-fever would
also favour in an especial way the continuance of the plague-
virus in certain spots of ground, although they would probably
never have originated it in this country.   Moreover, the products
of ordinary cadaveric decomposition would be so much pabulum
or nutriment for the continuance of the virus.   But all those
things being constant, the continuance of plague would largely
depend upon the manner in which the dead, after plague, or
after famine and fever, or in general, were disposed of.   The
soil of all England in 1348-9 was filled with multitudes of the
dead laid in trenches, and there were several general revivals of
plague in the fifty or sixty years following.   In London there
were plague-pits opened in the suburbs in many great epidemics
during three centuries.   Even when there was no epidemic the
dead were laid in the ground in such a manner that their resolution
was speedy, and the diffusion of the products unchecked.   But
it is undoubted that greater care in the disposal of the dead did
at length come into vogue.   Thus, in the Black Book of the
Corporation of Tewkesbury there is an entry under the year
1603, that all those dead of plague, "to avoid the perill, were
buried in coffins of bourde," the disease having carried off no
fewer than 560 the year before (1602) and being then in its
second season[1].   The reason given is "to avoid the peril," and
it is beyond question that burial in a coffin did in fact delay
decomposition (unless in peculiar circumstances which need not
be particularized), and kept the cadaveric products from passing
quickly and freely into the pores of the ground.   Again, if the
burial were in such coffins as the Chinese commonly use, the
decomposition would proceed almost as slowly as if the body
had been embalmed, and with as little risk of befouling the soil.
For a long time in England such burials were the privilege only
of the rich ; but as wealth increased by commerce they became
the privilege of all classes; and in the last great plague of London,
as I said in my former volume, " even at the worst time coffins
would seem to have been got for most."   Defoe's account of the
burials in heaps in plague-pits is so exactly like that of Dekker
for the plague of 1603, and of other contemporaries for the
plague of 1625, that one may reasonably suspect him to
have used these earlier accounts as his authority for the practice

[1] Rudder, *A New History of Gloucestershire*, 1779, p. 737.

in 1665, which he had no direct knowledge of. However, I do not contend that there were no such burials in 1665; just as one learns from Dekker that the coffin-makers in 1603 were busily employed and grew rich, although he also describes how a husband "saw his wife and his deadly enemy whom he hated" launched into the pit "within a pair of sheets." In ordinary times, as we learn from the tables of burial-dues, there were poorer interments without coffins as late as 1628, according to a document printed by Spelman, the name of the parish being withheld, and even as late as 1672 in the parish of St Giles's, Cripplegate. Spelman's object in writing in 1641 was to protest against the mercenary practices of the clergy in the matter of burial, recalling the numerous canons of the medieval Church directed against all such forms of simony; and incidentally he mentions that it was testified before the Commissioners that a certain parson "had made forty pound of one grave in ten yeeres, by ten pounds at a time"[1]—a "tenancy of the soil" short enough to satisfy even the so-called Church of England Burial Reform Association. The use of coffins in the burial of the very poorest is now so universal that we hardly realize how gradually it was introduced. I am unable to say when burial in a sheet or cerecloth ceased; but it became less and less the rule for the poorer classes throughout the 17th century. In 1666 was passed the Act for burial in woollen, which was re-enacted more strictly in 1678[2]. The motive of it was to encourage the native woollen manufactures, or to prevent the money of the country from being expended on foreign-made linen; and its clauses ordained that woollen should be substituted for linen in the lining of the coffin and in the shrouding of the corpse, but that no penalty should be exacted for burying in linen any that shall die of the plague. Whether it prohibited in effect the use of linen cere-cloths to enshroud corpses where no coffin was used does not appear clearly from the terms of the Act; but, as the intention was to discourage the use of linen, and to bring in the use of woollen, for all purposes of burial, it is probable that it served to put an end to coffinless burials altogether, wherever it was

---

[1] Spelman, *De Sepultura*. English ed. 1641, p. 28. He cites the burial fees paid to the parson as twice as much for coffined as for uncoffined corpses. This agrees on the whole with the evidence adduced in the former volume of this history, p. 335.

[2] 18 and 19 Car. II. cap. 4; 30 Car. II. (1), cap. 3. These Acts were repealed by 54 Geo. III., cap. 108.

enforced, inasmuch as the prescribed material was wholly un-suited for the purpose of a cerecloth.

The history of the London plague-pit between Soho and the present Regent Street shows that, after the last great plague of 1665–66, more caution was used against infection from the buried plague-bodies. Macaulay says it was popularly believed that the earth was deeply tainted with infection, and could not be disturbed without imminent risk to human life; and he asserts that no foundations were laid in the pest-field till two generations had passed and till the spot had long been sur-rounded with buildings, the space being left blank in maps of London as late as the end of George I.'s reign[1].

After 1666 the old churchyards were not less crowded than before, but more crowded, perhaps because coffined corpses occupied more space and decayed more slowly. On 17 October, 1672, Evelyn paid a visit to Norwich: "I observed that most of the churchyards (tho' some of them large enough) were filled up with earth, or rather the congestion of dead bodys one upon another, for want of earth, even to the very top of the walls, and some above the walls, so as the churches seemed to be built in pitts." The same day he had visited Sir Thomas Browne, the author of the famous essay on urn burial or cremation, (suggested to him by the digging up of forty or fifty funeral urns in a field at Old Walsingham). The essay is full of curious learning and equally curious moralizing. But Sir Thomas, though a physician, has not a word to say on so proximate a topic as the state of the Norwich churchyards, which came under his eyes and perhaps under his nose every day of his life[2].

The practice of burying in coffins, which came at length within the means of all classes, may seem too paltry a cause to assign, even in part, for so remarkable an effect as the absolute disappearance of plague after a duration of more than three

---

[1] *History of England*, I. 359.

[2] He has one or two relevant remarks: "But while we suppose common worms in graves, 'tis not easy to find any there; few in churchyards above a foot deep, fewer or none in churches, though in fresh-decayed bodies. Teeth, bones, and hair give the most lasting defiance to corruption. In an hydropsical body, ten years buried in the churchyard, we met with a fat concretion [adipocere] where the nitre of the earth and the salt and lixivious liquor of the body had coagulated large lumps of fat into the consistence of the hardest Castille soap, whereof part remaineth with us. The body of the Marquis of Dorset seemed sound and handsomely cereclothed, that after seventy-eight years was found uncorrupted. Common tombs preserve not beyond powder: a firmer consistence and compage of parts might be expected from arefaction, deep burial, or charcoal."

centuries. My view of the matter is that the virus would have died out of itself had it not been continually augmented, or fed by its appropriate pabulum, and that the gradual change in the mode of interment helped to check such augmentation or feeding.

But the more elaborate interment of the dead was itself an index of the greater spending power of the community, and it may be said that it was the better condition of the people, and not this one particular thing in it, which put an end to the periodical recurrences of plague. In all but its earliest outbursts in the fourteenth, and perhaps the fifteenth century, plague had been peculiarly an infection of the poor, being known as "the poor's plague." Perhaps the chief reason why the richer classes usually escaped it was that they fled from the plague-tainted place, leaving the poorer classes unable to stir from their homes, exposed to the infectious air, and all the more exposed that their habitual employments and wages would cease, their sustenance become precarious, their condition lowered, and their manners reckless. Again, it was not unusual for the plague to break out in a season of famine or scarcity, during which the ordinary risks of the labouring class would be aggravated. Famines ceased (except in Ireland, where there had been comparatively little plague), and scarcities became less common. The sieges and occupations of the Civil Wars in the middle of the 17th century, which undoubtedly were the occasion of the last outbursts of plague in many of the towns, were a brief experience, followed by unbroken tranquillity. Whatever things were tending to the removal of plague in all its old seats had free course thereafter.

On the other hand, one may make too much of the increase of well-being among the labouring class which coincided with the cessation of plague. As a check upon population plague worked in a very remarkable way. In London, as well as in towns like Newcastle and Chester, plague towards the end of its reign arose perhaps once in a generation and made a clean sweep of a fifth or a fourth part of the inhabitants, including hardly any of the well-to-do. It destroyed, of course, many bread-winners and many that were not absolutely sunk in poverty; but its broad effect was to cut off the margin of poverty as if by a periodical process of pruning. The Lord Mayor of London wrote to the Privy Council at the end of the great plague of 1625: "The great mortality, although it had

taken many poor people away, yet had made more poverty by decay of tradesmen"—a decay of trade which they might reasonably expect to recover from before long. No such ruthless shears was ever applied at intervals to the growing fringe of poverty in after times. The poor were a more permanent residue, pressing more upon each other; but they did not press more upon the rich, except through the poor rate; on the contrary, the separation of classes became more marked.

Perhaps I ought to give an illustration of this, so as not to leave so radical a change in the vague and disputable form of a generality. I shall take the instance of Chester; its circuit of walls, remaining from the Roman conquest, is something fixed for the imagination to rest upon amidst changes within and without them.

Passing over its medieval and its not infrequent Tudor experiences of epidemic sickness, let us come to the beginning of the 17th century. In two or three successive seasons from 1602 to 1605 it lost 1,313 persons by plague, as well as about 250 from other causes. The population was then mostly within the walls, and probably did not exceed 5000. There was a shipping quarter on the west side, with egress by the Water-gate to the landing-places on the Dee; a millers' quarter, with corn-market and hostelries, on the south, connecting by the South gate and bridge with a hamlet across the river along the road to Wales; a Liberty or Freedom of the city outside the walls on the east, along the road to Warrington and Manchester, with a Bar, a short distance out, as in London, to mark the limit of the mayor's jurisdiction; and on the north side, within the walls, the cattle-market and shambles, with the market for country produce, and a few straggling houses without the gate on the road leading to Liverpool. Chester was a characteristic county town, with its cathedral clergy, its garrison, its resident nobility and gentry, its professional classes, its tradesmen, market people and populace, with the addition of a shipping trade to Ireland and afterwards to foreign and colonial ports. Plague continuing from 1602 to 1605 cut off a fourth or a fifth of its population, and these the poorest. The gaps in the population would gradually have filled up, and the fringe of poverty grown again[1].

The plague came again in 1647, and cut off 2053 in the short space of twenty-three weeks from 22 June to 30 November. The bills of it are extant[2], and show on what parishes the plague fell most. All the parishes were originally within the walls but one, St John's, the ancient collegiate church of Mercia, built upon a rocky knoll in the south-east angle made by the walls with the river. The other nine parish churches and their graveyards were within the walls; but the parishes of three of them extended beyond the gates, just as the three parishes dedicated to St Botolph at the gates of London did. These three were St Oswald's, which included the Liberty on the east side, Trinity, which included the shipping quarter on the

---

[1] One may allege poverty on general grounds, as well as on particular. Thus, in 1636, the mayor was unpopular: "He was a stout man and had not the love of the commons. He was cruel, and not pitying the poor, he caused many dunghills to be carried away; but the cost was on the poor—it being so hard times might well have been spared." Ormerod, I. 203.

[2] Printed plague-bill, with MS. additions, Harl. MS. 1929.

west as well as the houses along the Liverpool road on the north, and St Mary's, which included the millers' suburb across the Dee on the south. Hollar's map, made a few years after the plague of 1647, shows very few houses beyond the walls, except in the ancient Liberty on the east. But it will appear from the following table that the parishes which had extended beyond the walls must either have been very crowded close up to the walls (as the Gate parishes were always apt to be), or there must have actually been a greater population outside the gates than the contemporary map shows :

Burials from Plague in the several Parishes of Chester in 23 weeks, June 22—Nov. 30, 1647.

5 parishes wholly within the walls.

	Total.	First week.	Worst (7th) week.
St Peter	75	0	14
St Bridget	85	7	9
St Martin	173	9	23
St Michael	133	26	9
St Olave	59	3	5

3 parishes extending beyond the walls.

St Oswald	396	11	37
St Mary	314	5	20
Trinity	232	1	32

1 parish wholly without the walls.

St John	358	2	26
Pesthouse	228	0	34
	2053	64	209

This was the last plague of Chester, but for a small outbreak in 1654. The next vital statistics that we get for the city are more than a century after, in 1774[1]. The population of 14,713 was then divided into two almost distinct parts, separated by the wall. The old city was being rebuilt, all but some ancient blocks of buildings held in the dead hand of the cathedral chapter ; it was becoming a model 18th century place of residence for a wealthy and refined class, who were remarkably healthy and not very prolific, the parishes wholly within the walls having 3502 inhabitants. The poorer class had gone to live mostly outside the walls in new and mean suburbs, the three parishes at the Gates and extending now far beyond the walls, together with the original extramural parish of St John's, having a population of 11,211. There was no town in Britain where the separation of the rich from the poor was more complete ; there was hardly another town of the size where the health of the rich was better ; and although the health of the populace was not so bad as in the manufacturing towns of Lancashire and Cumberland, close at hand, yet it is hardly possible to find so great a contrast as that between the clean and wholesome residential quarter within the walls and the mean fever-stricken suburbs as described by Haygarth in 1774 :

"The inhabitants of the suburbs," he says, "are generally of the lowest rank ; they want most of the conveniences and comforts of life ; their houses are small, close, crowded and dirty ; their diet affords very bad nourishment, and their cloaths are seldom changed or washed...These miserable wretches, even when they go abroad, carry a poisonous atmosphere round their bodies that is distinguished by a noisome and offensive smell, which is peculiarly disgustful even to the healthy and vigorous, exciting sickness and a sense of general debility. It cannot therefore be wondered that diseases should be produced where such poison is inspired with every breath."

[1] Haygarth, *Phil. Trans.*, LXVIII. 139.

The case of Chester shows by broader contrasts than anywhere else the change from the public health of plague-times to that of more modern times. But it can hardly be said to show the populace better off than before; it shows them changed into a proletariat, and separated from the richer classes by walls several feet thick. Such, at least, was the result after four generations of immunity from plague, a result which indicates, as I have said, that we may easily make too much of the improved well-being of the poorer classes as a cause of the cessation of plague.

An easy explanation of plague ceasing in London has long been current, and just because it is an easy explanation it will probably hold the field for many years to come. It is that the fire of 1666 burnt out the seeds of plague. Defoe, writing in 1723, ascribed this opinion to certain "quacking philosophers," but he would hardly have said so if he could have foreseen the respectable authority for it in after times. The plague had ceased in most of its provincial centres after the Civil Wars, and in some of them, such as York, from as early a date as 1604. It ceased in all the principal cities of Western Europe within a few years of its cessation in London. In London itself it ceased after 1666, not only in the City which was the part burned down in September of that year, but in St Giles's, where the Great Plague began, in Cripplegate, Whitechapel and Stepney, where it was always worst, in Southwark, Bermondsey and Newington, in Lambeth and Westminster. Nor can it be said that the City was the source from which the infection used to spread to the Liberties and out-parishes. All the later plagues of London, perhaps even that of 1563, began in the Liberties or out-parishes and at length invaded the City. The part of London that was rebuilt after 1666 contained many finer dwelling-houses than before, built of stone, with substantial carpentry, and elegantly finished in fine and rare woods. The fronts of the new houses did not overhang so as to obstruct the ventilation of the streets and lanes; but the streets, lanes, alleys and courts were somewhat closely reproduced on the old foundations. A side walk in some streets was secured for foot-passengers by means of massive posts, which, with the projecting signs of houses and shops, were at length removed in 1766. The improvements in the City after the fire were mostly in the houses of the richer

citizens. The City was the place of residence of the rich, with perhaps as many poorer purlieus in close proximity as the residential districts of London now have. But four-fifths of London at the time of the fire were beyond the walls of the City. It is in these extramural regions that the interest mostly lies for epidemical diseases. They remain, says Defoe in 1723, "still in the same condition they were in before." Unfortunately we know little of their condition, whether in the 17th century or in the 18th. But there must have been something in it most unfavourable to health; for we find from the Bills of Mortality that the cessation of plague made hardly any difference to the annual average of deaths, the increase of population being allowed for. This fact makes the disappearance of plague all the more remarkable.

Fevers to the end of the 17th century.

The epidemical seasons of 1685–86 were the last that Sydenham recorded; he was shortly after laid aside from active work by gout, and died in 1689. Morton, who made notes of fevers and smallpox until 1694, is more a clinical observer than a student of "epidemic constitutions"; and although his writings are of value to the epidemiologist, he does not help us to understand the circumstances in which epidemic diseases prevailed more at one time than another. To the end of the century there is no other medical source of information, and little besides generalities to be collected from any source. It is known that the years from 1693 to 1699 were years of scarcity all over the kingdom, that the fever-deaths in London reached the high figure of 5036 in 1694, and that there was a high mortality in many country parishes and market towns during the scarcity. But there are few particular illustrations of the type of epidemic sickness. There is, therefore, little left to do but to give the figures, and to add some remarks.

Fever Deaths in the London Bills, 1687—1700.

Year	Fever deaths	Spotted fever deaths	Deaths from all causes	Year	Fever deaths	Spotted fever deaths	Deaths from all causes
1687	2847	144	21460	1694	5036	423	24109
1688	3196	139	22921	1695	3019	105	19047
1689	3313	129	23502	1696	2775	102	18638
1690	3350	203	21461	1697	3111	137	20292
1691	3490	193	22691	1698	3343	274	20183
1692	3205	161	20874	1699	3505	306	20795
1693	3211	199	20959	1700	3675	189	19443

Tables from Short's Abstracts of Parish Registers.

Year	Registers examined	Registers with excess of death	Deaths in them	Births in them
		Country Parishes.		
1689	144	27	828	692
1690	146	17	532	324
1691	147	16	336	180
1692	147	10	207	146
1693	146	27	650	426
1694	148	18	465	348
1695	149	23	649	492
1696	150	19	503	344
1697	150	21	559	409
1698	152	12	397	289
1699	151	20	433	318
1700	160	29	890	739
		Market Towns.		
1689	25	12	1965	1415
1693	25	5	417	338
1694	25	6	1307	681
1695	25	3	309	246
1696	26	4	1020	708
1697	26	2	109	80
1698	26	4	575	423
1699	26	7	1181	867
1700	27	4	726	587

In the London figures the year 1694 stands out conspicuous by its deaths from all causes, and by its high total of fevers. The fever-deaths began to rise from their steady weekly level a little before Christmas, 1693, and remained high all through the year 1694, with a good many deaths from "spotted fever" in the worst weeks. Among the victims in London in February was Sir William Phipps, Governor of New England: his illness appeared at first to be a cold, which obliged him to keep his chamber; but it proved "a sort of malignant fever, whereof many about this time died in the city[1]." Pepys, writing to Evelyn on 10 August, 1694, calls it "the fever of the season," three being down with it at his house, but well advanced in their recovery. In that week and in the week following, the deaths in London from all causes touched the highest points of the year, the deaths from fever and spotted fever being a full quarter of them. Fever at its worst in London never made more than a quarter of the annual deaths from all causes; so that, if

---

[1] Cotton Mather's *Magnalia.* Ed. of 1853, I. 227.

we take it to have been the successor of the plague, it operated
in a very different way—with a greatly lessened fatality of all
that were attacked, with only a reminder of the old special
incidence upon the summer and autumn seasons, but with a
steadiness from year to year, and throughout each year, that
made the fever-deaths of a generation little short of one of those
enormous totals of plague-deaths that were rapidly piled up
during a few months, perhaps once or twice in a generation.

The following table from the London weekly Bills shows the
progress of the fever from the end of April, 1694, with the
number of deaths specially assigned to "spotted fever":—

London: Weekly Mortalities from fever and all causes, epidemic of 1694.

Week ending	Fever	Spotted fever	All deaths	Week ending	Fever	Spotted fever	All deaths
April 24	90	15	427	Aug. 28	111	20	510
May 1	77	10	369	Sept. 5	115	16	505
8	89	9	413	12	112	12	462
15	80	5	395	18	98	9	504
22	101	3	428	25	106	4	490
29	72	8	430	Oct. 2	124	8	533
June 5	112	12	469	9	125	10	553
12	113	12	434	16	114	9	552
19	113	11	430	23	104	3	511
26	99	14	396	30	118	3	528
July 3	94	11	423	Nov. 6	70	3	439
10	89	7	453	13	106	2	471
17	86	10	445	20	117	13	538
24	115	13	507	27	79	6	456
31	84	13	484	Dec. 4	87	6	475
Aug. 7	99	10	462	11	87	3	407
14	110	20	530	18	78	4	445
21	135	19	583	25	66	3	394

The year 1694, to which the epidemic of malignant fever
(as well as malignant smallpox) belongs, was one of the series
of "seven ill years" at the end of the 17th century (1693-99).
They were long noted, says Thorold Rogers, "for the distress of
the people and for the exalted profits of the farmer." The price
of wheat in the autumn and winter of 1693 was the highest since
the famine of 1661. In 1697-8 corn was again dear and much
of it was spoilt. At Norwich in 1698 wheat was sold at 44s. a
comb.

Harvests spoiled by wet weather or unseasonable cold appear
to have been the most general cause of the high prices of food.
In London there was no unusual sickness except in 1694; indeed
the other years to the end of the century show a somewhat low

mortality, the year 1696, which Macaulay marks as a time of severe distress among the common people owing to the calling in of the debased coinage[1], had the smallest number of deaths from all causes (18,638) since many years before, and for a century after allowing for the increase of population. But the deaths from "fever" were some three thousand every year, and the births, so far as registered, were, as usual, far below the deaths.

It was in the country at large that the effects of the "seven ill years" were chiefly felt. According to Short's abstracts of parish registers, there was unusual mortality at the beginning of the period and at the end of it; in his Chronology he mentions spotted fever, bloody flux and agues in 1693 (besides an influenza or universal slight fever recorded by Molyneux of Dublin), and again in 1697 and 1698 "purples, quinsies, Hungarian and spotted fever, universal pestilential spotted fever," from famine and bad food.

When we look for the evidence of this in England we shall have difficulty in finding it. Short's own abstracts give almost no colour to it; but there are other figures from the parish registers, scattered through the county histories and statistical works, which prove that the seven ill years must have checked population. Thus at Sheffield in the ten years 1691–1700 there was the greatest excess of burials over baptisms in the whole history of the town from 1561—namely, 2856 burials to 2221 baptisms (688 marriages). At Minehead, Somerset, a parish of some 1200 people occupied in weaving, the deaths and births were as follows in four years of the decennium:

	Baptised.	Buried.		Baptised.	Buried.
1691	57	75	1695	47	48
1694	34	55	1697	35	65

A glimpse of spotted or pestilential fever in Bristol during the years of distress at the end of the 17th century comes from Dr Dover, a man of no academical repute, but at all events an articulate voice. Passing from an account of the spotted pestilential fever at Guayaquil, "when I took it by storm," he goes on[2]:

---

[1] *History of England &c.,* IV. 707. Evelyn (*Diary,* 21 *May,* 1696) says the city was "very healthy," although the summer was exceeding rainy, cold and unseasonable.

[2] Thomas Dover, M.B., *The Ancient Physician's Legacy.* London, 1732, p. 98.

of
lg
ls
a
e
l
:

"About thirty-seven years since [written in 1732], this fever raged much in Bristol, so that I visited from twenty-five to thirty patients a day for a considerable time, besides their poor children taken into their workhouse, where I engaged myself, for the encouragement of so good and charitable an undertaking, to find them physick and give them advice at my own expense and trouble for the two first years. All these poor children in general had this fever, yet no more than one of them died of it of the whole number, which was near two hundred."

—an experience of typhus in children which was strictly according to rule. This had clearly been the occasion of a memorial addressed to the Mayor and Aldermen of Bristol, in 1696, praying that a capacious workhouse should be erected for children and the aged, which "will prevent children from being smothered or starved by the neglect of the parish officers and poverty of their parents, which is now a great loss to the nation[1]."

The year 1698 was the climax of the seven ill years. The spring was the most backward for forty-seven years, the first wheat in the ear being seen near London on 16th June. For four months to the end of August the days were almost all rainy, except from the 18th to the 26th July. Whole fields of corn were spoilt. In Kent there was barley standing uncut on 29th September, and some lay in the swathe until December. Much of the corn in the north of England was not got in until Christmas, and in Scotland they were reaping the green empty corn in January[2].

Fevers of the seven ill years in Scotland.

It is from Scotland that we hear most of the effects of the seven ill years in the way of famine and fever. Scotland was then in a backward state compared with England; and its northern climate, making the harvest always a few weeks later than in England, told especially against it in the ill years. Fynes Morryson, in the beginning of the 17th century, contrasts the Scotch manner of life unfavourably with the English, and Sir Robert Sibbald's account towards the end of that century is little better. Morryson says, "the excesse of drinking was then farre greater in generall among the Scots than the English." Sibbald remarks[3] on the drinking habits of the Scots common

[1] Broadsheet in the British Museum Library.
[2] Tooke, *Hist. of Prices*, Introd.
[3] *Scotia Illustrata.* Edin. 1684. Lib. II. p. 52.

people : their potations of ale or spirits on an empty stomach, especially in the morning, relaxed the fibres and induced "erratic fevers of a bad type, bastard pleurisies,...dropsies, stupors, lethargies and apoplexies." Morryson says : "Their bedsteads were then like cubbards in the wall, with doores to be opened and shut at pleasure, so as we climbed up to our beds. They used but one sheete, open at the sides and top, but close at the feete, and so doubled[1]." Sibbald says the peasantry had poor food and hard work, and were subject to many diseases —"heartburn, sleeplessness, ravings, hypochondriac affections, mania, dysentery, scrophula, cancer, and a dire troop of diseases which everywhere now invades the husbandmen that were formerly free from diseases." *Causa a victu est.* Therefore consumption was common enough. He has much to say of fevers,—of intermittents, especially in spring and autumn, catarrhal fevers, nervous fevers, comatose fevers, with delirium, spasms and the like symptoms, malignant, spotted, pestilential, hectic, &c. The continued fevers ranged in duration from fifteen to thirty-one days, recovery being ushered in with sweats, alvine flux and salivation. Purple fevers had sometimes livid or black spots mixed with the purple (mottling) ; in a case given, there were suppurations which appear to have been bubonic. There had been no plague in Scotland since 1647–48 ; but fevers, unless Sibbald has given undue prominence to them, would appear to have filled its place among the adults.

Another writer of this period, from whom some information is got as to fevers, was Dr Andrew Brown of Edinburgh. He is mainly a controversialist, and is on the whole of little use save for the history of the treatment of fevers. He came to London on a visit in 1687, attracted by the fame of Sydenham's method of curing fevers by antimonial emetics and by purgation: "Returning home as much overjoyed as I had gotten a treasure, I presently set myself to that practice"—of which he gave an account in his 'Vindicatory Schedule concerning the New Cure of Fever[2].' Continual fever, he says, takes up, with its pendicles, the half of all the diseases that men are afflicted with; and some part of what he calls continual fever must have been spotted: "As concerning the eruption of spots in fevers, these altogether resemble the marks made by stroaks on the skin, and these

[1] Fynes Morryson, *Itinerary*, 1614. Pt. III. p. 156.
[2] Edinburgh, 1691, p. 67.

marks are also made by the stagnation and coagulation of the blood in the small channels [according to the doctrine of obstructions]......They tinge the skin with blewness or redness."

The bitter controversy as to the treatment of fevers led Brown into another writing in 1699[1].

"The fevers that reign at this time [it was towards the end of the seven ill years] are for the most part quick and peracute, and cut off in a few days persons of impure bodies. And as I have used this method by vomiting and purging in many, and most successfully at this time, so I have had lately considerable experience thereof in my own family : wherein four of my children and ten servants had the fever, and blessed be God, are all recovered, by repeated vomiting with antimonial vomits and frequent purgings, except two servants, the one having gotten a great stress at work, who bragging of his strength did contend with his neighbour at the mowing of hay, and presently sickened and died the sixth day, and whom I saw not till the day before he died, and found him in such a condition that I could not give him either vomit or purge : and the other was his neighbour who strove with him, being a man of most impure and emaciate body, who had endured want and stress before he came to my service, and who got not all was necessary because he had not the occasion of due attendance, all my servants being sick at the time[2]."

This account of the experience which Dr Andrew Brown had lately had among his children and domestics in or near Edinburgh was written in 1699, and may be taken as relating to part of the wide-spread sickliness of the seven ill years in Scotland. Fletcher of Saltoun gives us a general view of the deplorable state of Scotland at the end of the 17th century, which was intensified by the succession of bad harvests[3]. The rents of cultivated farms were paid, not in money, but in corn, which gave occasion to many inequalities, to the traditional fraudulent practices of millers and to usury. The pasture lands for sheep and black cattle had no shelters from the weather, and no winter provision of hay or straw (roots were unheard of until long after), "so that the beasts are in a dying condition." The country swarmed with vagrants (a hundred thousand, he estimates, in ordinary times, but doubled in the dear years), who lived and multiplied in incest, rioted in swarms in the nearest hills in times of plenty, and in times of distress fell upon farmhouses in gangs

[1] *The Epilogue to the Five Papers, etc.* Edin. 1699, p. 22. This title refers to a controversy on the use of antimonial emetics in fevers. See Dr John Brown's essay on Dr Andrew Brown, in his *Locke and Sydenham*, new ed. Edinb., 1866.

[2] He adds that "the fever has several times before been in my family and among my servants and children." In mentioning the case of the Master of Forbes in August, 1691, whom he cured, he remarks that "the malicious said he was under no fever"; to disprove which Dr Brown refers to the symptoms of frequent pulse, watching and raving, continual vomiting, frequent fainting, and extreme weakness.

[3] Andrew Fletcher, *Two Discourses*. 1699.

C. II.

4

of forty or more, demanding food. Besides these there were great many poor families very meanly provided for by t Church boxes, who lived wholly upon bad food and fell ir various diseases. He had been credibly informed that sor families in the years of mere scarcity preceding the climax 1698–99 had eaten grains, for want of bread. "In the worst tin from unwholesome food diseases are so multiplied among po people that, if some course be not taken, the famine may ve probably be followed by a plague[1]."

We owe some details of these calamities in Scotland Patrick Walker, the Covenanter, who records them to sho how the prophecies of Divine vengeance on the land, uttere during the Stuart persecutions by Cargill and Peden, had bee in due time fulfilled[2]:

"In the year 1694, in the month of August, that crop got such a strok in one night by east mist or fog standing like mountains (and where remained longest and thickest the badder were the effects, which all our ol men, that had seen frost, blasting and mildewing, had never seen the like) tha it got little more good of the ground. In November that winter many wer smitten with wasting sore fluxes and strange fevers (which carried man off the stage) of such a nature and manner that all our old physicians ha never seen the like and could make no help; for all things that used to b proper remedies proved destructive. And this was not to be imputed t bad unwholesome victual; for severals who had plenty of old victual di send to Glasgow for Irish meal, and yet were smitten with fluxes and fever in a more violent and infectious nature and manner than the poorest in the land, whose names and places where they dwelt I could instance.

"These unheard-of manifold judgments continued seven years, not always alike, but the seasons, summer and winter, so cold and barren, and the wonted heat of the sun so much withholden, that it was discernible upon the cattle, flying fowls and insects decaying, that seldom a fly or gleg was to be seen. Our harvests not in the ordinary months, many shearing in November and December, yea some in January and February; the names of the places I can instruct. Many contracting their deaths, and losing the use of their feet and hands, shearing and working amongst it in frost and snow; and after all some of it standing still, and rotting upon the ground, and much of it for little use either to man or beast, and which had no taste or colour of meal. Meal became so scarce that it was at two shillings a peck, and many could not get it.

"Through the long continuance of these manifold judgments deaths and burials were so many and common that the living were wearied with burying of the dead. I have seen corpses drawn in sleds. Many got neither coffins nor winding-sheet.

"I was one of four who carried the corpse of a young woman a mile of way; and when we came to the grave, an honest poor man came and said, 'You must go and help me to bury my son, he is lien dead this

---

[1] The English Government took off the Customs duty upon victual imported from England to Scotland, and placed a bounty of 20*d*. per boll upon it.

[2] Patrick Walker, *Some Remarkable Passages in the Life and Death of Mr Daniel Cargill, &c.* Edinb. 1732. (Reprinted in *Biographia Presbyteriana*. Edinb. 1827, II. 25.)

two days; otherwise I will be obliged to bury him in my own yard.' We went, and there were eight of us had two miles to carry the corpse of that young man, many neighbours looking on us, but none to help us. I was credibly informed, that in the North, two sisters on a Monday's morning were found carrying the corpse of their brother on a barrow with bearing-ropes, resting themselves many times, and none offering to help them.

"I have seen some walking about at sunsetting, and next day at six o'clock in the summer morning found dead in their houses, without making any stir at their death, their head lying upon their hand, with as great a smell as if they had been four days dead; the mice or rats having eaten a great part of their hands and arms.

"The nearer and sorer these plagues seized, the sadder were their effects, that took away all natural and relative affections, so that husbands had no sympathy with their wives, nor wives with their husbands, parents with their children, nor children with their parents. These and other things have made me to doubt if ever any of Adam's race were in a more deplorable condition, their bodies and spirits more low, than many were in these years."

In the parish of West Calder, 300 out of 900 "examinable" persons wasted away.

Some facts and traditions of the Seven Ill Years were recorded nearly a century after in the Statistical Account of Scotland. From the Kirk Session records of the parish of Fordyce, Banffshire, it did not appear "that any public measures were pursued for the supply of the poor, nor anything uncommon done by the Session except towards the end. The common distribution of the collections of the church amounted only to about 1s. 2d. or 1s. 4d. weekly." The Kirk Session records bore witness to the numerous cases of immorality in the years before the famine that had been dealt with ecclesiastically, and to the entire and speedy cessation of such cases thereafter[1].

The account for the parish of Keithhall and Kinkell, Aberdeenshire, says that "many died of want, in particular ten Highlanders in a neighbouring parish, that of Kemnay; so that the Session got a bier made to carry them to the grave, not being able to afford coffins for such a number[2]." In the upland parish of Montquhitter, in the same county, the dear years reduced the population by one half or more. Until 1709 many farms were waste. Of sixteen families that resided on the estate of Lettertie, thirteen were extinguished. The account of this parish contains several stories of the distress, with the names of individuals[3]. It is clear, however, that all the parishes of Scotland were not equally distressed. The county of Moray and "some of the best land along the east coast of Buchan and Formartine [Aberdeenshire] abounded with seed and bread;" but transport to the upland parishes was difficult[4].

[1] Sir John Sinclair's *Statistical Account of Scotland*. 1st ed. III. 62.
[2] *Ibid*. II. 544.   [3] *Ibid*. VI. 122.
[4] In the remote parish of Kilmuir, Skye, the famine is referred to the year 1688, "when the poor actually perished on the highways for want of aliment." (*Ibid*. II. 551.) In Duthil and Rothimurchus, Invernessshire, the famine is referred to 1680, "as nearly as can be recollected:" "A famine in this and the neighbouring counties, of the most fatal consequence. The poorer sort of people frequented the churchyard to pull a mess of nettles, and frequently struggled about the prey, being the earliest spring greens....So many families perished from want that for six miles in a well-inhabited extent, within the year there was not a smoke remaining." (*Ibid*. IV. 316.) In the Kirk session records of the parish of Kiltearn, Rossshire, which I have seen in MS., there are various entries in the year 1697 relating to badges of lead to be worn by those licensed to beg from door to door: on 12 April, 34 such persons are named, and on 19 April, Robert Douglas was reimbursed for the cost of 35 badges. On 2 Aug., the number of poor who were to receive each from the heritors ten shillings Scots reads like "nighentie foure."

We may take it that these experiences in the reign of
William III. were peculiar to Scotland ; even Ireland, which had
troubles enough of the same kind in the 18th and 19th centuries,
was at that time resorted to as a place of refuge by the
distressed Scots.   Among the special and temporary causes in
Scotland were antiquated agricultural usage, an almost incredible
proportion of the people in a state of lawless vagrancy, such as
Henry VIII. and Elizabeth had to deal with a century and a
half before, a low state of morals, both commercial and private,
a tyrannical disposition of the employers, a sullen attitude of the
labourers, and a total decay of the spirit of charity.   An ancient
elder of the parish of Fordyce, who kept some traditions of the dear
years, remarked to the minister : " If the same precautions had
been taken at that time which he had seen taken more lately in
times of scarcity, the famine would not have done so much hurt,
nor would so many have perished."

The evil of vagrancy, for which Fletcher of Saltoun saw no
remedy but a state of slavery not unlike that which Protector
Somerset had actually made the law of England for a couple
of years, 1547–49, in somewhat similar circumstances, gradually
cured itself without a resort to the practices of antiquity or of
barbarism.

The union with England in 1707, by removing the customs
duties and opening the Colonial trade to Scots shipping (they
had a share in the East India trade already) gave a remarkable
impulse to the manufacture of linen and to commerce.   Such
was the demand for Scots linen that, it seemed to De Foe, " the
poor could want no employment " ; and it may certainly be
taken as a fact that the establishment on a free basis of
industries and foreign markets gave Scotland relief from the
pauperism and vagrancy, like those of Ireland in the 18th
and 19th centuries, that threatened for a time, and especially
in the Seven Ill Years, to retard the developement of the
nation.

For several years after the period of scarcity or famine
from 1693 to 1699, the history of fever in Britain presents little
for special remark.

A book of the time was Dr George Cheyne's *New Theory of
Continual Fever*, London, 1701.   His theory is that of Bellini
and Borelli, which accounted for everything in fevers on

mechanical principles, and ignored the infective element in them. Cheyne does not even describe what the fevers were; but in showing how the theory applies, he mentions incidentally the symptoms—quick pulse, pain in the head, burning heat, want of sleep, raving, clear or flame-coloured urine, and morbid strength. Equally theoretical is the handling of the subject by Pitcairn. Freind, in his essays on fevers[1], is mainly occupied with controversial matters of treatment, except in connexion with Lord Peterborough's expedition to Spain in 1705, as we shall see in a section on sickness of camps and fleets.

In the absence of clinical details from the medical profession, the following from letters of the time will serve a purpose:

On 18 September, 1700, Thomas Bennett writes to Thomas Coke from Paris giving an account of the fever of Coke's brother: His fever is very violent upon him, and he has a hickup and twitchings in his face; he is especially ill in the night, and has now and then violent sweats. He raved for eight days together and in all that time did not get an hour's sleep. He was attended by Dr Helvetius and other physicians. Lady Eastes, her son, and most of her servants are sick, but they are all on the mending hand; her steward is dead of a high fever, having been sick but five days[2]. These are Paris fevers, the symptoms suggesting typhus, especially the prolonged vigil in one of the cases. It is to be remarked that they occurred among the upper classes; and it appears that the universal fevers "of a bad type" in France in 1712 did not spare noble houses nor even the palace of Louis the Great[3].

The following from the London Bills will show the prevalence of fever from year to year[4].

---

[1] John Freind, M.D., *Nine Commentaries on Fevers*, transl. by T. Dale. London, 1730.

[2] *Cal. Coke MSS.* II. 405.

[3] Joannes Turner, *De Febre Britannica Anni* 1712. Lond. 1713, p. 3. "Vere proximè elapso, per Gallias passim ingravescere coeperunt febres mali moris in nobiles domos, et regiam praecipue infestae; quò Ludovicum Magnum ipsa infortunia ostenderent Majorem, et patientia Christianissima Maximum."

[4] From London, on 25 February, 1701, we hear of the illness from a violent fever of Mr Brotherton, at his house in Chancery Lane; he was member for Newton, and Mr Coke was advised to look after his seat. A letter of 18 April, 1701, from Chilcote, in Derbyshire, says that it has been a sickly time in these parts and that a certain lady and her daughter were both dead and to be buried the same day. In the same correspondence, cases of fever in London are mentioned on 18 June and 4 December the same year (1701). *Cal. Coke MSS.* II. 421, 424, 429, 441.

Year	Dead of Fever	Dead of Spotted Fever	Dead of all diseases
1701	2902	68	20,471
1702	2682	53	19,481
1703	3162	74	20,720
1704	3243	61	22,684
1705	3290	41	22,097
1706	2662	54	19,847
1707	2947	42	21,600
1708	2738	62	21,291
1709	3140	118	21,800
1710	4397	343	24,620
1711	3461	142	19,833
1712	3131	96	21,198
1713	3039	102	21,057
1714	4631	150	26,569
1715	3588	161	22,232
1716	3078	100	24,436
1717	2940	137	23,446
1718	3475	132	26,523
1719	3803	124	28,347
1720	3910	66	25,454

The London fever of 1709-10.

The "seven ill years" were followed by the fine summer and abundant harvest (although hardly more than half the breadth was sown) of 1699. Scarcity was not a cause of excessive sickness again until 1709-10; although the harvest of 1703 was unfavourable. The price of wheat in 1702 was 25s. 6d. per quarter, and continued low for a number of years, notwithstanding the war with France. In Marlborough's wars there were no war-prices for farmers, as in the corresponding circumstances a century after; on the contrary, corn and produce of all kinds were so cheap that farmers had difficulty in paying their rents. The bounty of five shillings per quarter on exported wheat had given a great impulse to corn-growing, so that the acreage of wheat sown was much more than the country in an ordinary year required, partly, no doubt, because the bread of the poorer classes was largely made from the coarser cereals. The period of abundance was broken by the excessively severe winter of 1708-9, one of three memorable winters in the 18th century. The frost lasted all over Europe from October to March, and was followed by a greatly deficient crop in 1709. The following shows the rise of the price of the quarter of wheat in England :

		s.	d.
1708	Lady-day	27	3
„	Michaelmas	46	3
1709	Lady-day	57	6
„	Michaelmas	81	9
1710	Lady-day	81	9

The export of corn was prohibited in 1709 and again in 1710.

An epidemic of fever began in London in the autumn of 1709 and continued throughout 1710, in which year the fever-deaths reached the highest total since 1694. But it was not altogether a fever of starvation or distress among the poor, and perhaps not mainly so. There is always the dual question in connexion with fever following bad seasons and high prices: how much of it was due to the scarcity, and how much to those states of soil and atmosphere upon which the failure of the crop itself depended. An authentic case of the malignant fever which began to rage in London in the autumn of 1709 will both serve to show the remarkable type of at least a portion, if not the whole of the epidemic, and to prove its incidence upon the houses of the rich.

The case is recorded by Sir David Hamilton[1]:

"About the 5th of October, 1709, the son of that worthy gentleman, William Morison, esquire, was seized with a fever; at which time, and for some weeks before, a malignant fever raged in London." He had a quick and weak pulse, great difficulty or hindrance of speech, and a stupidity; "whereto were added tremors, and startings of the tendons, a dry and blackish tongue, a high-coloured but transparent urine and coming away for the most part involuntarily, and a hot and dry skin." Dr Grew was called in, and prescribed alexipharmac remedies (cordials, sudorifics, etc.) "A few days after the patient's skin was stained or marked with red and purple spots, and especially upon his breast, legs and thighs. These symptoms, although a little milder now and then, prevailed for fourteen days; after that the spots vanished, and the convulsive motions so increased that the young gentleman seemed ready to sink under them for several days together." He was treated with the application of blisters, and with doses of bark. His strength and flesh were so wasted that the hip whereon he lay was seized with a gangrene. For ten or twelve days before his death, "he breathed and perspired so offensive a smell that they were obliged to smoke his chamber with perfumes; and even myself, whilst I inclined my body a little too near him, was, by receiving his breath into my mouth, seized all on a sudden with such a sickness and faintness that I was obliged to take the air in the open fields, and returning thence to drink plentifully of *mountain* wine at dinner." The examination after death was made by the celebrated anatomist Dr Douglas. There was still a heap of brown-coloured spots visible on the breast; "there was nothing contained in the more conspicuous vessels of the abdomen but grumes or clots of blackish blood, without any serum in the interstices." Hamilton adds: "We too seldom dissect the bodies of those dying in fevers."

[1] *Tractatus Duplex.* Lond. 1710. Engl. transl. 1737, p. 253.

The tremors, offensive sweats and offensive breath are distinctive of a form of typhus that became common towards the middle of the century, and was called putrid fever (not in the sense of Willis) or miliary fever from the watery vesicles of the skin that often attended it. But although Hamilton was writing on miliary fever (of the factitious variety) this case is not given as an example, but is appended to his sixteen cases of the latter, as an example of "a deadly fever with loss of speech from the beginning." Among earlier cases, those belonging to the epidemic of 1661 as described by Willis correspond closely with this case, which we may take as representing part of the malignant fever that then raged in London. We have an anatomical record from each; but in neither was there sloughing of the lymph-follicles of the intestine, or of the mesenteric glands, as in the enteric fever of our own time; while in both there were red or purple spots on the breast or neck, and on the limbs. The "loss of speech from the beginning" suggests Sydenham's "absolute aphonia" in the comatose fever of 1673–76, which resembled in other respects Willis's fever of the brain and nervous stock (mostly of children) in 1661. One of the synonyms of "infantile remittent" was "an acute fever with dumbness[1]." This seems to have been a common type of fever in the latter part of the 17th century and early part of the 18th. Some likeness to enteric fever may be found in it, but there is no warrant for identifying it with that fever. Its main features may be said to have been its incidence upon the earlier years of life, but not to the exclusion of adult cases, its remarkable ataxic symptoms, which led Willis to refer it to "the brain and nervous stock" (spinal cord), its comatose character, its spots, occasional miliary eruption, ill-smelling sweats and other foetid evacuations, its protracted course, and its hectic sequelae.

The weekly bills of mortality in London bear little evidence of unusual prevalence of fever in 1709, except in the weeks ending 13 and 20 September, when the fever-deaths were 96 and 75 (including "spotted fever"). But the unusual entry of "malignant fever" appears in three weekly bills, 19 July, 9 August and 23 August, one death being referred to it on each occasion. It was in the summer and autumn of 1710 that the fever reached a height in London, being attended with a very

---

[1] W. Butter, M.D., *A Treatise on the Infantile Remittent Fever.* Lond. 1782.

fatal smallpox. An essay on the London epidemic of 1710[1] is interesting chiefly for recording a probable case of relapsing fever, a form which was almost certainly part of the great febrile epidemic in London in 1727–29.

Mrs Simon, aged 20, had a burning fever, stifling of her breath, frequent vomiting and looseness, foul tongue, loss of sleep, restlessness, intermitting, low and irregular pulse. This terrible fever disappeared on the fourth day, and she thought herself recovered. But on the seventh day from her being taken ill the fever returned, she was light-headed, did not know her relatives, and was fevered in the highest degree. It looked like a malignant fever, but there were no spots.

The following table shows the very high mortality from fever (as well as from smallpox) in the epidemic to which the above case belonged.

London : Weekly deaths from fever, smallpox and all causes.

1710.

Week ending	Dead of fever	Dead of spotted fever	Dead of smallpox	Dead of all diseases
May 2	103	[illegible]	99	571
9	90	6	60	517
16	84	7	71	502
23	93	15	71	503
30	106	11	83	550
June 6	93	2	98	508
13	79	8	84	509
20	106	12	99	574
27	105	15	86	503
July 4	106	7	99	482
11	107	13	97	467
18	126	16	89	509
25	109	13	105	562
Aug. 1	91	12	79	444
8	92	11	72	463
15	98	10	58	459
22	105	10	63	463
29	111	16	71	495
Sept. 5	76	4	63	414
12[2]	107	12	57	520
19	115	9	83	548
26	81	11	46	456
Oct. 3	98	9	45	469
10	79	10	49	480
17	90	5	41	477
24	107	5	45	470
31	106	14	51	421
Nov. 7	71	6	55	425
14	92	2	41	390
21	70	4	25	345

[1] Philip Guide, M.D., *A Kind Warning to a Multitude of Patients daily afflicted with different sorts of Fevers.* Lond. 1710.
[2] One death from "malignant fever," two from scarlet fever.

Throughout England, in country parishes and in towns, the first ten years of the 18th century were on the whole a period of good public health. In Short's abstracts of the parish registers to show the excess of deaths over the births, those years are as little conspicuous as any in the long series. It was a time when there was a great lull in smallpox, and probably also in fevers. The figures for Sheffield may serve as an example[1]. It will be seen from the Table that the burials exceeded the baptisms in every decade from the Restoration to the end of the century: after that for twenty years the baptisms exceeded the burials, the marriages having increased greatly.

Vital Statistics of Sheffield.

Ten-year periods	Marriages	Baptisms	Burials
1661—70	585	2086	2266
1671—80	537	2240	2387
1681—90	540	2595	2856
1691—1700	688	2221	2856
1701—10	942	3033	2613
1711—20	991	3304	2765

Of particular epidemics, we hear of a malignant fever at Harwich in 1709. Harwich was then an important naval station, and the fever may have arisen in connexion with the transport of troops to and from the seat of war, just as camp- and war-fevers appeared at various ports in the next war, 1742–48.

There were rumours of a plague at Newcastle in 1710, which were contradicted by advertisement in the *London Gazette*[2]. But, as there was so much plague in the Baltic ports in 1710 it is possible that the Newcastle rumour may have been one of plague imported, and not a rumour suggested by the mortality from some other disease.

---

[1] Hunter's *Hallamshire*, ed. Gatty.

[2] Brand, *Hist. of Newcastle*, II. 308. Swift writes to Stella on 8 December, 1710: "We are terribly afraid of the plague; they say it is at Newcastle. I begged Mr Harley [the Lord President] for the love of God to take some care about it, or we are all ruined. There have been orders for all ships from the Baltic to pass their quarantine before they land; but they neglect it. You remember I have been afraid these two years." The orders referred to were probably the Order of Council of 9 Nov. 1710. Parliament met on the 25th Nov. and passed the first Quarantine Act (9 Anne, cap. II.). Swift had a good deal to say with Ministers on many subjects, and it is not impossible, however absurd, that his had been the first suggestion to Harley of a quarantine law. I had purposed including a history of quarantine in Britain, but can find no convenient context for it. I shall therefore refer the reader to the historical sketch which I have appended to the Article "Quarantine" in the *Encyclopaedia Britannica*, 9th ed.

To the same period of epidemic fever in London, about 1709–10, belongs also a curiously localized epidemic in an Oxford college, which reminds one somewhat of the circumstances of enteric fever in our time. It was told to Dr Rogers of Cork twenty-five or twenty-six years before the date of his writing (1734), by one who was a student at Oxford then: "There broke out amongst the scholars of Wadham College a fever very malignant, that swept away great numbers, whilst the rest of the colleges remained unvisited. All agreed that the contagious infection arose from the putrefaction of a vast quantity of cabbages thrown into a heap out of the several gardens near Wadham College[1]."

The next epidemic of fever in London was in 1714. Like that of 1710, it followed a great rise in the price of wheat, or perhaps it followed the unseasonable weather which caused the deficient harvest. Before the Peace of Utrecht wheat in England was as low as 33s. 9d. per quarter, in 1712, the peace next year sending it no lower than 30s. But at Michaelmas, 1713, it rose with a bound to 56s. 11d., doubtless owing to a bad harvest. The fever-deaths in London began to rise in the spring of 1714, reaching a weekly total of 103 in the week ending 20 April. All through the summer and autumn they continued very high, the weekly totals exceeding, on an average, those of the year 1710, as in the foregoing table, and having corresponding large additions of "spotted fever." The deaths from all causes in 1714 were a quarter more than those of the year before, the epidemic of fever being the chief contributor to the rise. This happened to be a very slack time in medical writing[2]; but, even in the absence of such testimony as we have for earlier and later epidemics of fever in London, we may safely conclude that the fever of 1714 was of the type of pestilential or malignant typhus, beginning in early summer and reaching a height in the old plague season of autumn.

A singular instance of what may be considered war-typhus

[1] *Essay on Epidemic Diseases.* Dublin, 1734, p. 34.

[2] Dr Guide a Frenchman, who had been in practice in London for many years, says in his *Kind Warning to a Multitude of Patients daily afflicted with different sorts of Fevers* (1710) "the British physicians and surgeons are lately fallen into an unhappy and terrible confusion and mixture of honest and fraudulent pretenders." Another writer of 1710, Dr Lynn, quoted in the chapter on Smallpox, implies that physicians were taking an unusually cynical view of their business. The most interesting essay of the time on fevers is by J. White, M.D. (*De recta Sanguinis Missione &c.* Lond. 1712), a Scot who had been in the Navy and afterwards in practice at Lisbon; but it throws no light upon the London fevers.

belongs to the winter of 1715–16. The political intrigues preceding and following the death of Queen Anne in 1714 culminated in the Jacobite rising in Scotland and the North of England in 1715. The Jacobites having been defeated at Preston on 13 November, prisoners to the number of 450 were brought to Chester Castle on the Sunday night before December 1st. A fortnight later (December 15th), Lady Otway writes of the 450 prisoners in the Castle:

"They all lie upon straw, the better and the worse alike. The king's allowance is a groat a day for each man for meat, but they are almost starved for want of some covering, though many persons are charitable to the sick." The winter was unusually severe, the snow lying "a yard deep." Many prisoners died in the Castle by "the severity of the season," many were carried off by "a very malignant fever." On February 16th Lady Otway writes again :—"So much sickness now in our Castle that they dye in droves like rotten sheep, and be 4 or 5 in a night throne into the Castle ditch ffor ther graves. The feavour and sickness increaseth dayly, is begun to spread much into the citty, and many of the guard solidyers is sick, it is thought by inffection. The Lord preserve us ffrom plague and pestilence[1]!"

Prosperity of Britain, 1715–65.

The fifty years from 1715 to 1765 were, with two or three exceptions, marked by abundant harvests, low prices and heavy exports of corn. This was undoubtedly a great time in the expansion of England, a time of fortune-making for the monied class, and of cheapness of the necessaries of life.

The well-being and comfort of the middle class were undoubtedly great; also there was something peculiar to England in the prosperity of towns and villages throughout all classes. In the very worst year of the period, the year 1741, Horace Walpole landed at Dover on the 13th September, having completed the grand tour of Europe. Like many others, he was delighted with the pleasant county of Kent as he posted towards London; and on stopping for the night at Sittingbourne, he wrote as follows in a letter :

"The country town delights me: the populousness, the ease, the gaiety, and well-dressed everybody, amaze me. Canterbury, which on my setting out I thought deplorable, is a paradise to Modena, Reggio, Parma, etc. I had before discovered that there was nowhere but in England the distinction of *middling people*. I perceive now that there is peculiar to us *middling houses*: how snug they are[2]!"

[1] Elizabeth, Lady Otway, to Benj. Browne, Dec. 1st and 15th, 1715, and Feb. 16, 1716. *Hist. MSS. Com.* x. pt. 4, p. 352 ; Hemingway's *Hist. of Chester*, II. 244.
[2] *Letters*, ed. Cunningham, I. 72.

Our history henceforth has little to record of malignant typhus fevers, or of smallpox, in these snug houses of the middle class, although not only the middle class, but also the highest class had a considerable share of those troubles all through the 17th century. But the 18th century, even the most prosperous part of it, from the accession of George I. to the beginning of the Industrial Revolution in the last quarter or third of it, was none the less a most unwholesome period in the history of England. The health of London was never worse than in those years, and the vital statistics of some other towns, such as Norwich, are little more satisfactory. This was the time which gave us the saying, that God made the country and man made the town. Praise of rural felicity was a common theme in the poetry of the time, as in Johnson's *London :*

> "There every bush with nature's music rings,
> There every breeze bears health upon its wings."

Both for the country and the town the history of the public health does not harmonize well with the optimist views of the 18th century. The historians are agreed that, under the two first Georges, during the ministries of Walpole, the Pelhams and Pitt, the prosperity of Britain was general. Adam Smith speaks of "the peculiarly happy circumstances of the country" during the reign of George II. (1727–60). Hallam characterizes the same reign as "the most prosperous that England had ever experienced." The most recent historian of England in the 18th century is of the same opinion[1]. The novels of Fielding give us the concrete picture of the period with epic fidelity, and the picture is of abundance and prodigality. Agriculture and commerce with the Colonies, India and the continent of Europe, were the sources of the country's wealth. Farming and stock-raising had been greatly improved by the introduction of roots and sown grasses.

[1] Lecky, *History of England in the Eighteenth Century*, VI. 204 :—" All the evidence we possess concurs in showing that during the first three-quarters of the century the position of the poorer agricultural classes in England was singularly favourable. The price of wheat was both low and steady. Wages, if they advanced slowly, appear .o have commanded an increased proportion of the necessaries of life, and there were all the signs of growing material well-being. It was noticed that wheat bread, and that made of the finest flour, which at the beginning of the period had been confined to the upper and middle classes, had become before the close of it over the greater part of England the universal food, and that the consumption of cheese and butter in proportion to the population in many districts almost trebled. Beef and mutton were eaten almost daily in villages."

In some country parishes the baptisms were three times the burials. But the public health during this period will not appear in a favourable light from what follows. More particularly there were three occasions, about the years 1718, 1728 and 1741, when a single bad harvest in the midst of many abundant ones brought wide-spread distress, with epidemics of typhus and relapsing fever; from which fact it would appear that the common people had little in hand. Thorold Rogers, among economists, was of the opinion that the prosperity was all on the side of the governing and capitalist classes, that the labourers were in "irremediable poverty" and "without hope," and that the law of parochial settlement, with the artificial fixing of wages by the Quarter Sessions and the bonuses out of the poor-rates, had the effect of keeping the mass of the people on the land "in a condition wherein existence could just be maintained[1]." I shall not attempt an independent judgment in economics, but proceed to those illustrations of national well-being which belong to my subject, leaving the latter to have their due weight on the one side of economical opinion or on the other. Besides the economical question there is of course also an ethical one. When the pinch came about 1766, there was the usual diversity of opinion expressed on the "condition of England" problem, one holding that the labourers were unfairly paid, another that the nation had been made "splendid and flourishing by keeping wages low," and that the distress was due to "want of industry, want of frugality, want of sobriety, want of principle" among the common people at large. "If in a time of plenty," wrote one austere moralist, "the labourers would abate of their drunkenness, sloth, and bad economy, and make a reserve against times of scarcity, they would have no reason to complain of want or distress at any time[2]." But there must have been something wrong in the economics and morals of their betters if it were the case that the working class as a whole, and not merely a certain number of individuals in it, was drunken, thriftless and slothful. The familiar proof of this is the apathy of the Church, broken by the Methodist revival of religion.

[1] *Six Centuries of Work and Wages*, pp. 398—415.
[2] *Gentleman's Magazine*, 1766.

The epidemic fevers of 1718–19.

In the fifty years from 1715 to 1765, the three worst periods of epidemic fever in England and Scotland correspond closely to the three periods of actual famine and its attendant train of sicknesses in Ireland, namely, the years 1718–19, 1727–29, and 1740–42. The three divisions of the kingdom suffered in common, Ireland suffering most. The first period, 1718–19, was an extremely slack tide in medical writing, insomuch that hardly any accounts of the reigning maladies remain, except those by Wintringham, of York, and Rogers, of Cork. The whole of the Irish history of fevers and the allied maladies is dealt with in a chapter apart. Of the Scots history, little is known for the first of the three periods beyond a statement that there was a malignant fever and dysentery in Lorn, Argyllshire, in January and February, 1717[1].

Wintringham gives the following account of the *synochus*, afterwards called typhus, which attracted notice in the summer of 1718 and became more common in the warm season of 1719: in each year it began about May, reached its height in July and lasted all August, carrying off many of those who fell into it.

It began with rigors, nausea and bilious vomiting, followed by alternate heats and chills, with great lassitude and a feeling of heaviness : then thirst and pungent heat, a dry and brown tongue, sometimes black. The patient slept little, did not sweat, and was mostly delirious, or anxious and restless, tossing continually in bed. About the 12th day it was not unusual for profuse and exhausting diarrhœa to come on. In a favourable case the fever ended in a crisis of sweating about the 16th day. Those who were of lax habit, unhealthy, hysteric, or cachectic, were apt to have tremors, spasms and delirium, while others were so prostrated as to have no control over their evacuations, lying in a stupor and raving when roused out of it. In these the fever would continue to the 20th day ; in some few it ended without a manifest crisis, and with a slow convalescence[2].

This applies to the city of York, but in what special circumstances we are not told. However, it happens that a physician of York, two generations after, in giving an account of the great improvement that had taken place in its public health, throws some light on its old-world state : " The streets

---

[1] Short.
[2] Clifton Wintringham, M.D., *Commentarium nosologicum, morbos epidemicos et aeris variationes in urbe Eboracensi locisque vicinis ab anno 1715 usque ad finem anni 1725 grassantes, complectens.* Londini, 1727.

have been widened in many places by taking down a number of old houses built in such a manner as almost to meet in the upper stories, by which the sun and air were almost excluded in the streets and inferior apartments[1]."

In London the fever-deaths, with the deaths from all causes, rose decidedly in 1718, and reached a very high figure in 1719, of which the summer was excessively hot. One cause, at least, was want of employment, especially among weavers in the East End[2]. But the epidemic fever of 1718–19 was not limited to the distressed classes; we have a glimpse of it, under the name of "spotted fever," in the family of the archbishop of Canterbury:

"On Friday night the archbishop of Canterbury's sixth daughter was interred in our chancel, with four others preceding, she dying on Monday after three days of the spotted fever. The fourth and seventh are recovered, and hoped past danger[3]."

The following table shows the fever-mortalities for London, from 1718 onwards, and, for comparison, the excessive mortalities in the epidemics of 1710 and 1714:

---

[1] W. White, M.D., *Phil. Trans.* LXXII. (1782), p. 35. The annual deaths under the old *régime* exceeded by a good deal the annual births: in the seven years 1728—35, according to the figures from the parish registers in Drake's *Eboracum*, the burials from all causes were 3488, and the baptisms 2803, an annual excess of 98 deaths over the births in an estimated population of 10,800 (birth-rate 37 per 1000, death-rate 46 per 1000). But in the seven years, 1770—76, the balance was the other way: the population had increased by two thousand (to 12,800), and the births were on an average 20 in the year more than the deaths (474 births, 454 deaths), the birth-rate being still 37 per 1000, and the death-rate fallen to 35 per 1000. But the correctness of these rates depends on the population being exactly given.

[2] "There has been very great mobbing by the weavers of this town, as they pretend, because they are starved for want of ⸺ and they pull the calico cloaths off women's backs wherever they see them. The Trainbands have been up since last Friday, and they were forced to fire at the mobb in Moor Fields before they would disperse, and four or five were shott and as many wounded." (Benjamin Browne to his father, 16 June, 1719: Mr Browne's MSS. *Hist. MSS. Com.* X. pt. 4, p. 351.) The calicoes which the London weavers tore from the backs of women were doubtless the Indian fabrics brought home by the ships of the East India Company. These imports were so injurious to home manufactures that an Act had been passed in 1700 prohibiting (with some exceptions) the use in England of printed or dyed calicoes or any other printed or dyed cotton goods. This prohibition was re-enacted in 1721, two years after the rioting at Moorfields. (7 Geo. I. cap. 7). Blomefield (*Hist. of Norfolk*, III. 437) says that at Norwich also there was tearing of calicoes, "as pernicious to the trade" of that city. On the 20th of September, 1720, a great riot arose there, the rabble cutting several gowns in pieces on women's backs, entering shops to seize all calicoes found there, beating the constables, and opposing the sheriff's power to such a degree that the company of artillery had to be called out.

[3] Ambrose Warren to Sir P. Gell, 16 Sept. 1718, *Hist. MSS. Com.* IX. pt. 2, p. 400 *b.*

London Mortalities from Fever, &c.

Year	Fevers	Spotted fevers	Smallpox	All causes
1710	4397	343	3138	24620
1714	4631	150	2810	26569
1718	3475	132	1884	26523
1719	3803	124	3229	28347
1720	3910	46	1442	25454
1721	3331	84	2375	26142
1722	3088	22	2167	25750
1723	3321	51	3271	29197
1724	3262	84	1227	25952
1725	3277	59	3188	25523
1726	4666	84	1569	29647
1727	4728	102	2379	28418
1728	4716	94	2105	27810
1729	5235	[The entry	2849	29722
1730	4011	ends.]	1914	26761
1731	3225		2640	25262
1732	2939		1197	23358
1733	3831		1370	29233
1734	3116		2688	26062
1735	2544		1594	23538
1736	3361		3014	27581
1737	4580		2084	27823
1738	3890		1590	25825
1739	3334		1690	25432
1740	4003		2725	30811

In country parishes, according to Short's abstracts of registers, there was no unusual sickness in 1718 and 1719. But in market towns the mortality rose greatly in 1719, which had an excessively hot summer; and that was the year when the *synochus* or typhus described by Wintringham reached its worst at York. The mortality kept high for several years after 1719.

Market Town

Year	Registers examined	Registers with excess of deaths	Deaths in same	Births in same
1716	30	8	1060	845
1717	30	9	1485	1290
1718	30	3	249	169
1719	30	6	1737	1320
1720	30	10	2186	1461
1721	33	9	1294	952
1722	33	11	1664	1345
1723	33	14	2532	2176

The high mortalities in 1721–23 were mostly from smallpox, exact figures of many of the epidemics in Yorkshire and elsewhere being given in the chapter on that disease. The country parishes shared in its prevalence :

C. II.

Country Parishes.

Year	Registers examined	Registers with excess of deaths	Deaths in same	Births in same
1721	174	35	793	586
1722	175	35	1015	775
1723	174	63	2021	1583

Besides smallpox, diarrhoeas and dysenteries in the autumn are given by Wintringham as the reigning maladies, fever not being mentioned.

The Epidemic Fevers of 1726–29: evidence of Relapsing Fever.

The four years 1726–29 were a great fever-period in London, the deaths having been as follows:

Year	Fever deaths	All deaths
1726	4666	29,647
1727	4728	28,418
1728	4716	27,810
1729	5335	29,722

In the last of those years the entry in the annual bills becomes "fever, malignant fever, spotted fever and purples."

The following are the weekly maxima of fever deaths and deaths from all causes during the four years, 1726–29; in nearly all the weeks the deaths from "convulsions" (generic name for most of the maladies of infants) contribute from a fourth to a third, or even more, of the whole mortality.

	Week ending	Fever deaths	All deaths		Week ending	Fever deaths	All deaths
1726				**1728**			
	Jan. 18	71	633		Feb. 6	112	748
	March 15	81	678		13	131	889
	May 31	103	611		20	121	850
	June 7	106	607		27	145	927
	Aug. 30	102	711		March 5	93	733
	Sept. 6	116	680		Aug. 27	138	525
	13	109	643		Sept. 3	131	562
	20	109	648		Dec. 10	122	734
1727				**1729**			
	Aug. 8	103	577		Sept. 9	109	676
	15	123	698		Nov. 4	213	908*
	22	132	730		11	267	993*
	29	130	789		18	166	783
	Sept. 5	150	764		Dec. 9	132	779
	12	134	795				
	19	165	798				
	26	163	715				
	Oct. 3	150	684				

* The sudden rise was due to influenza; but the fever mortality was high for weeks before and after.

These are high mortalities, whatever were the types of fever that caused them. That the old pestilential fever of London was one of them we need have no doubt. Dr John Arbuthnot, writing two or three years after, said, " I believe one may safely affirm that there is hardly any year in which there are not in London fevers with buboes and carbuncles [the distinctive pestilential marks]; and that there are many petechial or spotted fevers is certain[1]."

The essay of Strother also has a reference to "spotted fever" in its title, although the text throws very little light upon it[2]. But, for the rest, the " constitution " of 1727–29 is more than usually perplexing. There was an influenza at the end of 1729, which can be separated from the rest easily enough by the help of the London weekly bills of mortality ; and it is probable, unless Arbuthnot, Huxham and Rutty have erred in their dates, that one or more epidemics of catarrhal fever had occurred before that, in the years 1727 and 1728. The greatest difficulty is with a certain "little fever," or "hysteric fever," or "febricula," which gave rise to some writing and a good deal of talk. Strother does not specially treat of it, at least under that name, although he says that " many, especially women, have been subject to fits of vapours, cold sweats, apprehensions, and un-accountable fears of death; every small disappointment dejected them, tremblings and weakness attended them," etc. (p. 116); and again, "never was a season when apoplexies, palsies and other obstructions of the nerves did prevail so much as they do at present, and have done for some time past " (p. 102); while he had frequently seen hysterical and hypochondriacal symptoms, dejection of spirits and the like remaining behind the fever (p. 109). For some years before this, much had been heard in London of the vapours, the " hypo," the spleen, and the like, an essay by Dr Mandeville, better known by his 'Fable of the Bees,' having first made these maladies fashionable in the year 1711[2].

[1] John Arbuthnot, M.D., *Essay concerning the Effects of Air on Human Bodies.* Lond. 1733, p. 187.

[2] Edward Strother, M.D., *Practical Observations on the Epidemical Fever which hath reigned so violently these two years past and still rages at the present time, with some incidental remarks shewing wherein this fatal Distemper differs from Common fevers ; and more particularly why the Bark has so often failed : and methods prescribed to render its use more effectual. In which is contained a very remarkable History of a Spotted Fever.* London, 1729. This book was written before the influenza of the end of 1729. At p. 126 the author was writing on the 24th of May, 1728. The preface is undated.

[3] Bernard de Mandeville, M.D., *A Treatise of the Hypochondriack and Hysteric Diseases,* 3rd ed. 1730, 1st ed. 1711. It contains nothing about the " little fever."

5—2

In due time it began to be noticed that symptoms which many physicians made light of as a "fit of vapours" were really the beginning of a fever. Dr Blackmore, in an essay on the Plague written in 1721, admitted the ambiguity:

"For several days a malignant fever has so near a resemblance to one that is only hysterick, that many physicians and standers by, I am apt to believe, mistake the first for the last, and look upon a great and dangerous disease to be only the spleen, or a fit of the vapors, to the great hazard of the patient[1]."

In 1730, Dr William Cockburn, in a polemic against the physicians whom he styles "the academical cabal" (because they objected to his secret electuary for dysentery), professes to give a history of the mistakes of the faculty in London ove this "little fever," or "hysteric fever," which often became dangerous[2]:

"The present fever, with a variation in some of its symptoms, has now subsisted twelve years [or since 1718] not in England only, but all over Europe [Manningham says it was peculiarly English]. Few or no physicians suspected the reigning and popular disease to be a fever. Vapours, a nervous disease, and such general appellations it had from sundry physicians. Others, who discovered the fever, knew it was the low or slow fever, first mentioned by Hippocrates....The last were represented as ignorant for calling the distemper a fever, and affixing to it the name 'low' or 'slow,' a slow fever being, in their adversaries' opinion, altogether unheard of among physicians and never recorded in their books. Nothing was more monstrous than calling this distemper a fever, or confining persons afflicted with it to their bed, and dieting them with broth, or other liquid food of good nourishment, and what is easily concocted....'You are not hot, you are not dry; you are in good temper; and therefore you have no fever' was the common language of the town....They might have seen physicians practising for a destroying distemper, and yet, after seven years, they confess themselves ignorant of its very name."

At length, he continues, Blackmore admitted the ambiguity of diagnosis, while Mead, Freind and others, recognized that there was really such a thing as a slow, nervous fever, by no means free from danger to life. It is probably to this insidious fever that Strother refers:

"Thus, having gone on for six or seven days in a train of indolence, they have been surprized on the seventh day, and have died on the eighth lethargick or delirious, whereas, if they had taken due care, the fever would have run its course in fifteen days or more." It was the remissions, or inter-missions, he explains, that often misled patients, by which he seems to mean the clear intervals between relapses. "Others, wearied out with relapses, have hoped their recovery would as certainly ensue as it had hitherto, and

[1] Richard Blackmore, M.D., *A Discourse upon the Plague, with a prefatory account of Malignant Fever.* London, 1721, p. 17.
[2] W. Cockburn, M.D., *Danger of improving Physick, with a brief account of the present Epidemick Fever.* London, 1730.

have deferred asking advice until it was too late." These relapses, he thought, were brought on by venturing too soon into the air : "it is too well known that the fever has been cured, and patients have soon, after they have ventured into the air, relapsed and have again run the same circle of ill symptoms, if not worse than before." Bark failed conspicuously in these "remittents :" "it is therefore incumbent on me to examine into the reason of this *new phenomenon.* I call it *new,*" he explains, because bark had hitherto succeeded. "Perhaps we may find reason to lay some blame on the air for the frequent relapses....Periodical comas have of late been common ; so soon as the fit was over, the drowsiness abated till the fit returned."

Elsewhere he speaks of the frequent relapses as belonging to a "quartan," under which diagnosis bark had been tried. The fevers were less apt to "relapse" when treated by mild cathartics. Another symptom of this fever was jaundice : "If jaundice breaks forth on the fourth day of a fever, it is much better than if it comes at the conclusion of a fever....Jaundices are now very common after the cure of these fevers."

These indications, dispersed throughout the rambling essay of Strother, point somewhat plainly to relapsing fever[1]. But his theoretical pathology comes in to obscure the whole matter. He explains everything by obstructions. The jaundice was due to obstruction of the liver by "styptics," the hysteric symptoms to obstructions of the nerves; there were also theoretical obstructions of the mesentery, part of the matter being sometimes "thrown off into the mesenteric glands"; also "congestions" or phlegmons of the liver, spleen and pancreas. But it is when he comes to the bowels that his subjective morbid anatomy becomes truly misleading. There is nothing to show that Strother examined a single body dead of this fever. He says, however, in his *à priori* way : "The crisis of these slow fevers is generally deposited on the bowels...The lent fever is a symptomatical fever, arising from an inflammation, or an ulcer fixed on some of the bowels. A lent fever, depending on some fixed cause of the bowels, must be cured by having regard to those causes some of which I shall enumerate":—the first supposition being that the fever depends on phlegmons by congestion of "the liver, spleen, pancreas, or the mesentery"; the second, if it depends on extravasations in an equally comprehensive range of viscera ; the third, "if it depends on an ulcer, then all vulneraries must be administered internally ; but to speak truth, when the viscera are ulcerated, there remains but small hope of life"; the fourth supposition is worms, the fifth

[1] I am the more persuaded of the identity with relapsing fever of much that was called remittent in Britain, and even intermittent, after reading the highly original treatise by R. T. Lyons on *Relapsing or Famine Fever,* London, 1872, relating to the epidemics of it in India.

corruption of the humours. All this is paper pathology. There is not a single precise fact relating to ulcerated Peyer's patches, or to swollen mesenteric glands, or to enlarged spleen, which last would have been equally distinctive of relapsing as of enteric fever; it is "the viscera" that are ulcerated, or congested, or extravasated, or it is "some of the bowels," or the pancreas and liver obstructed as well as the spleen, the obstruction of the liver being invoked to explain the highly significant jaundice.

It is not quite clear whether Strother's fever with relapses and jaundice corresponded exactly to the little fever, hysteric fever, or nervous fever of the same years; but it is worthy of note that relapsing fever in Ireland a century later was called febricula or the "short fever." It was not until 1746 that the excellent essay upon it by Sir Richard Manningham was written. By that time a good deal was being said in various parts of Britain of a slow, nervous, or putrid fever, Huxham, in particular, identifying the nervous fever with Manningham's febricula or little fever[1]. Some have supposed that the nervous fever of the 18th century included cases of enteric fever, if it did not stand for that disease exclusively. Murchison takes Manningham's essay to be "an excellent description of enteric fever, under the title of febricula or little fever, etc.[2]" The following are brief extracts from his description, by which the reader will be able to form his own opinion on the question of identity[3].

At the beginning patients feel merely languid or uneasy, with flying pains, dryness of the lips and tongue but no thirst; in a day or two they find themselves often giddy, dispirited and anxious without apparent reason, and passing pale urine. They have transient fits of chilliness, a low, quick and unequal pulse, sometimes cold clammy sweats and risings in the throat. They go about until more violent symptoms come on, simulating those of quotidian, tertian or quartan fever; sometimes the malady simulates pleurisy. There may be attacks of dyspnoea, nausea and haemorrhage; the menses in women are checked. A loss of memory and a delirium occur at intervals for short periods. The malady is very difficult to cure and too often becomes fatal in the end. It will last thirty or forty days, unless it end fatally in stupor or syncope. A form of mania is a consequence of it, where it has been neglected or badly treated; "of late years this species of madness has been more than ordinarily frequent." All sorts were liable to it, but mostly valetudinarians, delicate persons, and those in the decline of life; the

[1] Huxham, *On Fevers*, chap. VIII.
[2] Murchison, *Continued Fevers of Great Britain*, 2nd ed. Lond. 1873, p. 423.
[3] Sir Richard Manningham, Kt., M.D. *Febricula or Little Fever, commonly called the Nervous or Hysteric Fever, the Fever on the Spirits, Vapours, Hypo, or Spleen.* 1746.

fatalities were "especially among the opulent families of this great metropolis[1]."

This fever-period in London corresponds on the whole closely with a series of unhealthy years in Short's tables from the registers of market towns and country parishes, and with high mortalities in the Norwich register. It was not specially a smallpox period, as the last unhealthy year, 1723, was. On the other hand the epidemiographists in Yorkshire, Devonshire and Ireland dwell most upon fevers of the nature of typhus, some of which were due to famine or dearth, and upon "agues."

Market Towns.

Year	Registers examined	No. with excess of deaths	Deaths in same	Births in same
1727	33	19	3606	2441
1728	34	23	4972	2355
1729	36	27	6673	3494
1730	36	16	3445	2529

Norwich.

Year	Buried	Baptized
1728	1417	774
1729	1731	843

Country Parishes.

Year	Registers examined	With excess of burials	Burials in same	Baptisms in same
1726	181	22	542	495
1727	180	55	1368	1091
1728	180	80	2429	1536
1729	178	62	2015	1442
1730	176	39	1302	1022
1731	175	24	700	614

The best epidemiologists of the time were not in London, but at York, Ripon, Plymouth, Cork and Dublin. Leaving the Irish history to a separate chapter, we shall find in the annals of Wintringham, Hillary and Huxham a somewhat detailed account of the fevers which caused the very high mortalities of the years 1727–29, with an occasional glimpse of the circumstances in which the fevers arose. Much of what follows relates to the same nervous, hysteric or "putrid" fever, with or without relapses, that has been described for London. Going back a

---

[1] It is clear that the nervous fever established itself as a distinct type in England in the earlier part of the 18th century, both in medical opinion and in common acceptation: thus Horace Walpole, writing from Arlington Street on 28 January, 1760, says: "I have had a nervous fever these six or seven weeks every night, and have taken bark enough to have made a rind for Daphne: nay, have even stayed at home two days." *Letters of Horace Walpole*, ed. Cunningham, iii. 281.

little, Wintringham says[1] that the continued fevers of 1720 were milder than those of the year before (which were synochus or typhus) and were often languid or nervous, with giddiness, stupor and nervous tremblings, a quick pulse, a whitish tongue, no thirst, and sweats of the head, neck and chest: this fever lasted twenty days or more, and ended in a general sweat. He had mentioned the "languid nervous fevers" first in the years 1716 and 1717, and he mentions them again as mixed with or following the synochus or typhus of 1727–28.

In April, 1727, there were fevers prevalent, remitting and intermitting, but with uncertain paroxysms; in May, a fever with pleuritic pains; in July, a putrid fever in some, but the chief diseases of that month were "remittents and intermittents," which were often attended by cutaneous eruptions, sometimes of dusky colour and dry, at other times full of clear serum; which, "as they depended upon a scorbutic taint, tormented the sick with pruritus." The sick persons in these remittents were for the most part drowsy and stupid, especially during the paroxysm; the fevers were followed by lassitude, debility, languor of spirits and hysteric symptoms.

Hillary[2], who practised at Ripon, not far from Wintringham, at York, records in 1726 the prevalence of remittents and intermittents: "some had exanthematous eruptions towards the latter end of the disease, filled with a clear or yellowish water, which went or dried away without any other inconvenience to the sick but an uneasy itching for a few days"—just as Wintringham had described a miliary fever for 1727. It is also under 1726 that he describes the same drowsy and nervous symptoms of Wintringham's summer fever of 1727:

"Ancient and weak hysterical people had nervous twitchings and catchings, and were comatous and delirious; some were very languid, sick and faint, and had tremors; the young and robust, who had more full pulses, were generally delirious, unless it was prevented or taken off by proper evacuations and cooling medicines. I found blistering to be of very great service in this fever, and the sick were more relieved by it than ever I observed in any other fever whatever. People of lax, weak constitutions were very low and faint, and had frequent, profuse, partial sweatings, which most commonly were cold and clammy." Huxham also, at the other end of England, says that in October and November, 1727, a slow nervous fever attacked not a few; and under the date of January, 1728, he confirms the Yorkshire experiences of the prevalence of angina.

[1] *Commentar. Nosol.* u. s.
[2] William Hillary, M.D., "An Account of the principal variations of the Weather and the concomitant Epidemical Diseases from 1726 to 1734 at Ripon." App. to *Essay on the Smallpox*, Lond. 1740.

There can be little doubt that England in 1727 was already suffering in a measure from the distress that was acutely felt in Ireland; it was much aggravated by the hard winter of 1728–29[1], but it had begun before that and was doubtless the indirect cause of the great prevalence of sickness. The exports of corn under the bounty system used to bring two or three millions of money into the country in a year. But in 1727 there was a debt balance of 70,757 quarters of wheat imported, and in 1728 the import exceeded the export by 21,322 quarters, the price rising at the same time from 4s. to 8s. per bushel[2]. Under the year 1727 Hillary says:

"Many of the labouring and poor people, who used a low diet, and were much exposed to the injuries and changes of the weather, died; many of whom probably wanted the necessary assistance of diet and medicines." And after referring, under the winter of 1727–28, to the prevalence of a fatal suffocative angina, which fell, by a kind of metastasis, on the diaphragm or pleura, and sometimes on the peritoneum, he proceeds (p. 16):—

"Nor did any other method, which art could afford, relieve them: insomuch that many of the little country towns and villages were almost stripped of their poor people, not only in the country adjacent to Ripon, but all over the northern parts of the kingdom: indeed I had no certain account of what distempers those who were at a distance died of, but suppose they were the same as those which I have mentioned, which were nearer to us. Bleeding, pectorals with volatiles, and antiphlogistic diluters and blistering, were the most successful. I observed that very few of the richer people, who used a more generous way of living, and were not exposed to the inclemencies of the weather, were seized with any of these diseases at this time....The quartans were very subject to turn into quotidians, and sometimes to continual, in which the sick were frequently delirious."

The Yorkshire accounts by Wintringham and Hillary for the second year of this epidemic period, the year 1728, are very full, as regards the symptoms or types of the fevers; but it would be tedious to cite them at length, and unnecessary to do so unless to answer the not inconceivable cavil that the fevers were not of the nature of typhus in one or other of its forms. The chief point is that the second year, towards Midsummer, brought a fever with the symptoms of *synochus*, and not rarely marked with small red spots like fleabites or with purple petechiae. In the autumn of 1729, Hillary noticed a fever of a slow type, which might go on as long as thirty days and end without a perfect crisis—the nearest approach to enteric fever in any of the descriptions. For the same years, 1727–29, Huxham, of

[1] Brand, *History of Newcastle*, ii. 517, says that the magistrates of that town made a collection for the relief of poor housekeepers in the remarkably severe winter of 1728–29, the sum raised being £362. 18s.
[2] Tooke, *History of Prices from 1793 to 1837.* Introd. chap. p. 40.

Plymouth, describes languid fevers of the "putrid" type, with profuse sweating, followed by typhus of a more spotted type. Like the Yorkshire observer, Huxham mentions also "intermittents" as mixed with the continued fevers.

The great prevalence of these fevers, "intermittents and other fevers," in the west of England in 1728-29 was known to Dr Rutty of Dublin, who speaks especially of "the neighbourhoods of Gloucester and London, and very mortal in the country places, but less in the cities." This is confirmed by Dover:

"I happened to live in Gloucestershire in the years 1728 and 1729, when a very fatal epidemical fever raged to such a degree as to sweep off whole families, nay almost whole villages. I was called to several houses where eight or nine persons were down at a time; and yet did not so much as lose one patient where I was concerned[1]."

Some of the cases of nervous or putrid fever in the epidemics of 1727-29 appear to have been marked by relapses in the country districts as well as in London. Huxham says under date of April, 1728, that those who had wholly got rid of the putrid fever were exceedingly apt to have relapses. Hillary does not mention relapses until March, 1733, when a fever, with many hysterical symptoms, which succeeded the influenza of that year, relapsed in several, "though seemingly perfectly recovered before." But he seems really to be contrasting relapsing fever and typhus when he points out that, whereas the inflammatory type of fever in the first year of the epidemic (1727) was greatly benefited by enormous phlebotomies, the fever patients in the two seasons following, when the fever was more of the nature of spotted typhus, could not stand the loss of so much blood, or, it might be, the loss of any blood[2]. This was precisely the remark made by Christison and others a century later, when the inflammatory synocha, which often had the relapsing type very marked, changed to the spotted typhus.

---

[1] *Ancient Physician's Legacy.* Lond. 1733, p. 144.

[2] "In the year 1727," says Hillary, "I ordered several persons to lose 120 to 140 ounces of blood at several times in these inflammatory distempers, with great relief and success; whereas, in this winter [1728] I met with few, and even the strong and robust, who could bear the loss of above 40 or 50 ounces of blood, at three or four times; but, in general, most of the sick could not bear bleeding oftener than twice, and then not to exceed 30 or 34 oz. at most, at two or three times; and especially those who had been afflicted with, and debilitated by, the intermitting fever in the autumn before,—these could not bear blooding oftener than once, or twice at most, and in very small quantities too, though the acuteness of the pain, and the other symptoms in all, seemed at first to indicate much larger evacuations that way; but the first bleeding often sunk the pulse and strength of the patient so much that I durst not repeat it more than once, and in some not at all." Hillary, u. s. p. 26.

From the year 1731 we begin to have annual accounts (soon discontinued) of the reigning maladies in Edinburgh, on the same plan as Wintringham's, Hillary's and Huxham's, with which, indeed, they are sometimes collated and compared[1]. The fevers of Edinburgh and the villages near were as various as those of Plymouth, according to Huxham, and singularly like the latter. Thus, in the winter of 1731–32, there was much worm fever, comatose fever, or convulsive fever among children, but not limited to children, marked by intense pain in the head, raving in some, stupor in others, tremulous movements, leaping of the tendons, and all the other symptoms described by Willis for the fever of 1661, a fatal case of October, 1732, in a boy of ten, recorded by St Clair one of the Edinburgh professors, reading exactly like the cases of Willis already given[2]. St Clair's case, which was soon fatal, had no worms; but in the general accounts, both for the winter of 1731–32 and the autumn of 1732, it is said that many of the younger sort passed worms, both *teretes* and *ascarides*, and recovered, the fatalities among children being, as usual, few. In March and April, 1735, there were again "very irregular fevers of children." Huxham records exactly the same "worm-fever" of children at Plymouth in the spring of 1734—a fever with pains in the head, languor, anxiety, oppression of the breast, vomiting, diarrhoea, and a comatose state (*affectus soporosus*), which attacked the young mostly, and was often attended by the passage of worms. He gives the same account of the seasons as Gilchrist—the years 1734 and 1735 marked by almost continual rains, the country more squalid than had been known for some years[3].

But it is the nervous fever that chiefly engrosses attention both in Scotland and in England. In 1735, Dr Gilchrist, of Dumfries, made it the subject of an essay, returning to the subject a few years after[4]. "As *our* fever," he says, "seems to be peculiar to this age, it is not a little surprising that much more has not been said upon it." He is not sure whether its frequency of late years may not be owing to the manner of living (it was the time of the great drink-craze, which Huxham

[1] *Edin. Med. Essays and Obs.* I–VI. This annual publication was the original of the *Transactions* of the Royal Society of Edinburgh.
[2] *Ibid.* I. 40; II. 27; II. 287 (St Clair's case); IV.
[3] Huxham, *De aere et morbis.*
[4] Ebenezer Gilchrist, M.D., "Essay on Nervous Fevers." *Edin. Med. Essays and Obs.* IV. 347, and VI. (or V. pt. 2), p. 505.

also connects with the reigning maladies) and to a long cou
of warm, rainy seasons; the winters for some years had be
warm and open, and the summers and harvests rainy. It v
only the poorer sort and those a degree above them who we
subject to this fever; he knew but few instances of it among
those who lived well, and none amongst wine-drinkers. It w
in some insidious in its approach; those who seemed to be in
danger the first days for the most part died. In others tl
onset was violent, with nausea, heat, thirst and delirium. Amor
the symptoms were looseness, pains in the belly, local sweatin
tickling cough, leaping of the tendons. Sometimes they wer
in continual cold clammy sweats; at other times profuse sweat
ran from them, as if water were sprinkled upon them, the ski
feeling death cold.

At Edinburgh, from October, 1735, to February, 1736, the
fever became very common, and was often a relapsing fever.

"The sick had generally a low pulse on the first two or three days, with
great anxiety and uneasiness, and thin, crude urine. Delirium began
about the fourth day, and continued until the fever went off on the seventh
day. Sometimes the disease was lengthened to the fourteenth day. The
approach of the delirium could always be foretold by the urine becoming
more limpid, and without sediment....A large plentiful sweat was the crisis
in some. Others were exposed to relapses, which were very frequent, and
rather more dangerous than the former fever[1]."

These evidences, beginning with Strother's for London in
1728 and extending to the Edinburgh record of 1735, must
suffice to identify true relapsing fever. In the chapter on Irish
fevers we shall find clear evidence of relapsing fever in Dublin
in 1739, before the great famine had begun.

Huxham's account of the fevers at Plymouth, in Devonshire
generally, and in Cornwall about the years 1734–36 is of the
first importance. It is highly complex, owing to the prevalence
of an affection of the throat, so that one part of the constitution
is "anginose fever." This has been dealt with in the chapter
on Scarlatina and Diphtheria. Another part was true typhus.
In his account of the nervous fever we are introduced, as in the
Yorkshire annals, 1726–27, to a phenomenon that was almost
distinctive of the low, nervous or putrid fever from about 1750
to 1760 or longer, namely, the eruption of red, or purple, or
white watery vesicles, from which it got the name of miliary
fever. Huxham's annals are full of this phenomenon about the

[1] *Ibid.* v. pt. 1, p. 30.

years 1734–36[1]. The red pustules, or white pustules, with attendant ill-smelling sweats, are mentioned over and over again. He thought them critical or relieving: "Happy was then the patient who broke out in sweats or in red pustules." These fevers are said to have extended to the country parts of Devonshire, after they had ceased in Plymouth, and to Cornwall in August, 1736. In Plymouth itself the type of fever changed after a time to malignant spotted fever, synochus, or true typhus.

The malignant epidemic seemed to have been brought in by the fleet; it had raged for a long time among the sailors of the fleet lying at Portsmouth, and had destroyed many of them. In March, 1735, it was raging among the lower classes of Plymouth. About the 10th day of the fever, previously marked by various head symptoms, there appeared petechiae, red or purple, or livid or black, up to the size of vibices or blotches, or the eruption might be more minute, like fleabites. A profuse, clammy, stinking sweat, or a most foetid diarrhoea wasted the miserable patients. A black tongue, spasms, hiccup, and livid hands presaged death about the 11th to 14th day. So extensive and rapid was the putrefaction of the bodies that they had to be buried at once or within twenty-four hours. It was fortunate for many to have had a mild sweat and a red miliary eruption about the 4th or 5th day; but for others the course of the disease was attended with great risk. In April the type became worse, and the disease more general. There was rarely now any constriction of the throat. Few pustules broke out; but in place of them there were dusky or purple and black petechiae, and too often livid blotches, with which symptoms very many died both in April and May. In July this contagious fever had decreased much in Plymouth, and in September it was only sporadic there. With a mere reference to Hillary's account of somewhat similar fevers at Ripon in 1734–5 (with profuse sweats, sometimes foetid, great fainting and sinking of spirits, starting of the limbs and beating of the tendons, hiccup for days, etc.[2]) we may pass to a more signal historical event, the great epidemic of fever in 1741–42, of which the Irish part alone has hitherto received sufficient notice[3].

[1] *Obs. de aere et morbis;* also his essay *On Fevers.*
[2] Hillary, App. to *Smallpox,* 1740, pp. 57, 66.
[3] Mr. Lecky (*History of England in the 18th Century,* II.), says that the famine and fever of 1740-41, which he describes as an important event in the history of

The epidemic fever of 1741–42.

The harvest of 1739 had been an abundant one, and the export of grain had been large. At Lady-day the price of wheat had been 31s. 6d. per quarter, and it rose 10s. before Lady-day, 1740. An extremely severe winter had intervened, one of the three memorable winters of the 18th century. The autumn-sown wheat was destroyed by the prolonged and intense frost, and the price at Michaelmas, 1740, rose to 56s. per quarter, the exportation being at the same time prohibited, but not until every available bushel had been sold to the foreigners. The long cold of the winter of 1739–40 had produced much distress and want in London, Norwich, Edinburgh and other towns. In London the mortality for 1740 rose to a very high figure, 30,811, of which 4003 deaths were from fever and 2725 from smallpox. In mid-winter, 1739–40, coals rose to £3. 10s. per chaldron, owing to the navigation of the Thames being closed by ice; the streets were impassable by snow, there was a "frost-fair" on the Thames, and in other respects a repetition of the events preceding the London typhus of 1685–86. The *Gentleman's Magazine* of January, 1740, tells in verse how the poor were "unable to sustain oppressive want and hunger's urgent pain," and reproaches the rich,—"colder their hearts than snow, and harder than the frost"; while in its prose columns it announces that "the hearts of the rich have been opened in consideration of the hard fate of the poor[1]." The long, hard winter was followed by the dry spring and hot summer of 1740, during which the sickness (in Ireland at least) was of the dysenteric type. In the autumn of 1740 the epidemic is said to have taken origin both at Plymouth and Bristol from ships arriving with infection among the men—at the former port the king's ships 'Panther' and 'Canterbury,' at the latter a merchant ship. At Plymouth it was certainly raging enormously from June to the end of the year—"febris nautica pestilentialis jam saevit maxime," says Huxham; it continued

Ireland, "hardly excited any attention in England." It was severely felt, however, in England; and if it excited hardly any attention, that must have been because there were so many superior interests which were more engrossing than the state of the poor.

[1] *Gent. Magaz.* X. (1740), 32, 35. Blomefield, for Norwich, says that many there would have perished in the winter of 1739–40 but for help from their richer neighbours.

there all through the first half of 1741, "when it seemed to become lost in a fever of the bilious kind." It was in the dry spring and very hot summer of 1741 that the fever became general over England. Wall says that it appeared at Worcester at the Spring Assizes among a few; at Exeter also it was traced to the gaol delivery; and it was commonly said that the turmoil of the General Election (which resulted in driving Walpole from his long term of power) helped its diffusion. But undoubtedly the great occasion of its universality was a widely felt scarcity. The rise in the price of wheat was small beside the enormous leaps that prices used to take in the medieval period, having been at no time double the average low price of that generation. It was rather the want of employment that made the pinch so sharp in 1741. The weaving towns of the west of England were losing their trade; of "most trades," also, it was said that they were in apparent decay, "except those which supply luxury[1]." Dr Barker, of Sarum, the best medical writer upon the epidemic, says:

"The general poverty which has of late prevailed over a great part of this nation, and particularly amongst the woollen manufacturers in the west, where the fever has raged and still continues to rage with the greatest violence, affords but too great reason to believe that this has been one principal source of the disease[2]."

He explains that the price of wheat had driven the poor to live on bad bread. This is borne out by a letter from Wolverhampton, 27 November, 1741[3]. The writer speaks of the extraordinary havoc made among the poorer sort by the terrible fever that has for some time raged in most parts of England and Ireland. At first it seldom fixed on any but the poor people, and especially such as lived in large towns, workhouses, or prisons. Country people and farmers seemed for the most part exempt from it, "though we have observed it frequently in villages near market towns"; whereas, says the writer, the epidemic fevers of 1727, 1728 and 1729 were first observed to begin among the country people, and to be some time in advancing to large towns. This writer's theory was that the fever was caused by bad bread, and he alleges that

---

[1] W. Allen, *Landholder's Companion*, 1734. Cited by Tooke.
[2] *An Inquiry into the Nature, Cause and Cure of the present Epidemic Fever... with the difference betwixt Nervous and Inflammatory Fevers, and the Method of treating each*, 1742, p. 54.
[3] John Altree, *Gent. Magaz.* Dec. 1741, p. 655.

horse-beans, pease and coarse unsound barley were almost the only food of the poor. To this a Birmingham surgeon took exception[1]. Great numbers of the poor had, to his knowledge, lived almost entirely upon bean-bread, but had been very little afflicted with the fever. Besides, every practitioner knew that the fever was not confined to the poor. He pointed out that in Wolverhampton, whence the bad-bread theory emanated, the proportion of poor to those in easier circumstances was as six to one, poverty having increased so much by decay of trade that many wanted even the necessaries of life. The Birmingham surgeon was on the whole inclined to the theory of "the ingenious Sydenham, that the disease may be ascribed to a contagious quality in the air, arising from some secret and hidden alterations in the bowels of the earth, passing through the whole atmosphere, or to some malign influence in the heavenly bodies"—these being Sydenham's words as applied to the fever of 1685–6.

Barker, also, draws a parallel between the epidemic of 1741 and that of 1685–86: the Thames was frozen in each of the two winters preceding the respective epidemics, and the spring and summer of 1740 and 1741 were as remarkable for drought and heat as those of 1684 and 1685.

In London the deaths from fever in 1741 reached the enormous figure of 7528, the highest total in the bills of mortality from first to last, while the deaths from all causes were 32,119, in a population of some 700,000, also the highest total from the year of the great plague until the new registration of the whole metropolitan area in 1838. It will be seen from the following table (on p. 81) of the weekly mortalities that the fever-deaths rose greatly in the autumn, but, unlike the old plague, reached a maximum in the winter.

The effects of the epidemic of typhus upon the weaving towns of the west of England, in which the fever lasted, as in London, into the spring of 1742, were seen at their worst in the instance of Tiverton. It was then a town of about 8000 inhabitants, having increased little during the last hundred years. Judged by the burials and baptisms in the parish register it was a more unhealthy place since the extinction of plague than it had been before that. It was mostly a community of weavers, who had not been in prosperous circum-

[1] White, *ibid.* 1742, p. 43.

Mortality by Fever in London, 1741—42.

1741	Week ending	Fever	All causes		Week ending	Fever	All causes
	March 10	123	660	Sept.	1	171	675
	17	103	564		8	190	691
	24	112	624		15	182	760
	31	105	573		22	199	748
	April 7	123	670		29	189	733
	14	128	687	Oct.	6	207	784
	21	89	580		13	192	787
	28	123	622		20	232	793
	May 5	104	495		27	234	850
	12	141	587	Nov.	3	250	835
	19	129	573		10	228	772
	26	153	600		17	182	670
	June 2	138	512		24	214	806
	9	138	483	Dec.	1	224	768
	16	115	536		8	203	748
	23	127	494		15	191	761
	30	154	513		22	179	775
	July 7	149	523		29	180	702
	14	162	551	**1742**			
	21	130	485	Jan.	5	221	893
	28	151	621		12	184	760
	Aug. 4	128	512		19	184	826
	11	142	541		26	151	724
	18	172	636	Feb.	2	132	675
	25	192	665		9	103	533
					16	108	675
					25	103	641

Effects of the Epidemic of 1741-42 on Provincial Towns.
(Short's Abstracts of Parish Registers.)

Year	Registers examined	With burials more than baptisms	Baptisms in the same	Burials in the same
1740	27	6	1409	1940
1741	27	14	3787	6205
1742	26	6	1721	3345

stances for sometime past. In 1735 the town had been burned down, and in 1738 it was the scene of riots. The hard winter of 1739–40 brought acute distress, and in 1741 spotted fever was so prevalent that 636 persons were buried in that year, being 1 in 12 of the inhabitants. At the height of the epidemic ten or eleven funerals were seen at one time in St Peter's churchyard. Its population twenty years after is estimated to have declined by two thousand, and at the end of the 18th century it was a less populous place than at the beginning[1].

[1] Dunsford, *Historical Memorials of Tiverton.* The accounts of the great weaving towns of the South-west are not unpleasing until we come to the time when they

Other parts of the kingdom may be represented by Norwich, Newcastle and Edinburgh. The record of baptisms in Norwich is almost certainly defective; in only two years from 1719 to 1741, is a small excess of baptisms over burials recorded, namely, in 1722 and 1726, while in a third year, 1736, the figures are exactly equal. In 1740 there are 916 baptisms to 1173 burials, and in 1741, 851 baptisms to 1456 burials; while in 1742, owing to an epidemic of smallpox, the deaths rose to 1953, or to more than double the recorded births[1]. The distress was felt most in East Anglia in 1740. Blomefield, who ends his history in that year, says there was much rioting throughout the kingdom, "on the pretence of the scarcity and dearness of grain." At Wisbech Assizes fourteen were found guilty, but were not all executed. In Norfolk two were convicted and executed accordingly. At Norwich the military fired upon the mob and killed seven persons, of whom only one was truly a rioter[2]. It was also in the severe winter of 1739–40 that the distress began in Edinburgh. The mills were stopped by ice and snow, causing a scarcity of meal; the harvest of 1740 was bad, riots took place in October, and granaries were plundered[3]. The deaths from fever were many in 1740, but were nearly doubled in 1741, with a significant accompaniment of fatal dysentery[4]:

Edinburgh Mortalities, 1740–41.
(Population in 1732, estimated at 32,000.)[5]

	1740	1741
All causes	1237	1611
Consumption	278	349
Fever	161	304
Flux	3	36
Smallpox	274	206
Measles	100	112
Chincough	26	101
Convulsions	22	16

were overtaken by decay of work and distress, from about 1720 onwards. The district, says Defoe, was "a rich enclosed country, full of rivers and towns, and infinitely populous, in so much that some of the market towns are equal to cities in bigness, and superior to many of them in numbers of people." Taunton had 1100 looms. Tiverton in the seven years 1700–1706 had 331 marriages, 1116 baptisms, 1175 burials (a slight excess), and an estimated population of 8693, which kept nearly at that level for about twenty years longer (from 1720 to 1726 the marriages were 284, the baptisms 1070 and the burials 1175).

[1] *Gent. Magaz.* XI. (1742), p. 704.
[2] Blomefield, *History of Norfolk*, III. 449.
[3] Arnot, *History of Edinburgh*, 1779, p. 211.
[4] *Gent. Magaz.* 1741, p. 705. [5] *Edin. Med. Essays and Obs.* I. Art. 1.

The last four items are of children's maladies, for which Edinburgh was worse reputed even than London.

At Newcastle the deaths in the register in 1741 were 320 more than in 1740, in which year they were doubtless excessive, as elsewhere. But there is a significant addition: "There have also been buried upwards of 400 upon the Ballast Hills near this town[1]."

The symptoms of the epidemic fever of 1741–42 are described by Barker, of Salisbury, and Wall, of Worcester[2]. It began like a common cold, as was remarked also in Ireland. On the seventh day spots appeared like fleabites on the breast and arms; in some there were broad purple spots like those of scurvy. Miliary eruptions were apt to come out about the eleventh day, especially in women. In most, after the first six or seven days, there was a wonderful propensity to diarrhoea, which might end in dysentery. The cough, which had appeared at the outset, went off about the ninth day, when stupor and delirium came on. Gilchrist, of Dumfries, describes the fever there in November, 1741, as more malignant than the "nervous fever" which he had described in 1735. It came to an end about the fourteenth day; the sick were almost constantly under a coma or raving, and they died of an absolute oppression of the brain; a profuse sweat about the seventh day was followed by an aggravation of all the symptoms[3]. An anonymous writer, dating from Sherborne, uses the occasion to make an onslaught upon blood-letting[4].

---

[1] *Gent. Magaz.* 1742, p. 186.

[2] John Wall, M.D., *Medical Tracts*, Oxford, 1780, p. 337. See also *Obs. on the Epid. Fever of* 1741, 3rd ed., by Daniel Cox, apothecary, with cases.

[3] *Edin. Med. Essays and Obs.* VI. 539.

[4] "And here I cannot but observe how many ignorant conceited coxcombs ride out, under a shew of business, with their lancet in their pocket, and make diseases instead of curing them, drawing their weapon upon every occasion, right or wrong, and upon every complaint cry out, 'Egad! I must have some of your blood,' give the poor wretches a disease they never might have had, drawing the blood and the purse, torment them in this world," etc.—*An Essay on the present Epidemic Fever,* Sherborne, 1741. The practice of blood-letting in continued fevers received a check in the second half of the 18th century, but it was still kept up in inflammatory diseases or injuries. Even in the latter it was freely satirized by the laity. When the surgeon in *Tom Jones* complained bitterly that the wounded hero would not be blooded though he was in a fever, the landlady of the inn answered: "It is an eating fever, then, for he hath devoured two swingeing buttered toasts this morning for breakfast." "Very likely," says the doctor, "I have known people eat in a fever; and it is very easily accounted for; because the acidity occasioned by the febrile matter may stimulate the nerves of the diaphragm, and thereby occasion a craving which will not be easily distinguishable from a natural appetite....Indeed I think the gentleman in a very dangerous way, and, if he is not blooded, I am afraid will die."

Sanitary Condition of London under George II.

The great epidemic of fever in 1741–42 was the climax of a series of years in London all marked by high fever mortalities. If there had not been something peculiarly favourable to contagious fever in the then state of the capital, it is not likely that a temporary distress caused by a hard winter and a deficient harvest following should have had such effects. This was the time when the population is supposed to have stood still or even declined in London. Drunkenness was so prevalent that the College of Physicians on 19 January, 1726, made a representation on it to the House of Commons through Dr Freind, one of their fellows and member for Launceston :

"We have with concern observed for some years past the fatal effects of the frequent use of several sorts of distilled spirituous liquor upon great numbers of both sexes, rendering them diseased, not fit for business, poor, a burthen to themselves and neighbours, and too often the cause of weak, feeble and distempered children, who must be, instead of an advantage and strength, a charge to their country[1]."

"This state of things," said the College, "doth every year increase." Fielding guessed that a hundred thousand in London lived upon drink alone ; six gallons per head of the population per annum is an estimate for this period, against one gallon at present. The enormous duty of 20s. per gallon served only to develope the trade in smuggled Hollands gin and Nantes brandy. In the harvest of 1733 farmers in several parts of Kent were obliged to offer higher wages, although the price of grain was low, and could hardly get hands on any terms, "which is attributed to the great numbers who employ themselves in smuggling along the coast[2]."

The mean annual deaths were never higher in London, not even in plague times over a series of years, the fever deaths keeping pace with the mortality from all causes, and, in the great epidemic of typhus in 1741, making about a fourth part of the whole. The populace lived in a bad atmosphere, physical and moral. As Arbuthnot said in 1733, they "breathed their own steams"; and he works out the following curious sum :

"The perspiration of a man is about $\frac{1}{34}$ of an inch in 24 hours, consequently one inch in 34 days. The surface of the skin of a middle-sized man is about 15 square feet ; consequently the surface of the skin of 2904 such

[1] Munk, *Roll of the College of Physicians*, II. 53.
[2] *Gentleman's Magaz.* III. 1733, Sept., p. 492.

men would cover an acre of ground, and the perspir'd matter would cover an acre of ground 1 inch deep in 34 days, which, rarefi'd into air, would make over that acre an atmosphere of the steams of their bodies near 71 foot high." This, he explains, would turn pestiferous unless carried away by the wind; "from whence it may be inferred that the very first consideration in building of cities is to make them open, airy, and well perflated[1]."

In the growth of London from a medieval walled city of some forty or sixty thousand inhabitants to the "great wen" of Cobbett's time, these considerations had been little attended to so far as concerned the quarters of the populace. The Liberties of the City and the out-parishes were covered with aggregates of houses all on the same plan, or rather want of plan. In the medieval period the extramural population built rude shelters against the town walls or in the fosse, if it were dry, or along the side of the ditch. The same process of squatting at length extended farther afield, with more regular building along the sides of the great highways leading from the gates. Queen Elizabeth's proclamation of 1580 was designed to check the growth of London after this irregular fashion; but as neither the original edict nor the numerous copies of it, reissued for near a hundred years, made any provision for an orderly expansion of the capital, these prohibitions had merely the effect of adding to the hugger-mugger of building, "in odd corners and over stables." The outparishes were covered with houses and tenements of all kinds, to which access was got by an endless maze of narrow passages or alleys; regular streets were few in them, and it would appear from the account given by John Stow in 1598 of the parish of Whitechapel that even the old country highway, one of the great roads into Essex and the eastern counties, had been "pestered[2]." The "pestering" of the field lanes in the suburban parishes with poor cottages is Stow's frequent theme[3].

[1] *Effects of Air on Human Bodies*, 1733, pp. 11, 17. His excellent remarks on the need of fresh air in the treatment of fevers, two generations before Lettsom carried out the practice, are at p. 54. The curious calculation above cited was copied by Langrish, and usually passes as his.

[2] "Also without the bars both sides of the street be pestered with cottages and alleys even up to Whitechapel Church, and almost half a mile beyond it, into the common field: all which ought to be open and free for all men. But this common field, I say, being sometime the beauty of this city on that part, is so encroached upon by building of filthy cottages, and with other purprestures, enclosures and laystalls (notwithstanding all proclamations and Acts of Parliament made to the contrary) that in some places it scarce remaineth a sufficient highway for the meeting of carriages and droves of cattle. Much less is there any fair, pleasant or wholesome way for people to walk on foot, which is no small blemish to so famous a city to have so unsavoury and unseemly an entrance or passage thereunto." Stow's *Survey of London*, section on "Suburbs without the Walls."

[3] The line of an old field walk can still be followed from Aldermanbury Postern to Hackney, Goldsmiths' Row being one of the wider sections of it.

The borough of Southwark, as part of the City, may have been better than most: " Then from the Bridge straight towards the south a continual street called Long Southwark, built on both sides with divers lanes and alleys up to St George's Church, and beyond it through Blackman Street towards New Town or Newington "—the mazes of courts and alleys on either side of the Borough Road which may be traced in the maps long after Stow's time.   So again in St Olave's parish along the river bank eastwards from London Bridge—"continual building on both sides, with lanes and alleys, up to Battle Bridge, to Horsedown, and towards Rotherhithe." In the Western Liberty, the lanes that had been laid out in Henry VIII.'s time, Shoe Lane, Fetter Lane and Chancery Lane, served as three main arteries to the densely populated area between Fleet Street and Holborn, but for the rest it was reached by a plexus or *rete mirabile* of alleys and courts, notorious even in the 19th century.   In like manner Drury Lane and St Martin's Lane were the main arteries between High Holborn and the Strand.   One piazza of Covent Garden was a new centre of regular streets, to which the haberdashers and other trades were beginning to remove from the City, for greater room, about 1662. The Seven Dials were a wonder when they were new, about 1694, and had the same intention of openness and regularity as in Wren's unused design for the City after the fire.   The great speculative builder of the Restoration was Nicholas Barbone, son of Praise-God Barbones. He built over Red Lion Fields, much to the annoyance of the gentlemen of Gray's Inn[1], and his manner of building may be inferred from the following:

" He was the inventor of this new method of building by casting of ground into streets and small houses, and to augment their number with as little front as possible, and selling the ground to workmen by so much per foot front, and what he could not sell build himself. This has made ground-rents high for the sake of mortgaging; and others, following his steps, have refined and improved upon it, and made a superfoetation of houses about London[2]."

In these mazes of alleys, courts, or "rents" the people were for the most part closely packed. Overcrowding had been the rule since the Elizabethan proclamation of 1580, and it seems to have become worse under the Stuarts.   On February 24, 1623,

[1] Luttrell's *Diary* 10 June, 1684.
[2] Roger North's " Autobiography," in *Lives of the Norths*, new ed. 3 vols., 1890, III. 54.

certain householders of Chancery Lane were indicted at the Middlesex Sessions for subletting, "to the great danger of infectious disease, with plague and other diseases." In May, 1637, one house was found to contain eleven married couples and fifteen single persons; another house harboured eighteen lodgers. In the most crowded parishes the houses had no sufficient curtilage, standing as they did in alleys and courts. When we begin to have some sanitary information long after, it appears that their vaults, or privies, were indoors, at the foot of the common stair[1]. In 1710, Swift's lodging in Bury Street, St James's, for which he paid eight shillings a week ("plaguy deep" he thought), had a "thousand stinks in it," so that he left after three months. The House of Commons appears to have been ill reputed for smells, which were specially remembered in connexion with the hot summer of the great fever-year 1685[2].

The newer parts of London were built over cesspools, which were probably more dangerous than the visible nuisances of the streets satirized by Swift and Gay. There were also the "intramural" graveyards; of one of these, the Green Ground, Portugal Street, it was said by Walker, as late as 1839; "The effluvia from this ground are so offensive that persons living in the back of Clement's Lane are compelled to keep their windows closed." But that which helped most of all to make a foul atmosphere in the houses of the working class, an atmosphere in which the contagion of fever could thrive, was the window-tax. It is hardly possible that those who devised it can have foreseen how detrimental it would be to the public health; it took nearly a century to realize the simple truth that it was in effect a tax upon light and air.

[1] Willan, 1801: "The passage filled with putrid excremental or other abominable effluvia from a vault at the bottom of the staircase." See also Clutterbuck, *Epid. Fever at present prevailing.* Lond. 1819, p. 60. Ferriar, of Manchester, writing of the class of houses most apt to harbour the contagion of typhus, says, "Of the new buildings I have found those most apt to nurse it which are added in a slight manner to the back part of a row, and exposed to the effluvia of the privies."

[2] C. Davenant to T. Coke, London, 14 Dec. 1700. *Cal. Coke MSS.*, II. 411, "I heartily commiserate your sad condition to be in the country these bad weeks; but I fancy you will find Derbyshire more pleasant even in winter than the House of Commons will be in a summer season. For, though it be now sixteen years ago [1685], I still bear in memory the evil smells descending from the small apartments adjoining to the Speaker's Chamber, which came down into the House with irresistible force when the weather is hot."

The Window-Tax.

Willan, writing of fever in London in 1799, mentions that even the passages of tenement houses were "kept dark in order to lessen the window-tax," and the air therefore kept foul[1]. Ferriar, writing of Manchester in the last years of the 18th century, mentions, among other fever-dens, a large house in an airy situation which had been built for a poor's-house, but abandoned: having been let to poor families for a very trifling rent, many of the windows and the principal entrance were built up, and the fever then became universal in it[2]. The Carlisle typhus described by Heysham for 1781 began in a house near one of the gates, tenanted by five or six very poor families; they had "blocked up every window to lessen the burden of the window-tax[3]." John Howard's interest having been excited in the question of gaol-fever, he noted the effects of the window-tax not only in prisons but in other houses. The magistrates of Kent appear to have paid the tax for the gaols in that county from the county funds; but in most cases the burden fell on the keepers of the gaols.

"The gaolers," says Howard, "have to pay it; this tempts them to stop the windows and stifle their prisoners;" and he appends the following note: "This is also the case in many work-houses and farm-houses, where the poor and the labourers are lodged in rooms that have no light nor fresh air; which may be a cause of our peasants not having the healthy ruddy complexions one used to see so common twenty or thirty years ago. The difference has often struck me in my various journeys[4]."

Such impressions are known to be often fallacious; but in the history of the window-tax, which we shall now follow, it will appear that there was a new law, with increased stringency, in the years 1746–1748, corresponding to the "twenty or thirty years ago" of Howard's recollection.

The window-tax was originally a device of the statesmen of the Revolution "for making good the deficiency of the clipped money." By the Act of 7 and 8 William and Mary, cap. 18, taking effect from the 25th March, 1696, every inhabited house owed duty of two shillings per annum, and, over and above such duty on all inhabited houses, every dwelling-house with ten windows owed four shillings per annum, and every house with

[1] *Report on the Diseases in London,* 1796–1800. Lond. 1801.
[2] John Ferriar, M.D., *Medical Histories and Reflections.* London 1810, II. 217.
[3] Heysham, *Jail Fever at Carlisle in* 1781. Lond. 1782, p. 33.
[4] John Howard, *State of the Prisons.*

twenty windows eight shillings. In 1710 houses with from twenty
to thirty windows were made to pay ten shillings, and those with
more than thirty windows twenty shillings. Various devices
were resorted to to check the evasions of bachelors, widows
and others. A farmer had to pay for his servants, recouping
himself from their wages. A house subdivided into tenements
was to count as one; which would have made the tax difficult
to gather except from the landlord. The machinery of collection was a board of commissioners, receivers-general and collectors.

But in the 20th of George II. (1746) the basis of the law
was changed. The tax was levied upon the several windows
of a house, so much per window, so that it fell more decisively
than before upon the tenants of tenement-houses, and not on
the landlords. The two-shillings house duty was continued;
but the window-tax became sixpence per annum for every
window of a house with ten, eleven, twelve, thirteen or fourteen
windows, or lights, ninepence for every window of a house with
fifteen, sixteen, seventeen, eighteen or nineteen windows, and
one shilling for every window of a house with twenty or more
windows. An exemption in the Act in favour of those receiving parochial relief was decided by the law officers of the
Crown not to apply to houses with ten or more windows or
lights, which would have included most tenement-houses; on
the other hand they ruled that hospitals, poor-houses, workhouses,
and infirmaries were not chargeable with the window duty. To
remove doubts and check evasions another Act was made in
21 George II. cap. 10. All skylights, and lights of staircases,
garrets, cellars and passages were to count for the purpose of
the tax; also certain outhouses, but not others, were to count
as part of the main dwelling whether they were contiguous or
not. The 11th paragraph of the Amendment Act shows how
the law had been working in the course of its first year: "No
window or light shall be deemed to be stopped up unless such
window or light shall be stopped up effectually with stone or
brick or plaister upon lath," etc.

This remained the law down to 1803, when a change was
made back to the original basis of rating houses as a whole,
according to the number of their windows, the rate being
considerably raised and fixed according to a schedule. The
tax for tenement houses was at the same time made recoverable

from the landlord. The window-tax thus became a form of the modern house-tax, rated upon windows instead of upon rental, and so lost a great part of its obnoxious character.

The law of 1747–48, which taxed each window separately, and was enforced by a galling and corrupt machinery of commissioners, receivers-general and collectors paid by results, could not fail to work injuriously; for light and air, two of the primary necessaries of life, were in effect taxed. Even rich men appear to have taken pleasure in circumventing the collectors[1]. But it was among the poor, and especially the inhabitants of tenement houses, that the effect was truly disastrous; a tax on the skylights of garrets and on the lights of cellars, staircases and passages, taught the people to dispense with them altogether. Towards the end of the 18th century the grievance became now and then the subject of a pamphlet or a sermon.

Gaol-Fever.

Besides these ordinary things favouring contagious epidemic fever both in town and country, there were two special sources of contagion, the gaols and the fleets and armies. I shall take first the state of the gaols, which has been already indicated in speaking of the window-tax. In the opinion of Lind, a great part of the fever, which was a constant trouble in ships of the navy, came direct from the gaols through the pressing of newly discharged convicts.

The state of the prisons in the first half of the 18th century was certainly not better than Howard found it to be a generation after; it was probably worse, for the administration of justice was more savage. About the beginning of the century, many petitions were made to Parliament by imprisoned debtors, complaining of their treatment, and a Bill was introduced in 1702. Sixty thousand were said to be in prison for debt[2]. On 25

---

[1] *Notes and Queries*, 4th ser. XII. 346. Jenkinson, who was a Minister under George II., was reputed to have set an example of stopping up windows in his mansion near Croydon:

You e'en shut out the light of day
To save a paltry shilling.

Others had boards painted to look like brickwork, which could be used to cover up windows at pleasure.

[2] Petition, undated, but placed in a collection in the British Museum among broadsides of the years 1696–1700. In 1725 the imprisoned debtors at Liverpool petitioned Parliament for relief, alleging that they were reduced to a starving condi-

February, 1729, the House of Commons appointed a committee
"to inquire into the state of the gaols of this Kingdom"; but
only two prisons were reported on, the Fleet and the Marshalsea,
in London, the inquiries upon these being due to the energy
of Oglethorpe, then at the beginning of his useful career. The
committee found a disgraceful state of things:—wardens, tip-
staffs and turnkeys making their offices so lucrative by extortion
that the reversion of them was worth large sums, prisoners
abused or neglected if they could not pay, some prisoners kept
for years after their term was expired, the penniless crowded
three in a bed, or forty in one small room, while some rooms
stood empty to await the arrival of a prisoner with a well-filled
purse. On the common side of the Fleet Prison, ninety-three
prisoners were confined in three wards, having to find their own
bedding, or pay a shilling a week, or else sleep on the floor.
The "Lyons Den" and women's ward, which contained about
eighteen, were very noisome and in very ill repair. Those who
were well had to lie on the floor beside the sick. A Portuguese
debtor had been kept two months in a damp stinking dungeon
over the common sewer and adjoining to the sink and dunghill;
he was taken elsewhere on payment of five guineas. In the
Marshalsea there were 330 prisoners on the common side,
crowded in small rooms. George's ward, sixteen feet by fourteen
and about eight feet high, had never less than thirty-two in it "all
last year," and sometimes forty; there was no room for them
all to lie down, about one-half of the number sleeping over the
others in hammocks; they were locked in from 9 p.m. to 5 a.m.
in summer (longer hours in winter), and as they were forced
to ease nature within the room, the stench was noisome beyond
expression, and it seemed surprising that it had not caused a
contagion; several in the heat of summer perished for want of
air. Meanwhile the room above was let to a tailor to work in,
and no one allowed to lie in it. Unless the prisoners were
relieved by their friends, they perished by famine. There was
an allowance of pease from a casual donor who concealed his
name, and 30 lbs. of beef three times a week from another
charitable source. The starving person falls into a kind of
hectic, lingers for a month or two and then dies, the right of
his corpse to a coroner's inquest being often scandalously re-

tion, having only straw and water at the courtesy of the serjeant. *Commons'
Journals*, xx. 375.

fused[1]. The prison scenes in Fielding's *Amelia* are obviously faithful and correct.

Oglethorpe's committee had done some good since they first met at the Marshalsea on 25th March, 1729, not above nine having died from that date to the 14th May; whereas before that a day seldom passed without a death, "and upon the advancing of the spring not less than eight or ten usually died every twenty-four hours." Two of the chief personages concerned were found by a unanimous vote of the House of Commons to have committed high crimes and misdemeanours; but when they were tried before a jury on a charge of felony they were found not guilty.

About a year after these reports to the Commons there was a tragic occurrence among the Judges and the Bar of the Western Circuit during the Lent Assizes of 1730. The Bridewell at Taunton was filled for the occasion of the Assizes with drafts of prisoners from other gaols in Somerset, among whom several from Ilchester were said to have been more than ordinarily noisome. Over a hundred prisoners were tried, of whom eight were sentenced to death (six executed), and seventeen to transportation. As the Assize Court continued its circuit through Devon and Dorset several of its members sickened of the gaol fever and died: Piggot, the high-sheriff, on the 11th April, Sir James Sheppard, serjeant-at-law, on 13th April at Honiton, the crier of the court and two of the Judge's servants at Exeter, the Judge himself, chief baron Pengelly, at Blandford, and serjeant-at-law Rous, on his return to London, whither he had posted from Exeter as soon as he felt ill[2]. It is said that the infection afterwards spread within the town of Taunton, where it arose, "and carried off some hundreds"; but the local histories make no mention of such an epidemic in 1730, and no authority is cited for it[3]. Something of the same kind is

---

[1] *Commons' Journals*, 20 March, 17$\frac{28}{29}$, 14 May, 1729, 24 March, 17$\frac{29}{30}$.

"Mrs Mary Trapps was prisoner in the Marshalsea and was put to lie in the same bed with two other women, each of which paid 2s. 6d. per week chamber rent; she fell ill and languished for a considerable time; and the last three weeks grew so offensive that the others were hardly able to bear the room; they frequently complained to the turnkeys and officers, and desired to be removed; but all in vain. At last she smelt so strong that the turnkey himself could not bear to come into the room to hear the complaints of her bedfellows; and they were forced to lie with her on the boards, till she died."

[2] *Political State of Great Britain*, XXXIX. April, 1730, pp. 430-431, 448.

[3] *Gent. Magaz.*, XX. 235. This authority is twenty years after the event, the incident having been recalled in 1750, on the occasion of the Old Bailey catastrophe.

believed to have happened at a gaol delivery at Launceston in 1742, but the circumstances are vaguely related, and it does not appear that any prominent personage in the Assize Court died on the occasion[1].

The great instance of a Black Assize in the 18th century, comparable to those of Cambridge, Oxford and Exeter in the 16th[2], was that of the Old Bailey Sessions in London in April, 1750. It has been fully related by Sir Michael Foster, one of the justices of the King's Bench, who had himself been on the bench at the January sessions preceding, and was the intimate friend of Sir Thomas Abney, the presiding judge who lost his life from the contagion of the April sessions[3].

"At the Old Bailey sessions in April, 1750, one Mr Clarke was brought to his trial; and it being a case of great expectation, the court and all the passages to it were extremely crowded; the weather too was hotter than is usual at that time of the year[4]. Many people who were in court at this time were sensibly affected with a very noisome smell; and it appeared soon afterwards, upon an enquiry ordered by the court of aldermen, that the whole prison of Newgate and all the passages leading thence into the court were in a very filthy condition, and had long been so. What made these circumstances to be at all attended to was, that within a week or ten days at most, after the session, many people who were present at Mr Clarke's trial were seized with a fever of the malignant kind; and few who were seized recovered. The symptoms were much alike in all the patients, and in less than six weeks time the distemper entirely ceased. It was remarked by some, and I mention it because the same remark hath formerly been made on a like occasion [Oxford, 1577], that women were very little affected: I did not hear of more than one woman who took the fever in court, though doubtless many women were there.

"It ought to be remembered that at the time this disaster happened there was no sickness in the gaol more than is common in such places. This circumstance, which distinguisheth this from most of the cases of the like kind which we have heard of, suggesteth a very proper caution: not to presume too far upon the health of the gaol, barely because the gaol-fever is not among the prisoners. For without doubt, if the points of cleanliness and free air have been greatly neglected, the putrid effluvia which the prisoners bring with them in their clothes etc., especially where too many are brought into a crowded court together, may have fatal effects on people who are accustomed to breathe better air; though the poor wretches, who are in some measure habituated to the fumes of a prison, may not always be sensible of any great inconvenience from them.

"The persons of chief note who were in court at this time and died of the fever were Sir Samuel Pennant, lord mayor for that year, Sir Thomas Abney, one of the justices of the Common Pleas, Charles Clarke, esquire,

---

[1] Huxham.

[2] See the former volume of this History, pp. 375–386.

[3] *A Report &c. and of other Crown Cases.* By Sir Michael Foster, Knt., some time one of the Judges of the Court of King's Bench. 2nd ed. London, 1776, p. 74.

[4] The *Gentleman's Magazine* however says (1750, p. 235): "There being a very cold and pi cing east wind to attack the sweating persons when they came out of court."

one of the barons of the exchequer, and Sir Daniel Lambert, one of the aldermen of London. Of less note, a gentleman of the bar, two or three students, one of the under-sheriffs, an officer of Lord Chief Justice Lee, who attended his lordship in court at that time, several of the jury on the Middlesex side, and about forty other persons whom business or curiosity had brought thither."

The same thing was remarked here as at Exeter in 1586 that those who sat on the side of the Court nearest to the dock were most attacked by the infection[1]. When the cases of fever began to occur, after the usual incubation of "a week or ten days," there was much fear of the infection spreading, so that many families, it is said, retired into the country[2]. But Pringle wrote on 24 May, "However fatal it has been since the Sessions, it is highly probable that the calamity will be in a great measure confined to those who were present at the tryal[3];" and Justice Foster gives no hint of anyone having taken the fever who was not present in court.

The tragedy of gaol-fever at the Old Bailey in 1750 secured increased attention to the subject of scientific ventilation. The great bar to fresh air indoors throughout the 18th century was the window-tax. It bore particularly hard on prisoners, for the gaolers had to pay the window-tax out of their profits, and they naturally preferred to build up the windows. Scientific ventilation of gaols was something of a mockery in these circumstances; but it is the business of science to find out cunning contrivances, and ingenious ventilators were devised for Newgate, the leading spirit in this work being the Rev. Dr Hales, rector of a parish near London, and an amateur in physiology at the meetings of the Royal Society.

A ventilating apparatus had been erected at Newgate about a year before the fatal sessions of 1650, but it does not seem to have answered. It consisted of tubes from the various wards meeting in a great trunk which opened on the roof. A committee of the Court of Aldermen in October 1750 resolved, after consulting Pringle and Hales, to add a windmill on the leads over the vent, and that was done about two years after. Pringle, who inspected the ventilator on 11 July, 1752, says that

---

[1] See Bancroft, *Essay on the Yellow Fever, with observations concerning febrile contagion etc.* Lond. 1811.

[2] *Gent. Magaz.* 1750, p. 274: "Many families are retired into the country, and near 12,000 houses empty"—an impossible number.

[3] Sir John Pringle, *Observations on the Nature and Cure of the Hospital and Jayl Fever.* Lette. to Mead, May 24. London, 1750.

a considerable stream of air of a most offensive smell issued from the vent; and it appeared that no fewer than seven of the eleven carpenters who were working at the alterations on the old ventilator caught gaol-fever (of the petechial kind), which spread among the families of some of them[1]. Pringle and Hales were of opinion that the wards furnished with tubes were less foul than the others; and they claimed, on the evidence of the man who took care of the apparatus, that only one person had died in the gaol in two months, whereas, before the windmill was used, there died six or seven in a week[2]. But Oglethorpe had claimed an improvement of the same kind at the Marshalsea in 1729 merely from having the prisoners saved from hunger; and Lind, who was a most matter-of-fact person, did not think that the ingenious contrivances for ventilation had answered their end[3].

Howard's visitations of the prisons, which began in 1773 and were continued or repeated during several years following, brought to light many instances of epidemic sickness therein, which was nearly always of the nature of gaol-typhus. The following is a list compiled from his various reports, the two or three instances of smallpox infection being given elsewhere.

Wood Street Compter, London. About 100 in it, chiefly debtors. Eleven died in beginning of 1773; since then it has been visited by Dr Lettsom at the request of the aldermen.

Savoy, London. On 15 March, 1776, 119 prisoners. Many sick and dying. Between that date and next visit, 25 May, 1776, the gaol-fever has been caught by many.

Hertford. Inmates range from 20 to 30. In the interval of two visits, the gaol-fever prevailed and carried off seven or eight prisoners and two turnkeys. (The interval probably corresponded to the admission of an unusual number of debtors.)

Chelmsford. Number of inmates varies from 20 to 60, about one-half debtors. A close prison frequently infected with the gaol-distemper.

Dartford, County Bridewell. A small prison. About two years before visit of 1774 there was a bad fever, which affected the keeper and his family and every fresh prisoner. Two died of it.

Horsham, Bridewell. The keeper a widow: her husband dead of the gaol-fever.

---

[1] One of the cases was that of an apprentice: "Some of the journeymen working in Newgate had forced him to go down into the great trunk of the ventilator in order to bring up a wig which one of them had thrown into it. As the machine was then working, he had been almost suffocated with the stench before they could get him up." Pringle, "Ventilation of Newgate," *Phil. Trans.* 1753, p. 42.

[2] Thomas Stibbs to Sir John Pringle, Jan. 25, 1753. *Ibid.* p. 54.

[3] "Ventilators some years since when first introduced, it was thought, would prove an effectual remedy for and preservative against this infection in jails; great expectations were formed of their benefit, but several years' experience must now have fully shewn th. ventilators will not remove infection from a jail." Lind, *Means of Preserving the Health of Seamen in the Royal Navy.* New ed. Lond. 1774, p. 29.

Petworth, Bridewell. Allowance per diem a penny loaf (7½ oz.). Th. Draper and Wm. Godfrey committed 6 Jan., 1776: the former died on 11 Jan., the other on 16th. Wm. Cox, committed 13 Jan., died 23rd. "None of these had the gaol-fever. I do not affirm that these men were famished to death; it was extreme cold weather." After this the allowance of bread was doubled, thanks to the Duke of Richmond.

Southwark, the new gaol. Holds up to 90 debtors and felons. "In so close a prison I did not wonder to see, in March, 1776, several felons sick on the floors." No bedding, nor straw. The Act for preserving the health of prisoners is on a painted board.

Aylesbury. About 20 prisoners. First visit Nov., 1773, second Nov., 1774: in the interval six or seven died of the gaol-distemper.

Bedford. About twenty years ago the gaol-fever was in this prison; some died there, and many in the town, among whom was Mr Daniel, the surgeon who attended the prisoners. The new surgeon changed the medicines from sudorifics to bark and cordials; and a sail-ventilator being put up the gaol has been free from the fever almost ever since. (This was the gaol which is often said to have started Howard on his inquiries when he was High Sheriff.)

Warwick. Holds up to fifty-seven. The late gaoler died in 1772 of the gaol-distemper, and so did some of his prisoners. No water then; plenty now.

Southwell, Bridewell. A small prison. A few years ago seven died here of the gaol-fever within two years.

Worcester. Has a ventilator. Mr Hallward the surgeon caught the gaol-fever some years ago, and has ever since been fearful of going into the dungeon; when any felon is sick, he orders him to be brought out.

Shrewsbury. Gaol-fever has prevailed here more than once of late years.

Monmouth. At first visit in 1774, they had the gaol-fever, of which died the gaoler, several of his prisoners, and some of their friends.

Usk (Monmouth) Bridewell. The keeper's wife said that many years ago the prison was crowded, and that herself, her father who was then keeper, and many others of the family had the gaol-fever, three of whom, and several of the prisoners, died of it.

Gloucester, the Castle. Many prisoners died here in 1773; and always except at Howard's last visit, he saw some sick in this gaol. A large dunghill near the stone steps. The prisoners miserable objects: Mr Raikes and others took pity on them.

Winchester. The former destructive dungeon was down eleven steps, and darker than the present. Mr Lipscomb said that more than twenty prisoners had died in it of the gaol-fever in one year, and that the surgeon before him had died of it.

Liverpool. Holds about sixty, offensive, crowded. Howard in March, 1774, told the keeper his prisoners were in danger of the gaol-fever. Between that date and Nov., 1775, twenty-eight had been ill of it at one time.

Chester, the Castle. Dungeon used to imprison military deserters. Two of them brought by a sergeant and two men to Worcester, of which party three died a few days after they came to their quarters. (For fever in this prison in 1716 see the text, p. 60.)

Cowbridge. The keeper said, on 19 August, 1774, that many had died of the gaol-fever, among them a man and a woman a year before, at which time himself and daughter were ill of it.

Cambridge, the Town Bridewell. In the spring of 1779, seventeen women were confined in the daytime, and some of them at night, in the workroom, which has no fireplace or sewer. This made it extremely offensive, and occasioned a fever or sickness among them, which so alarmed the Vice-Chancellor that he ordered all of them to be discharged. Two or three of them died within a few days.

Exeter, the County Bridewell. Between first visit in 1775 and next on 5 Feb., 1779, the surgeon and two or three prisoners have died of the gaol-fever. In 1755 a prisoner discharged from the gaol went home to Axminster, and infected his family, of whom two died, and many others in that town afterwards.

Exeter, the High Gaol for felons. Mr Bull, the surgeon, stated that he was by contract excused from attending in the dungeons any prisoners that should have the gaol-fever.

Winchester, Bridewell. Close and small. Receives many prisoners from other gaols at Quarter Sessions. It has been fatal to vast numbers. The misery of the prisoners induced the Duke of Chandos to send them for some years 30 lbs. of beef and 2 gallon loaves a week.

Devizes, Bridewell. Two or three years ago the gaol-fever carried off many. An infirmary added since then.

Marlborough. The rooms offensive. Saw one dying on the floor of the gaol-fever. One had died just before, and another soon after his discharge.

Launceston. Small, with offensive dungeons. No windows, chimneys, or drains. No water. Damp earthen floor. Those who serve there often catch the gaol-fever. At first visit, found the keeper, his assistant and all the prisoners but one sick of it (on 19 Feb., 1774, eleven felons in it). Heard that, a few years before, many prisoners had died of it, and the keeper and his wife in one night. A woman confined three years by the Ecclesiastical Court had three children born in the gaol.

Bodmin, Bridewell. Much out of repair. The night rooms are two garrets with small close-glazed skylight 17 in. × 12 in. A few years ago the gaol-fever was very fatal, not only in the prison but also in the town.

Taunton, Bridewell. Six years ago, when there was no infirmary provided, the gaol-fever spread over the whole prison, so that eight died out of nineteen prisoners.

Shepton Mallet. Men's night room close, with small window. So unhealthy some years ago that the keeper buried three or four in a week.

Thirsk. Prisoners had the gaol-fever not long ago.

Carlisle. During the gaol-fever which some years ago carried off many of the prisoners, Mr Farish, the chaplain, visited the sick every day.

I shall add some medical experiences of gaol-fever in London from the notes of Lettsom[1]:—

May, 1773. A person released from Newgate "in a malignant or jail-fever" was brought into a house in a court off Long Lane, Aldersgate Street; soon after which fourteen persons in the same confined court were attacked with a similar fever: one died before Lettsom was called in, one was sent to hospital, eleven attended by him all recovered, though with difficulty. Two deaths in Wood Street Compter: 1. Rowell, an industrious, sober workman, who had supported for many years a wife and three children; some of these having been lately sick, he fell behind with his rent, a little over three guineas; he offered all he had (more than enough) to the landlord, but the latter preferred to throw the man and his family into the Compter, where Rowell died of fever. 2. Russell, once a reputable tradesman on Ludgate Hill, fell into a debt of under three guineas, sent to the Compter with his wife and five children, took fever and died; attended in his sickness in a bare room by his eldest daughter, elegant and refined, aged seventeen; his son, aged fourteen, took the fever and recovered.

[1] J. C. Lettsom, M.D., *Medical Memoirs of the General Dispensary in London,* 1773-4. Lond. 1774.

There was one Black Assize at this period, at Dublin in April 1776. A criminal, brought into the Court of Sessions without cleansing, infected the court and alarmed the whole city. Among others who died of the contagion were Fielding Ould, High Sheriff, the counsellors Derby, Palmer, Spring and Ridge, Mr Caldwell, Messrs Bolton and Eriven, and several attorneys and others whose business it was to attend the court[1].

There were two notorious outbreaks of malignant fever among foreign prisoners of war, one in 1761[2] and another in 1780[3], the first among French and Spaniards at Winchester and Portchester, the second among Spaniards at Winchester.

Howard found so little typhus in the gaols in his later visits that it seemed as if banished for good. But it was heard of frequently about 1780–85—at Maidstone, at Aylesbury, at Worcester, costing the lives of some of the visiting physicians.

Circumstances of severe and mild Typhus.

The circumstances of the gaol distemper bring out one grand character of typhus which will have to be stated formally before we go farther. Ordinary domestic typhus was not a very fatal disease. Haygarth says that of 285 attacked by it in the poorer quarters of Chester in the autumn of 1774, only twenty-eight died. Ferriar, in Manchester, had sometimes an even more favourable experience than that: "The mortality of the epidemic was not great,...out of the first ninety patients whom I attended, only two died." This was before the House of Recovery was opened; so that the low mortality was of typhus in the homes of the people.

The fever was often an insidious languishing, without great heat, and marked most by tossing and wakefulness, which might pass into delirium; when it went through the members of a family or the inmates of a house, there would be some cases concerning which it was hard to say whether they were cases of typhus or not. Misery and starvation brought it on, and often it was itself but a degree of misery and starvation. "I have found," says Ferriar, "that for three or four days before the

---

[1] *Gent. Magaz.* 1776, April 22. p. 187.
[2] Lind, *Two Papers on Fevers and Infection.* Lond. 1763. pp. 90, 106. Many cases had buboes both in the groins and the armpits.
[3] Carmichael Smyth, *Description of the Jail Distemper among Spanish Prisoners at Winchester in 1780.* Lond. 1795.

appearance of typhus in a family consisting of several children, they had subsisted on little more than cold water." " It has been observed," says Langrish, " that those who have died of hunger and thirst, as at sieges and at sea, etc., have always died delirious and feverish." The fever was on the whole a distinct episode, but in many cases it had no marked crisis. "Those women who recovered," says Ferriar, " were commonly affected with hysterical symptoms after the fever disappeared ; " and again : "Fevers often terminate in hysterical disorders, especially in women ; men, too, are sometimes hysterically inclined upon recovering from typhus, for they experience a capricious disposition to laugh or cry, and a degree of the globus hystericus." These were probably the more case-hardened people, inured to their circumstances, their healthy appetite dulled by the practice of fasting or "clemming," or by opium, and their blood accustomed to be renovated by foul air. If the limit of subsistence be approached gradually, life may be sustained thereat without any sharp crisis of fever, or with only such an interlude of fever as differs but little from a habit of body unnamed in the nosology.

The worst kind of typhus, often attended with delirium, crying and raving, intolerable pains in the head, and livid spots on the skin, ending fatally perhaps in two or three days, or after a longer respite of stupor or waking insensibility, was commonly the typhus of those not accustomed to the minimum of wellbeing —the typhus of hardy felons newly thrown into gaol, of soldiers in a campaign crowded into a hospital after a season in the open air, of sailors on board ship mixing with newly pressed men having the prison atmosphere clinging to them, of judges, counsel, officials of the court and gentlemen of the grand jury brought into the same atmosphere with prisoners at a gaol-delivery, of the wife and children of a discharged prisoner returned to his home, of the gaol-keeper, gaol-chaplain, or gaol-doctor, of the religious and charitable who visited in poor localities even where no fever was known to be, and most of all of country people who crowded to the towns in search of work or of higher wages or of a more exciting life.

It was in these circumstances that the most fatal infections of typhus took place. Such extraordinary malignancy of typhus happened often when the type of sickness (if indeed there was definite disease at all) among the originally ailing

failed to account for it; it was the great disparity of condition that accounted for it. There were, however, more special occasions when a higher degree of malignancy than ordinary was bred or cultivated among the classes at large who were habitually liable to typhus. But even the old pestilential spotted fever which used to precede, accompany, and follow the plague itself, was fatal to a comparatively small proportion of all who had it. Thus, towards the end of the great London plague of 1625, on 18th October, Sir John Coke writes to Lord Brooke: "In London now the tenth person dieth not of those that are sick, and generally the plague seems changed into an ague[1]." One in ten is probably too small a fatality for the old pestilential fever; but that is the usually accepted proportion of deaths to attacks in the typhus fever of later times. The rate of fatality is got, naturally, by striking an average. But in truth an aggregate of typhus cases, however homogeneous in conventional symptoms or type-characters, was not always really homogeneous. We have seen that ninety cases of typhus could occur in the slums of Manchester with only two deaths. On the other hand there were outbreaks of gaol-fever in which half or more of all that were attacked died; and I suspect that the average fatality in typhus of one in ten was often brought up by an admixture of cases of healthy and well-conditioned people who caught a much more malignant type of fever from their contact with those inured to misery. To strike an average is in many instances a convenience and a help to the apprehension of a truth; but for the average to be instructive, the members of the aggregate must be more or less comparable in their circumstances. It has been truly said that there is no common measure between Lazarus and Dives as regards their subjective views of things; it is not a little strange to find that they are just as incommensurable in their risk of dying from the infection of typhus fever. The rule seems to be that the degree of acuteness or violence of an attack of typhus was inversely as the habitual poor condition of the victim. In adducing evidence of the tragic nature of typhus infection conveyed across the gulf of misery to the other side, I shall endeavour to keep strictly to the scientific facts, leaving the moral, if there be a moral (and it is not always obvious), to point itself.

Let us take first the common case of country-bred people

[1] *Cal. Coke MSS.* Hist. MSS. Commiss. i. 218.

migrating to the towns. Any lodging in a crowded centre of industry and trade would be high-rented compared with the country cottage which they had left, and they would naturally gravitate to the slums of the city.

"Great numbers of the labouring poor," says Ferriar of Manchester, "who are tempted by the prospect of large wages to flock into the principal manufacturing towns, become diseased by getting into dirty infected houses on their arrival. Others waste their small stock of money without procuring employment, and sink under the pressure of want and despair....The number of such victims sacrificed to the present abuses is incredible." And again:

"It must be observed that persons newly arrived from the country are most liable to suffer from these causes, and as they are often taken ill within a few days after entering an infected house, there arises a double injury to the town, from the loss of their labour, and the expense of supporting them in their illness. A great number of the home-patients of the Infirmary are of this description. The horror of these houses cannot easily be described; a lodger fresh from the country often lies down in a bed filled with infection by its last tenant, or from which the corpse of a victim to fever has only been removed a few hours before[1]."

Two instances from the same author will show the severe type of the fever.

The tenant of a house in Manchester, who was herself ill of typhus along with her three children, took in a lodger, a girl named Jane Jones, fresh from the country. The lodger fell ill, but the fact was kept concealed from the visiting physician until her screams discovered her: "She was found delirious, with a black fur on the lips and teeth, her cheeks extremely flushed, and her pulse low, creeping, and scarcely to be counted." Treatment was of no use; she "passed whole nights in shrieking," and in her extremity, she was saved, as Ferriar believed, by affusions of cold water. Another case, exactly parallel, proved fatal in three days:

"In 1792 I had two patients ill of typhus in an infected lodging-house. I desired that they might be washed with cold water; and a healthy, ruddy young woman of the neighbourhood undertook the office. Though apparently in perfect health before she went into the sick chamber, she complained of the intolerable smell of the patients, and said she felt a head-ache when she came down stairs. She sickened, and died of the fever in three days[2]."

These are instances of country-bred people, plunging abruptly into the fever-dens of cities and catching a typhus

---

[1] *Med. Hist. and Reflect.* ut infra.

[2] The following case, which happened five or six years ago, shows disparity of conditions in a twofold aspect. A lady from a city in the north of Scotland travelled direct to Switzerland to reside for a few weeks at one of the hotels in the High Alps. Within an hour or two of the end of her journey she began to feel ill, and was confined to her room from the time she entered the hotel. An English physician diagnosed the effects of the sun; the German doctor of the place, from his reading only, diagnosed typhus fever, which proved to be right, the patient dying with the most pronounced signs of malignant typhus. An explanation of the mystery was soon forthcoming. The lady had been a district visitor in an old and poor part of the Scotch city; she had, in particular, visited in a certain tenement-house in a court, from which half-a-dozen persons had been admitted to the Infirmary with typhus (an unusual event) at the very time when she was ill of it on the Swiss mountain.

severe in the direct ratio of their ruddy, healthy condition. Another class of cases is that of persons carrying the atmosphere of a gaol into the company of healthy and otherwise favourably situated people.   Howard gives a case : at Axminster a prisoner discharged from Exeter gaol in 1755 infected his family with the gaol-distemper, of which two of them died, and many others in that town.   The best illustrations of the greater severity and fatality of typhus among the well-to-do come from Ireland, in times of famine, and will be found in another chapter.   But it may be said here, so that this point in the natural history of typhus fever may not be suspected of exaggeration, that the enormously greater fatality of typhus (of course, in a smaller number of cases) among the richer classes in the Irish famines, who had exposed themselves in the work of administration, of justice, or of charity, rests upon the unimpeachable authority of such men as Graves, and upon the concurrent evidence of many.

Ship-Fever.

The prevalence of fevers in ships of war and transports from the Restoration onwards can be learned but imperfectly, and learned at all only with much trouble.   Sir Gilbert Blane, who was not wanting in aptitude and had the archives of the Navy Office at his service, goes no farther back than 1779, from which date an account was kept of the causes of death in the naval hospitals.   But the deaths on board ships of the fleet were not systematically recorded until 1811, when the Board of Admiralty instructed all commanders of ships of war to send to the Naval Office an annual account of all the deaths of men on board[1].   The sources of information for earlier periods are more casual.

The war with France, which dated from the accession of William III. and continued until the Peace of Ryswick in 1697, led to numerous conflicts with French and Spaniards in the West Indies, and to naval expeditions year after year. The loss of life from sickness in the British ships for a few years at the end of the century was such as can hardly be realized by us.   Some part of it happened on the outward voyages, but by far the greater part of it was from the poison of yellow fever

[1] Blane, *Select Dissertations.* London, 1822, p. 1.

which had entered the ships in the anchorages of West Indian
colonies. It was probably to that cause that the enormous
mortality in the fleet under Sir Francis Wheeler was owing.
After some ineffective operations against the French in the
Windward Islands in the winter of 1693–4, he sailed for North
America with the intention of attacking Quebec. This he
failed to do, having sailed from Boston for home on the 3rd of
August without entering the St Lawrence. The reason of the
failure was probably the extraordinary fatality which Cotton
Mather, of Boston, professes to have heard from the admiral
himself, namely, that he lost by a malignant fever on the
passage from Barbados to Boston 1300 sailors out of 2100, and
1800 soldiers out of 2400[1].

Another instance comes from Carlisle Bay, Barbados. The
slave ship 'Hannibal' arrived there in November, 1694, during a
disastrous epidemic of yellow fever. Phillips, the captain, whose
journal of the voyage is published[2], had great difficulty in
saving his crew from being pressed into the king's ships, which
were short of men owing to the yellow fever. Captain Sherman,
of the 'Tiger,' who convoyed the 'Hannibal' and other
merchantmen back to England in April, 1695, told Phillips
that he buried six hundred men out of his ship during the two
years that he lay at Barbados, though his complement was but
220, "still pressing men out of the merchant ships that came in,
to recruit his number in the room of those that died daily."

These and other similar experiences of yellow fever in the
West Indies, which might be collected from the naval history,
do not come properly into this chapter; and I pass from
them to ship-fever proper, having indicated how much of the
loss of life abroad was due to yellow fever.

Some light is thrown upon the state of health on board ships
of war on the home station by Dr William Cockburn, physician
to the fleet, afterwards the friend of Swift, who calls him
"honest Dr Cockburn." He had a secret remedy for dysentery,
which he succeeded in getting adopted by the Admiralty,
greatly to his own emolument for many years after. Dining on

[1] Mather's *Magnalia*. 2 vols. Hartford, 1853, i. 226 "Life of Sir William
Phipps." "Whereof there died, ere they could reach Boston, as I was told by Sir
Francis Wheeler himself ['but a few months ago'], no less than 1300 sailors out of
21, and no less than 1800 soldiers out of 24." He had brought 1800 troops with him
from England to Barbados in transports.
[2] Churchill's Collection, VI. 173.

board one of the ships at Portsmouth, in 1696, with Lo
Berkeley of Stratton, he brought up the subject of his electuary
and arranged for a public trial of it next day on board the
'Sandwich.' An uncertain number, which looks to have been
about seven in Cockburn's own account, but became seventy
the pamphlet which advertised the electuary after his death
were available for the trial and were speedily cured. Cockburn
three essays on the health of seamen[1] leave no doubt as to the
extensive prevalence of scurvy and the causes thereof; while
his references to "malignant fever," although they are, as usual
brought in to illustrate some doctrinal or theoretical point
give colour to the belief that ship-typhus may have been as
common then as we know it to have been in the ships at
Portsmouth and Plymouth, on the more direct testimony of
Huxham in 1736, and of Lind twenty years later.

A naval surgeon of the time of William III. and Anne, was
induced by his enthusiasm for blood-letting in fevers to record
some of his experiences on board ship[2]. It was usually the
lustiest, both of the young, strong and healthy people, and likewise of the elder sort, that died of fevers, the symptoms which
proved so mortal having been delirium, phrenitis, coma or
stupor, whether they occurred in the συνόχοι (of Sydenham) or
in the συνεχεῖς (of the same author):

"I had observed in a ship of war whose complement was near 500, in a
Mediterranean voyage in the year 1694, where we lost about 90 or 100 men,
mostly by fevers, that those who died were commonly the young, but almost
always the strongest, lustiest, handsomest persons, and that two or three
escaped by means of such [natural] haemorrhagies, which were five or six
pounds of blood"—the point being that the amount of blood drawn by
phlebotomy should be in proportion to the robustness and body-weight of the
patient.

In 1703 and 1704 he was surgeon to two of Her Majesty's
ships "where a delirium, stupor and phrenitis" were found as
symptoms of the fevers. In the summer of 1704, cruising in the
latitudes of Portugal and Spain, the men brought on board from
Lisbon unripe lemons with which they made great quantities of
punch. This was the evident cause of a cholera morbus and
dysentery: "after this we had a pretty many taken with the

[1] W. Cockburn, M.D. *An Account of the Nature, Causes, Symptoms and Cure of the Distempers that are incident to Seafaring People.* 3 Parts. London, 1696-97.
[2] J. White, M.D. *De recta Sanguinis Missione, or, New and Exact Observations of Fevers, in which Letting of Blood is shew'd to be the true and solid Basis of their Cure, &c.* London, 1712. His chief point, that the strongest and lustiest were most obnoxious to malignant fevers, had been urged by Cockburn in 1696.

synochus putris, and some with the *causus*" [malignant fever]. Most of these fevers went off by a crisis in sweating, "which was so large I had good reason to believe it judicatory." In several the fevers left on the 9th, 10th or 11th day, and in almost all by the 14th. "About the latter end of July, and in August, there were many taken with a delirium and stupor or coma, and some with the phrenitis in their fever." Among the symptoms was one which we find described for fevers on board ship on the West Coast of Africa at the same time— "soreness all over as if from blows with a cane," a symptom afterwards associated with dengue. "Sometimes the bones (as they term it) don't pain them much." In some cases there were petechial spots as well as a stupor. In the month of August "the fevers with a stupor and phrenitis" came on apace. The treatment was to take ten ounces of blood every day from the second to the eighth day of the fever, to give tartar emetic in five-grain doses at the outset, and to administer cathartic glysters in the second half of the fever. "Seeing the lustiest men now ran no more hazard of their lives than any other who were usually taken with this fever, nor indeed so much, in the beginning of September I resolved, after all the phlebotomy was done in these fevers, to try the cathartic sooner." Many of these who had accustomed themselves to the liberal use of spirituous liquors miscarried in the phrenitis.

White left the navy in 1704 and settled in practice at Lisbon, where he saw much fever. He had seen epidemics break out in British ships of war at anchor in the Tagus, crowded with men and prisoners. One case he mentions in a Lisbon woman, with continual synochus, stupor, and petechiae on the fifth day: "This was contagious, for she got it by going often to assist a gunner of a man-of-war, who came to her house with this distemper upon him: for many at the same time on board that ship were sick of that disease." Among the causes of fever on board ship he mentions the effluvia of the bilge-water.

Exposed to these emanations were "a multitude of people breathing and constantly perspiring in a close place, such as a ship's *allop* or lower deck next the hould, where is the entry to a certain vacant space near the ship's center, which leadeth to the bottom, for gathering all the water together which the ship draweth by leakage, and is called the well. Several times there is occasion for some people to go down to examine the quantity of the water, and in some ships to bore an augur hole to let in as much as will preserve a good air. I have often known two or three men killed at

a time, as it is said; and the reason may be understood from what I said of the general effects of that fluid in ordinary fever [he is now writing on heat apoplexy], where there is not above two or three inches, but just as much as may make a surface, almost equal to the square of the well, of stagnant salt water which had been a long while in gathering; and the air over the whole *allop* extremely rarified, and here not at all ventilated[1]."

We owe it to the accident of the celebrated Dr Freind having accompanied Lord Peterborough's expedition to Spain in 1705 that some account has been preserved of the sickness among the troops ashore and afloat[2].

The expedition of some 8000 men being then in its second year, fever and dysentery were by far the most common diseases, so common that "we can hardly turn, whether at sea or in camp, without finding them as if our inseparable companions and as if domesticated among us." In the summer of the previous year there had been much fever both in the ships of the fleet and in the camp before Barcelona: "It was of the continual kind, though it usually remitted in the day time, and seemed to approach nearly to the stationary one which Sydenham has described in the years 1685 and 1686." He then gives symptoms, which were on the whole those of the hospital fever to be afterwards described from Pringle's medical account of the campaigns in 1743–48. Persons of a robust habit were affected more than others, and more severely, and carried off sooner. The others were generally taken away by a lingering death. "Some, when the fever seemed to have been wholly gone off lay four or five days without pain or sickness, though weak;

---

[1] Lind (*Two Papers on Fevers and Infection*, London, 1763, p. 113) gives an instance where the poisonous effluvia of the ship's well did not spread through the 'tween decks: "The following accident happened lately [written in 1761] in the Bay of Biscay. In a ship of 60 guns, by the carpenter's neglecting to turn the cock that freshens the bilge-water, which had not been pumped out for some time, a large scum, as is usual, or a thick tough film was collected a-top of it. The first man who went down to break this scum in order to pump out the bilge-water was immediately suffocated. The second suffered an instantaneous death in like manner. And three others, who successively attempted the same business, narrowly escaped with life: one of whom has never since perfectly recovered his health. Yet that ship was at all times, both before and after this accident, remarkably healthy." It was the contention of Renwick, a naval surgeon who wrote in 1794, that it was the stirring of the bilge-water in being discharged from the ship's well, or the adding of fresh water to the foul, that caused the offensive emanations. "Hence the first cause of febrile sickness in all ships recently commissioned." Renwick made so much of the foul bilge-water as a cause that he thought the fevers ought to be termed "bilge-fevers." *Letter to the Critical Reviewer*, p. 42.

[2] These particulars are not given in Freind's special work on Peterborough's campaign, which deals only with the military and political history, but in his *Nine Commentaries on Fever* (Engl. ed. by Dale, London, 1730), and in a Latin letter to Cockburn, dated Barcelona, 9 Sept. 1706, which was first printed in *Several Cases in Physic*. By Pierce Dod, M.D. London, 1746.

afterwards being suddenly seized with convulsions of the nerves they in a short time expired"—perhaps the phenomenon of relapse, which Lind recorded for ship-fever fifty years after and was seen among the troops landed from Corunna in 1809. In some few the parotids, or abscesses formed about the groin, carried off the disease.

He then gives the case of a lieutenant on board the 'Barfleur.' At first he was restless and delirious; on the 7th and 8th days he had *subsultus tendinum;* on the 8th day his tongue was sometimes fixed, and his eyes sparkled; on the 9th day, he was wholly deprived of his understanding; he pulled off the fringe of the bed and plucked the flocks; when he had before faultered in his speech, he was sometimes seized with hiccough. But on the 10th day, after 12 oz. of blood had been drawn from the jugular vein, his delirium went off on a sudden, and he began to mend, making a perfect recovery.

Until the middle of the 18th century there are few other notices of ship-fever, but it is probable that Huxham's accounts of a very malignant typhus among the crews of ships of war at Plymouth in 1735 (as well as at Portsmouth according to report), and again in 1741, are to be taken as samples of what might have been recorded on many occasions[1].

Fever and Dysentery of Campaigns: War Typhus, 1742-63.

The war in Ireland after the accession of William III. produced two remarkable instances of war-sickness, which are fully given in another chapter. The campaigns of Marlborough against the armies of Louis XIV., from 1704 to the Treaty of Utrecht in 1713, appear to have found no historian from the medical side, nor does the duke refer to these matters in his dispatches or letters, beyond a remark in a letter to his wife from near Munich, 30 July, 1704, a fortnight before the battle

---

[1] Smollett joined the 'Cumberland' as surgeon's mate in 1740, before she sailed with the fleet sent out under Vernon and others to Carthagena. His account in *Roderick Random* of the sick-bay of the 'Thunder' as she lay at the Nore is doubtless veracious: "When I observed the situation of the patients, I was much less surprised that people should die on board, than that any sick person should recover. Here I saw about fifty miserable distempered wretches, suspended in rows, so huddled one upon another that not more than fourteen inches space was allowed for each with his bed and bedding; and deprived of the light of the day, as well as of fresh air; breathing nothing but a noisome atmosphere of the morbid steams exhaling from their own excrements and diseased bodies, devoured with vermin hatched in the filth that surrounded them, and destitute of every convenience necessary for people in that helpless condition." Chap. xxv. He wrote a separate account of the fatal Carthagena expedition in a compendium of voyages.

of Blenheim : " There having been no war in this country for above sixty years, these towns and villages are so clean that you would be pleased with them[1]."

The war of 1742–48, in which George II. joined Austria against France, produced the first good accounts of war typhus, on land and on board ship, in the writings of Pringle[2]. After the battle of Dettingen, 27 June, 1743, the men were exposed all night in the wet fields ; during the next eight days five hundred of them were attacked with dysentery, and in a few weeks near half the army were either ill of it or had recovered from it. The dysentery continued all July and part of August, while the army lay at Hanau. The village of Feckenheim, a league from the camp, was used as a hospital, some 1500 being quartered in it, most of them ill at first of dysentery. The latrines appear to have been ill designed and badly kept. " A malignant fever began among the men, from which few escaped : for however mild or bad soever the flux was for which the person was sent to hospital, this fever almost surely supervened. The petechial spots, blotches, parotids, frequent mortifications, and the great mortality, characterized a pestilential malignity : in this it was worse than the true plague....Of 14 mates employed about the hospital five died ; and, excepting one or two, all the rest had been ill and in danger. The hospital lost nearly half of the patients ; but the inhabitants of the village of Feckenheim, where the sick were, having first received the bloody flux, and afterwards the fever by contagion, were almost utterly destroyed[3]." The survivors from the sick troops in Feckenheim were removed to Neuwied, where they were relieved ; " but the rest, who were mixed with them, caught the infection." The mixed troops were sent still down the Rhine in bilanders, during which voyage " the fever became so virulent that above half the number died in the boats, and many of the remnant soon after their arrival." A parcel of tents sent in these bilanders to the Low Countries were given to a Ghent tradesman to refit ; he employed twenty-three journeymen upon them, " but these unhappy men were quickly seized with

[1] Coxe's *Life of Marlborough.* Bohn's ed. I. 183.
[2] Grainger's essay, *Historia febris anomalae Bataviae annorum*, 1746, 1747, 1748, *etc.* Edin. 1753, is chiefly occupied with an anomalous "intermittent" or "remittent" fever with miliary eruption, and with dysentery.
[3] For a full discussion of the relation of dysentery to typhus, see Virchow, "Kriegstypus und Ruhr." *Virchow's Archiv*, Bd. LII. (1871), p. 1.

this fever, whereof seventeen died." They had no other communication with the infected but through the tents.

"These," says Pringle, "are instances of high malignity. The common course of the infection is slow, and only catching to those constantly confined to the bad air. Sometimes one will have this fever about him for several days before it confines him to his bed; others I have known complain for weeks of the same symptoms without any regular fever at all; and some, after leaving the infectious place, have afterwards fallen ill of it[1]."

After the battle of Fontenoy on 11 May, 1745, the army was in good health: "the smallpox was the only new disease; it came with the recruits from England, but did not spread; and indeed we have never known it of any consequence in the field."

On the Jacobite rebellion breaking out in Scotland later in the same year, some of the returning troops were ordered to disembark at Newcastle, Holy Island and Berwick. They had a long voyage, so that a kind of remitting fever which some of them had acquired in the autumn in the Low Countries was "by the crowds and the foul air of the hold soon converted into the jail distemper and became infectious." At Newcastle most of the nurses and medical attendants of the extemporized hospital were seized with it, of whom three apothecaries, four apprentices and two journeymen died. But the most remarkable experience was on Holy Island. Of ninety-seven men taken out of the ships there, ill of the gaol-fever, forty died, "and the people of the place receiving the infection, in a few weeks buried fifty, the sixth part of the inhabitants of that island." At Nairn and Inverness there was a singular experience in the spring of 1746. The ships which brought Houghton's brigade to Nairn carried also thirty-six deserters to be tried by court-martial at the headquarters at Inverness: these men had deserted to the French in Flanders, had been found on board of a captured French transport carrying men to aid the Pretender, and had been thrown into gaol in England till an opportunity arose of sending them to their trial. Three days after the landing at Nairn of the force with which these deserters sailed, six of the officers were seized with fever and many of the men,

[1] Sir John Pringle, *Obs. on the Nature and Cure of Hospital and Jayl Fever,* Lond. 1750 (Letter to Mead); and his *Obs. on Diseases of the Army,* Lond. 1752 (fullest account).

of whom eighty were left sick at Nairn; in the ten days that the regiment remained at Inverness it sent one hundred and twenty more to hospital, ill of the same fever, which became frequent also among the inhabitants of the town. "Though the virulence of the distemper diminished afterwards in their march to Fort Augustus and Fort William, yet the corps continued sickly for some time." From the middle of February, 1746, when the army crossed the Forth, to the end of the campaign, there were two thousand sick in hospital, including wounded, of which number near three hundred died, mostly of the contagious fever [1].

After the Peace of Aix-la-Chapelle in 1748, the English troops embarked at Willemstad for home; "but the wind being contrary, several of the ships lay above a month at anchor, and, after all, meeting with a tedious and stormy passage, during which the men kept mostly below deck, the air was corrupted and produced the jail or hospital fever." The ships that came to Ipswich were in the worst state, about four hundred men having been landed sick there, most of them ill of this contagious fever. The infection was at first as active and the mortality as great on shore as on board; but the virulence of the fever was at length subdued by dispersing the sick and convalescents as much as possible [2].

Monro gives a similar account of the camp sickness among the British troops during the campaigns in North Germany in 1760–63. In the autumn of 1760, before he joined the forces, there had been much malignant fever and dysentery: the camp at Warburg was near the battlefield (31 July, 1760), where many of the dead were scarce covered with earth; there were also many dead horses, and in a time of heavy rains, the camp, with the neighbouring villages and fields, was filled with the excrements of a numerous army. Not only the soldiers, but the inhabitants of the country, who were reduced to the greatest misery and want, were infected, and whole villages almost laid waste. When Monro joined at Paderborn in January, 1761, he found the hospitals overcrowded, and the malignancy of the fever thereby much increased, so that a great many died. "The 1st and 3rd regiments suffered most, owing to all the sick of each regiment being put into a particular hospital by themselves,

[1] Pringle, *Diseases of the Army*, pp. 40–45.
[2] *Ibid.* p. 68.

which kept up the infection, so that they lost one-third of those left ill of this fever, and many of the nurses and people who attended them were seized with it." He distributed the sick men of the Coldstreams among the houses in the town, and lost few in comparison with the 1st and 3rd regiments. The contagion, under this bold policy, did not spread.

Two points in the symptoms are noteworthy: first the occurrence of suppurating buboes of the groins and armpits in several; and, secondly, the frequency of round worms.

"In this fever it was common for patients to vomit worms, or to pass them by stool, or, what was more frequent, to have them come up into the throat or mouth, and sometimes into their nostrils, while they were asleep in bed, and to pull them out with their fingers. The same thing happened to most of the British soldiers brought to the hospitals for other feverish disorders as well as this."

He cannot explain the commonness of round worms in the sick, unless it was from the great quantity of crude vegetables and fruits eaten, and the bad water. Patients in convalescence often suffered from deafness, and from suppurating parotids. Some had frequent relapses into the fever, " which seemed to be owing to the irritation of these insects," namely the worms. Most of those who fell into profuse, kindly, warm sweats recovered, the sweats lasting from twelve to forty-eight hours, and carrying off the fever. He never saw any miliary eruptions, and only sometimes petechiae, or small spots, or marbling as in measles[1].

Ship-Fever in the Seven Years' War and American War.

Ship-fever would appear to have been at its worst after the middle of the 18th century. Dr James Lind joined Haslar Hospital in 1758, and brought to the naval medical service the same high qualities which Pringle and Monro brought to that of the army[2]. The smaller ships, such as the 'Saltash' sloop, the 'Richmond' frigate, and the 'Infernal' bomb were full of fever of the most malignant kind; of 120 men in the 'Saltash,' 80 were infected with a contagion much more virulent and dangerous than that in the guard-ships. The explanation was

[1] Donald Monro, M.D. *Diseases of British Military Hospitals in Germany, from Jan.* 1761 *to the Return of the Troops to England in* 1763. Lond. 1764. The same campaign called forth also Dr Richard Brocklesby's *Œconomical and Medical Observations from* 1758 *to* 1763 *on Military Hospitals and Camp Diseases etc.* London, 1764.

[2] *Essay on Preserving the Health of Seamen,* Lond. 1757 ; *Two papers etc.* u. s.

that the smaller ships were receiving vessels for the larger ships, and were manned from the gaols; drafts from them carried the infection to the guard-ships and to the ships fitting out for foreign service. Malignant fever also arose on the voyage home from America[1]. In September and October 1758, after the reduction of Louisburg, several of the ships arriving at Spithead were infected with a malignant fever; three hundred men were received from them at Haslar Hospital (some with scurvy), of whom twenty-eight died. The 'Edgar,' having been manned at the Nore from gaols, sailed for the Mediterranean, and lost sixty men from fever and scurvy. The 'Loestoffe,' having lain in the St Lawrence for eight months in perfect health, took on board six convalescent men from Point Levi Hospital before sailing for home; in forty-eight hours, fifty out of her two hundred men were seized with fevers and fluxes, and six died on the voyage home. The 'Dublin' on the homeward voyage from Quebec buried nineteen, and on her arrival reported ninety men sick of fever, fluxes and scurvy. The 'Neptune' was said to have lost one hundred and sixty men in a few months, and reported 136 sick. The 'Cambridge,' with 650 men in health, sent three of her crew to the 'Neptune' laid up, to prepare her for the dock; of these three, one on the fifth day became spotted and died, and another narrowly escaped with life. The 'Diana' developed fever during a rough passage home from America. The 'St George,' having sailed from Spithead in 1760, met with rough weather and had to return on account of sickness. On the other hand, Hawke's fleet of twenty ships of the line with fourteen thousand men, which defeated the French in November 1759, kept the Bay of Biscay for four months in the most perfect health.

From 1 July, 1758, to 1 July, 1760, there were 5743 admissions to Haslar Hospital, the chief diseases being as follows:

Fevers	2174
Scurvy	1146
Consumption	360
Rheumatism	350
Fluxes	245

Of the fevers some were of an intermittent type, but by far the most were continued ship-typhus. Relapses were common, even to the sixth or seventh time. The fever varied a good

[1] In 1755 a pestilential sickness raged in the North American fleet, the 'Torbay' and 'Munich' being obliged to land their sick at Halifax.

deal in malignity, but never produced buboes, livid blotches or mortifications, and seldom parotids. Twenty-four men received from January to March 1760 out of the 'Garland' had most of them petechial spots accompanied with other symptoms of malignity, and of these, five died or 20 per cent. But of 105 received during the same months from the 'Postilion' and 'Liverpool' only eight died, and those mostly of a flux. The infection had little tendency to spread among the attendants at Haslar. In the first six months only one nurse died ; in 1759, two labourers and two nurses died, one of the nurses by infection, having concealed some infected shirts under her bed, the other by decay of nature. Of more than a hundred persons employed in various offices about the sick there died only those five in the course of eighteen months.

Although Lind's account of ship-fever in the British navy is bad enough, he has collected some far worse particulars of foreign ships. Febrile contagion destroyed two-thirds of the men in the Duc d'Anville's fleet at Chebucto (now Halifax), in 1746, the complete destruction of which was afterwards accomplished by the scurvy. It was ship-fever which ravaged the Marquis d'Antin's squadron in 1741, the Count de Roquesevel's in 1744, and the Toulon squadron in 1747. He takes the following from Poissonnier's *Traité de Maladies des Gens de Mer:* The fleet commanded by M. Dubois de la Mothe sailed in 1757 from Rochefort for Louisburg, Canada, having some men sickly. The ships touched at Brest, and sent 400 ashore sick. They sailed from Brest on 3 May, and arrived at Louisburg on 28 June. There was then sickness in only two ships, but in a short time it appeared in all the fleet. On 14 October the fleet sailed from Louisburg for home, embarking one thousand sick, and leaving four hundred supposed dying. In less than six days from sailing most of the thousand sick were dead. When the fleet arrived at Brest on 22 November there were few seamen well enough to navigate the ships ; 4000 men were ill, the holds and decks being crowded with the sick. The hospitals at Brest were already occupied, two ships from Quebec shortly before having sent a thousand men to them. Fifteen hospitals were soon filled, attended by five physicians and one hundred and fifty surgeons. Two hundred almoners and nurses fell victims. The infection passed to the lower class of the citizens, the havoc became general, and houses everywhere were filled with the dying and the dead. At length it got among the prisoners in the hulks. This dreadful infection began to abate in March, 1758, and ceased in April, having carried off in less than five months upwards of 10,000 people in the hospitals alone, besides a great number of the Brest townspeople. The stench was intolerable. No person could enter the hospitals without being immediately seized with headache ; and every kind of indisposition quickly turned to fatal fever, as in the old plague times. The state of the bodies showed the degree of malignity that had been engendered : the lungs were engorged with blood, and looked gangrenous ; the intestines often contained a green offensive liquor, and sometimes worms. Lind's other instances are chiefly of the Dutch East Indiamen that anchored at Spithead with fever on board. In Nov., 1770, the 'Yselmonde' bound to Batavia, came to anchor at Spithead, and buried a number of men every day ; two custom-house officers caught the fever and died. He gives two other instances of Dutch ships bound to

C. II.   8

Batavia, which came in to Portsmouth with fever[1]. The Dutch were said to send annually 2000 soldiers to Batavia, and to lose three-fourths of them by the ship-fever before they arrived. In 1769 Lind saw ship-fever in the Russian fleet at Spithead.

Brownrigg, of Whitehaven, gives a good instance of the diffusion of typhus in a newly-commissioned ship of war, and thence to the civil population, which bears out Lind's favourite notion that the gaols and the press-gang had far-reaching effects. In the year 1757 a sloop of war had been hastily manned at the Nore to protect the shipping between the Irish and Cumberland ports. She reached Whitehaven in May, with fever on board. The men were landed and lodged in small houses. Brownrigg found about forty lying on the floor of three small rooms, very close together, many of them in a dying state; seven days after he was himself seized with fever, and had a narrow escape with life. The ship's surgeon died of it, his mate recovered with difficulty, two surgeons of the town died of it, and two more in Cockermouth. The contagion spread widely among the inhabitants of Whitehaven, Cockermouth and Workington[2].

Lind showed to Howard in one of the wards of Haslar Hospital a number of sailors ill of the gaol fever; it had been brought on board their ship by a man who had been discharged from a prison in London, and it spread so much that the ship had to be laid up[3].

With the outbreak of the American War we begin to hear of still more disastrous epidemics of fever in the English fleets. Some instances from Robertson's full collection must suffice[4]. The 'Nonsuch' left England in March, 1777, and fifty of her men were carried off by fever before December; in that month, the 'Nonsuch,' 'Raisonable' and 'Somerset' had each from 130

---

[1] The *Gentleman's Magazine* for December, 1772 (p. 589), records the following: "The bodies of two Dutchmen who were thrown overboard from a Dutch East Indiaman, where a malignant fever raged, were cast up near the Sally Port at Portsmouth; they were so offensive that it was with difficulty that anyone could be got to bury them."

[2] W. Brownrigg, M.D. *Considerations on preventing Pestilential Contagion.* London, 1771, p. 36.

[3] Lind writes in his book on the Health of Seamen, "The sources of infection to our armies and fleets are undoubtedly the jails: we can often trace the importers of it directly from them. It often proves fatal in impressing men on the hasty equipment of a fleet. The first English fleet sent last war to America lost by it alone two thousand men."

[4] R. Robertson, M.D. *Observations on Jail, Hospital or Ship Fever from the 4th April, 1776, to the 30th April, 1789, made in various parts of Europe and America and on the Intermediate Seas.* London, 1789. New edition.

to 150 men on the sick list, chiefly fever in the 'Somerset,' and scurvy in the other two. In April, 1778, the 'Venus,' with a crew of 240, was at Rhode Island very sickly; the surgeon told Robertson that they had lost about fifty men of fever, which still continued to rage on board: they became sickly from being crowded with prisoners and cruising with them on board in bad weather. The 'Somerset' had buried 90 men of the fever since she left England, 70 of them being of the best seamen. On arriving at Spithead in October, 1779, Robertson found much fever in the Channel Fleet which had lately come in, especially in the 'Canada,' 'Intrepid,' 'Shrewsbury,' London' and 'Namur,' three or four of which were put past service, so much were they disabled by sickness. At Gibraltar Hospital from 12 January to 31 March, 1780, there were admitted 570 men from twenty-seven ships, of whom 57 died; of 110 sick from the 'Ajax,' 18 died; of 437 Spanish prisoners, 37 died. Next year, in May, 1781, at Gibraltar, the 'Bellona' had buried 27 men since she left England, and had 108 on the sick list. The 'Cumberland' had buried 15; of the 'Marlborough's' men, 40 had died at the hospital. Robertson had to purchase at his own expense vegetable acids, fruit and vegetables for the sick.

Some statistics remain of the loss of men in the navy by sickness in the Seven Years' War (1756–62) and in the American War[1]. The House of Commons had ordered a return of the number of seamen and marines raised and lost in the former; but the return was too general to be of much use, the number "lost" having included all those men who had been sent to hospital and never returned to their ships, all those who had been discharged as unserviceable, and all deserters. The number raised was 184,899, and the number "lost" 133,708, besides 1512 killed. The Return by the Navy Board for the period of the American War was more specific, showing only the number of the dead and killed.

Seamen and Marines raised, dead or killed, during the American War, 29 Sept., 1774, to 29 Sept., 1780 :

Year	Raised	Dead	Killed
1774	345	—	—
1775	4,735	—	—
1776	21,565	1679	105
1777	37,457	3247	40
1778	31,847	4801	254
1779	41,831	4726	551
1780	28,210	4092	293
	175,990	18,545	1243

[1] Given by Blane in a Postscript to his paper "On the Comparative Health of the British Navy, 1779–1814" in *Select Dissertations*, London, 1822, p. 62.

Fully a tenth part of the men raised were lost by sickness. Fever was the chief sickness, and as it happened rarely that more than one in ten cases of fever died, it will be easy to form an approximate estimate of the proportion of all the men raised for the ships that were on the sick list at one time or another with fever—nearly the whole, one might guess.

During the three last years of the period Haslar Hospital was constantly full of typhus fever. Admiral Keppel's fleet arrived at Spithead on 26 October, 1778, and soon began to be infected with contagious fever; before the end of December, 3600 men had been sent to Haslar, which could make up at a pinch 1800 beds. But the great epidemic at Portsmouth was the next year, 1779, when the very large Channel Fleet under Sir Charles Hardy came in. During the month of September, 2500 men were received into hospital, and more than 1000 ill of fevers remained on board for want of room in the hospitals. In the last four months of 1779, 6064 sick were sent to Haslar, which had 2443 patients on 1 January, 1780. There was an additional hospital at Foston, holding 200, as well as two hospital ships holding 600. The infection was virulent during the winter, when Portsmouth was crowded with ships; and in the first five months of 1780, when 3751 cases of fever were admitted during the decline of the epidemic, one in eight died. The following shows how much fever preponderated at Haslar Hospital in 1780. In 8143 admissions on the medical side, the chief forms of sickness were as follows[1]:

Continued Fevers	5539
Scurvy	1457
Rheumatism	327
Flux	240
Consumption	218
Smallpox	42

Blane gives the instance of the 'Intrepid,' one of the Channel Fleet under Hardy in 1779: "Almost the whole of her crew either died at sea or were sent to the hospital upon arriving at Portsmouth. This ship, after refitting, was pretty healthy for a little time; but probably from the operation of the old adhering infection, she became extremely sickly immediately after joining our fleet and sent 200 men to the hospital after arriving in the West Indies. Most of these were ill of dysentery[2]." During a voyage of three weeks of the 'Alcide' and 'Torbay' from the Windward Islands to New York in September, 1780, nearly a half of the men were unfit. In the 'Alcide' it was a fever that raged, in the 'Torbay' it was a dysentery[3].

[1] Blane, u. s. p. 47, from information supplied by Dr John Lind, of Haslar Hospital.
[2] *Diseases incident to Seamen*, p. 18.   [3] *Ibid.* p. 34.

These experiences of fever in the ships of the Royal navy continued to the end of the 18th century. In Trotter's time, as in Lind's, receiving ships were a source of contagion to others, one ship of the kind, the 'Cambridge' having diffused fever among many ships of the Channel Fleet by men drafted from her[1].

Ship typhus was also an incident of the voyages of the East India Company's ships, which nearly always carried troops. In the voyage of the 'Talbot,' 22 March—25 August, 1768, with 240 persons on board, "towards the end of July a fever of a very bad kind made its appearance, attended with delirium, low pulse, petechiae or livid vibices and hæmorrhages from the nose, of which one died and three or four escaped hard." The sick were isolated, and the infection did not spread. Such outbreaks of typhus were not uncommon at sea, although the loss of life from them was small beside that from the fevers of Madagascar, Sumatra, Batavia and Bengal. The ship typhus usually began on board among the soldiers. The most notable point is that relapses were common, as Lind also observed at Haslar Hospital; some on board the 'Lascelles' in 1783 (150 attacks among 151 soldiers) had relapsed seven times. It does not appear, however, that the best class of merchantmen suffered greatly from fevers. Dr Clark, who compiled a report of the practice in fevers in the ships of the East India Company from 1770 to 1785, had reason to congratulate the Company on the general healthiness of their fleet:

"When ships set out at a proper season, when they are not too much crowded, when the weather is favourable, and no mismanagement appears, fewer lives are lost in these long voyages than in the most healthy country villages. And in perusing the medical journals I have the peculiar pleasure of finding that many ships have arrived in India without the loss of a single life by disease," e.g. the 'Valentine' in 1784, seven months out, with 300 souls, no deaths, and the 'Barrington' in 1789, no deaths outward bound[2].

[1] Trotter, *Medicina Nautica*, I. 61. His general abstracts of the health of the fleet in the first years of the French War, 1794–96, give many instances of ship-typhus.

[2] John Clark, M.D. *Observations on the Diseases which prevail in Long Voyages to Hot Countries, &c.* London, 1773. 2nd ed. 2 vols, 1792.

John Lorimer, M.D., published in *Med. Facts and Observations*, VI. 211, a "Return of the ships' companies and military on board the ships of the H. E. I. C. for the years 1792 and 1793."

	Outward voyages		Homeward voyages		In port
	Crew	Military	Crew	Invalids	
Number of men	2657	3919	2701	1075	—
Sick	1253	1751	1058	282	1533
Dead	28	50	51	27	96

On the other hand, these English reports give incidentally the most unfavourable accounts of the Dutch East Indian ships. Three Dutch ships, then in Praya Bay, St Jago (Cape de Verde Islands), had buried 70 to 80 men each, and had some hundreds of sick on board. Another report says: "Before we left Table Bay several Dutch ships arrived, some of which had buried 80 people in the voyage from Holland. None lost less than 40 men. I am informed that some of their ships last year buried 200 men"—the causes of the sickness being overcrowding, filth, and the slowness of the voyages. One experience of the very worst kind happened to an English expedition consisting of the 100th regiment, the 98th regiment, the second battalion of the 42nd, and four additional companies. They had formed part of the force for the reduction of the Cape of Good Hope, whence they re-embarked for Bombay. During the voyage from Saldanha Bay a contagious fever and scurvy broke out among the troops, who were crowded and badly clothed; dead men were thrown overboard by dozens, and the regiments were reduced to a third of their original numbers. Six officers of the 100th regiment died, and an equal if not greater proportion of those of the 98th and 42nd.

The other chief occasion of ship typhus was the emigration to the American and West Indian colonies from Britain and Ireland. The Irish emigration was especially active from the beginning of the 18th century, owing to rack-renting and other causes. Madden[1] professed to know that one-third of the Irish who went to the West Indies (perhaps he should have included Carolina) perished either on the voyage or by diseases caught in the first weeks after landing; and as we know that typhus attended the Irish emigration in the 19th century, we may infer that the same was the cause of mortality in the 18th.

The trouble from ship-fever in the navy was so great all through the 18th century that many ingenious shifts were tried to overcome it. Towards the end of the century, the favourite device was fumigation with the vapour of mineral acids; one such plan, for which the Admiralty paid a good sum, ended in the burning of several ships to the water's edge. An earlier plan was ventilation of the hold and 'tween decks by means of

---

[1] *Reflections and Resolutions for the Gentlemen of Ireland*, p. 28. Cited by Lecky.

Sutton's pipes[1], which found a strong advocate in the Rev. Stephen Hales, of the Royal Society[2].

Twice in the course of a paper to that learned body[3] he asserts that the noxious, putrid, close, confined, pestilential air of ships' holds and 'tween decks "has destroyed millions of mankind"; on the other hand, according to the testimony of a captain of the navy, Sutton's pipes had kept his ship free from fever. Lind caps this with the case of H.M.S. 'Sheerness,' bound to the East Indies. She was fitted with Sutton's pipes, the dietary being at the same time so arranged that the men had salt meat only once a week. After a very long passage of five months and some days she arrived at the Cape of Good Hope without having had one man sick. "As the use of Sutton's pipes had been then newly introduced into the king's ships, the captain was willing to ascribe part of such an uncommon healthfulness in so long a run to their beneficial effects; but it was soon discovered that, by the neglect of the carpenter, the cock of the pipes had been all this while kept shut[4]."

Ship-fever was at length got rid of by more homely and more radical means than scientific ingenuity. Lind had shown one root of the evil to lie in the pressing of men just out of gaol. Admiral Boscawen, by his unaided wits, discovered another means of checking it. He avoided the mixing of fresh hands with crews seasoned to their ships, unless when some evident utility or necessity of service made it proper; "and upon this principle he used to resist the solicitation of captains, when they requested to carry men from one ship to another when changing their command[5]." Towards the end of the 18th century many reforms were made in the naval service—in the dietary, in the allowance of soap, in keeping the bilges clean, in the use of iron and lead instead of timber; so that Blane dates from the year 1796 a new era in the health of the navy[6].

[1] Sutton, "Changing Air in Ships," *Phil. Trans.* XLII. 42; W. Watson, M.D. *ibid.* p. 62; H. Ellis, *ibid.* XLVII. 211.
[2] *Ibid.* XLIX. 332, "Ventilation of a Transport."
[3] *Ibid.* pp. 333, 339.
[4] Lind, *Essay on the Most Effectual Means of Preserving the Health of Seamen in the Royal Navy.* New Ed. London, 1774, p. 29.
[5] Blane, *Diseases incident to Seamen*, 1785, p. 243.
[6] *Id.* "On the Comparative Health of the British Navy from the year 1799 to the year 1814, with Proposals for its farther Improvement." *Select Dissertations*, 1822, p. 1.

The " Putrid Constitution " of Fevers in the middle third of the 18th Century.

Resuming the history of fevers among the people at large from the great typhus epidemic of 1741–42 to the end of the century, we find the conditions somewhat different in the earlier and later divisions of the period. The time of prosperity, when England exported large quantities of wheat in every year except two or three, is reckoned from 1715 to 1765; after the latter date England gradually ceased to be an exporting country, owing to various causes, including the increase of pasture farming and the growth of industrial populations in the northern counties. The year 1765 marks the beginning of what has been called the Industrial Revolution; and it is also an important point of time in the history of the fevers of the country, for it is in the generation after that we obtain all the best information on what may be called industrial typhus, in the writings of a group of physicians who were at once philanthropic and exact. But there was an earlier period of fever, which is somewhat difficult to the historian. It is perhaps the last period in which Sydenham's language of " epidemic constitutions " seems to be appropriate, whether it be that the writers of the time were still under his influence, or because the prevalent maladies could not well be accounted for in any other way. The constitution in question was a "putrid" one. It coincided with the great outburst of putrid or gangrenous sore-throat, to be described elsewhere; and it included an extensive prevalence of fevers which were also called putrid or nervous, and sometimes called miliary. Fevers of the same kind, and with the same miliary rash, are described by earlier writers, such as Huxham. Perhaps the most correct view of the matter is to consider this type of fever as corresponding roughly to the middle third of the century, and as having been interrupted by the typhus epidemic of 1741–42, during a time of special distress. Besides the great outburst of putrid or malignant sore-throat, there was also a disastrous murrain of cattle for several years; and at Rouen there was a remarkable fever which some English writers of the time took to be the highest manifestation of the same " putrid " constitution that they discovered also in the English and Irish fevers.

The fever at Rouen which Le Cat specially described to the Royal Society was an outbreak from the end of November, 1753, to February, 1754. This outbreak was only one of a series; but as it attacked a great number of persons of distinction and made great havock among them, it attracted unusual notice and was regarded as something new, the rumour spreading over Europe that Rouen had been visited by plague. The same fever, however, had occurred there in previous years; and allied forms of sickness, of the same gangrenous character, including gangrenous sore-throat, could be traced back for twenty or thirty years. It will suffice to mention of these the malignant fever which appeared in 1748 and continued in 1749, 1750 and 1751. There was a fixed pain in the head, pain about the heart, a low fever with delirium, often miliary eruptions, continual faint sweating, drowsiness, scanty or suppressed urine, abdominal distension. After death the stomach was found "inflamed" at places, as well as the small intestine. In some cases there were ulcerations which almost penetrated the coats. The lungs were engorged with blood. In one case, of a young woman aged twenty, the mesentery was filled with obstructed glands and the intestines mortified in different places. In another, almost the whole mesentery was mortified and there was an anthrax or carbuncle at the upper fore part of the armpit. At the same time some cases of smallpox, with miliary eruption, also had ulcerations of the stomach, with inflammatory spots on other parts of it and of the intestine, the mesenteric glands being enlarged and hard. Some of the cases at the Hôtel Dieu in 1750 were traced to infection from bales of horse-hair; but the type of the disease in those cases did not differ essentially from that of other cases. Some rapidly fatal cases in the winter of 1752–53 had suppurative inflammation about the heart. (In 1739 there had been deaths from continued fever at the Hôtel Dieu, after an illness of six or seven days, marked by frequent faintings, small abscesses being found after death in the substance of the heart near the auricles.) The fever among the upper classes in the winter of 1753–54 was marked, in its most mortal form, by lowness, continued fever, pain in the head, cough, sore-throat, nausea, dry black tongue, delirium, sweats, stupor, some oppression of the heart, spitting of blood, sometimes swelling of the belly, these symptoms being followed often by miliary eruption, and sometimes by a slight flux with blood. Many were affected with a dejection of spirits, and with a feeling of terror which made them tremble at the ordinary sound of the voice. The fever ran a full course of thirty or forty days (the miliary eruption coming about the 21st day), while death usually ensued about the 25th. The appearances after death were remarkable (many bodies were opened): "In some a part of the villous coat of the stomach and of the small guts was inflamed; and the rest of these organs were filled with an eruption of the miliary crystalline kind, except that it was larger; and there was likewise an obstruction in the glands of the mesentery. In others a strong inflammation had seized the whole stomach and a small portion of the oesophagus, but the intestines were free...In those cases where the delirium had continued long and violent, we found either ulceration on the stomach, or its villous coat separated, together with a great inflammation, and even some gangrenous spots, on the other coats of that organ." Some recovered by critical abscesses. Others who escaped death by the poison carried its terrible effects for many months; their limbs and joints were feeble, and they were troubled with vertigo, lassitude and fears[1].

Exactly covering the period of these fevers at Rouen, there were low putrid fevers in London, in Worcestershire, in Ireland, and among the English colonists in Barbados. It was certainly

[1] Le Cat, *Phil. Trans.* XLIX. 49.

not a mere fashion in medicine which produced the accounts of a similar fever, for these accounts came from places far apart and were independent of each other. Dr Fothergill, of Lombard Street, published in the *Gentleman's Magazine* every month for five years a short account of the weather and prevalent diseases of London, beginning with April, 1751, and ending with December, 1755. He had the weekly bills of mortality before him, and he makes various comments upon them; but his accounts of prevalent diseases are from his own observation and by way of illustrating the bills. His first reference to a fever is under October, 1751: "A slow continual fever, with acute pain in the forehead: not many attacked, few mortally." The year 1752 was remarkably free from fevers until November, when we read of a fatal fever which had rheumatic symptoms at first (as at Rouen in 1744), attacking the head later, with coma-vigil and a dark-coloured ichor on the tongue and lips. It continued into January and February, 1753, proving fatal to several. In the summer and autumn months there were fevers of the low, depressed kind, sometimes called "remittents," with copious sweats, or "slow, remitting, dangerous fever," or "slow, treacherous, remittent fever, too often fatal." The references to it are most numerous in the months from November, 1753, corresponding to Le Cat's Rouen narrative. It was slow and imperceptible in its approach, the sick often going about ill for a week before seeking advice; it was attended with profuse sweats which never relieved, and was fatal to many. It continued more or less through the summer, and from August, 1754, it is again prominent. In September, it was the most alarming form of disease, and was then commonly vehement in its access, with lassitude, and pain in the head and back; unrelieving sweats are again mentioned, with dry tongue, delirium, coma-vigil, and death about the 14th–15th day. Fothergill was at a loss to know whether he should order blood to be drawn, owing to the low depressed nature of the fever. In February, 1755, the fever is still "too much of the nature of those which prevailed in the preceding months to allow a repetition of bleeding." In April it is called the petechial and miliary fever, the miliary eruption being of a white sort with a very noisome scent; the petechial spots turned livid, black and gangrenous; few patients escaped who had been sweated at the beginning. The fever was truly malignant, the patient restless from the outset, the sweats

weakening. Fothergill's last entries of it are important, under the months of May and June, 1755. In May, 1755, the fevers were "for the most part allied to that dangerous remittent which has for some years past more or less prevailed in different places of this kingdom." In June: "It does not appear that either in the hospitals or any part of the city a disease has broken out of so dangerous a nature as has been reported. The same kind of fever that has long continued in this city with some small variations in its type, still remains, but it is by no means more frequent than it has been in the preceding months, nor is it attended with more unfavourable symptoms."

It is impossible to say how general over England this fever may have been in the years 1751–57. Our fullest accounts come from Worcestershire; but the putrid fever is heard of more widely. Thus a short Latin piece in the *Gentleman's Magazine*, dated 14 April, 1755, is on the putrid fever lately epidemic, and not yet extinct, in some parts of the county of Somerset and adjoining places; its signs were contagiousness, pains of the head and loins, nausea and vomiting, diarrhoea, quick weak pulse, purple spots, delirium and coma[1]. Grainger, writing from Edinburgh in 1753, declares his motive for publishing an account of the anomalous fever of the Netherlands in 1746–48 to be that the same had lately been raging over almost the whole of Britain.

We have some particulars for Kidderminster, which can hardly have been exceptional for an industrial town, and according to the accounts were true also for villages and market towns near. Kidderminster was, in the year 1756, a town of about four thousand inhabitants, mostly hand-loom weavers of worsted and silk. There were no power-looms anywhere in England at that time; and the condition of the Kidderminster weavers' houses was doubtless what that of the Tiverton community had been fifteen years before. Many of the weavers, we are told, are lodged in small nasty houses, for the most part crowded with looms and other utensils[2]. Many of these houses were built on a low flat of the river Stour, whence rose putrid

---

[1] "Its cause seemed to be something contagious mixed with the contents of the stomach and intestines, especially the bile and alvine faeces, which absorbed thence contaminates the whole body and affects especially the cerebral functions." *Gent. Magaz.*, Article signed "S," 1755, p. 151.

[2] James Johnstone, M.D., senior, *Malignant Epidemic Fever of 1756.* London, 1758.

vapours after floods. Its situation had served to render the town specially unhealthy before, as in the epidemic of 1727–29[1].

The first notice by Dr Johnstone is of a low miliary fever from Midsummer 1752 to the end of the year. This was a comparatively mild affair, although it carried off several. But after Christmas it was succeeded by a fever which would then have been classed as of the putrid kind. The first great season was in 1753, it ceased in the fine years 1754–55, but came back in 1756 and 1757. It began with languor, lowness, flutterings, faintness, vague pains in the limbs, a low quick pulse, giddiness and slight sickness. Some had a propensity to loose stools and to profuse hurtful sweats; some bled at the nose, others coughed and spit blood; some had pain in the throat, and crimson-red tongue, the sweat and breath of the sick had a strong, offensive, putrid smell. In some of the worst cases livid petechiae, large livid blotches, and dark brown spots occurred over the trunk and limbs. The successful treatment was by mineral acids, bark, port wine, and vesication. "This malignant fever was very often (though not constantly) complicated with, and in general bore great analogy to the malignant sore-throat which at this time prevailed in many parts of England." The fever which prevailed during that remarkable year (1753) was very evidently contagious, for whole families were either all together or one after another seized with it. One of the most distinctive symptoms was a tendency to trembling of the whole body, as well as leaping of the tendons at the wrists. In some the tonsils were beset with aphthous sloughs, and towards the decline there would be aphthae of the mouth, but symptomatic only, and not the dominant lesion as in the ulcerous sore-throat. About the 15th day the fever was generally at its height. The miliary eruptions were critical to the few that had them; the flat livid petechiae appeared at all times of the disorder. Johnstone then compares the fever with that described by Le Cat at Rouen in the winter of the same year; and although he had been unable to satisfy his curiosity by opening any body dead of the fever, he felt sure that these dreadful symptoms arose from

[1] Nash, *Hist. of Worcestershire*, II. 39, found evidence in the Kidderminster registers that the fevers of 1727, 1728 and 1729 had "very much thinned the people, and terrified the inhabitants." Watson, "On the Medical Topography of Stourport," *Trans. Proc. Med. Assoc.*, II., had heard or read somewhere that fever was so bad in Kidderminster in the first part of the 18th century that farmers were afraid to come to market.

some affection of the stomach and small guts, at first erysipelatous, afterwards gangrenous, and at last truly sphacelous.

Johnstone's statement that the putrid fever in Worcestershire
in 1752–53 was often complicated with and bore great analogy
to the malignant sore-throat is borne out by Huxham's accounts
for Plymouth during the same season :

> "In all sorts of fevers," he writes, "there was a surprising disposition to
> eruptions of some kind or other [including miliary], to sweats, soreness
> of throat and aphthae." It is hardly possible to make out all his cases of
> "malignant anginose fever" to have been scarlet fever with sore-throat.
> Thus there occurred stench, swelling, and samious haemorrhages "commonly
> in those that died of malignant anginose fever above described. I have
> known the whole body swell vastly, even to the ends of the fingers and toes,
> with a cadaveric lividity, though almost quite cold, and an intolerable
> stench, even before the person was actually dead, blood issuing at the same
> time from the ears, nose, mouth and guts[1]."

The first years of this putrid or miliary fever were not
seasons of scarcity, there having been no failure of the crops since
1741 (unless in Ireland, in the province of Ulster mostly, in
1744); on the contrary, many of the seasons had been unusually
fine and abundant, the exports from England of wheat, barley,
malt and rye in the three years 1748, 1749 and 1750 amounting
to four million quarters. Prices were at the same time favourable
to the poorer classes[2]. But there had been a destructive murrain
for several years (30,000 cows are said to have died in Cheshire
in 1751), and the harvest of 1756 was a failure.

To the month of February, 1756, the season had been very
forward, but the early promise of spring was blighted by cold,
a wet summer and autumn ensued, the fruit crop was ruined,
and the corn harvest spoiled by long, heavy rains. A dearth,
bread-riots, &c. ensued[3]; but it is to be noted that the revival of
the dangerous malignant contagious fever began at Kidderminster
as early as April, becoming much worse after harvest. "Many
for weeks or months laboured under an uncommon depression
of spirits, felt their strength abate, with great lassitude, and very
often a great proneness to faint away." As the summer advanced
the fever became truly epidemic not only in Kidderminster but
in many other parts of the West and North-west of England.

---

[1] Huxham, *Dissertation on the Malignant Ulcerous Sore-Throat.* Lond. 1757,
p. 60.

[2] Tooke, *History of Prices.* Introduction.

[3] In Shrewsbury gaol, in 1756, thirty-seven colliers were confined for rioting
during the dearth. Four of them died in gaol, ten were condemned to death, of
whom two were executed. Phillips, *History of Shrewsbury*, 1779, p. 213.

It went through whole families, who succumbed either all together or one member after the other, and was carried from place to place by the attendants on the sick. "It prevailed chiefly in poor families, where numbers were lodged in mean houses, not always clean, but sordid and damp. It seemed to affect such poor families most where there was reason to think a sufficiency of the necessaries of life, on account of the dearth, had for some time been scantily supplied; yet the other poor persons, given to the intemperate use of malt liquors and ardent spirits, were observed to be very much liable to its influence. And not a few persons in easy circumstances of life were affected with this fever like others."

Frost in October checked it, and then measles of a malignant type had its turn among the children, the whooping-cough succeeding the measles. From November to Christmas the putrid fever, which chiefly affected persons from ten to fifty, and more women than men, returned with increased force. In fatal cases, the face was ghastly, sunken and livid (the facies Hippocratica), the patient sweated profusely, but seldom became cold till death was at hand. There was an abominable cadaverous stench in the breath, perspiration and stools. In these cases death took place from the 12th to the 14th day.

The intense and long frost of the opening months of 1757 nearly put a stop to the fever at Kidderminster.

"But in other neighbouring villages and market towns it has since the spring hitherto (Dec. 1757) been very frequent in places that were little affected with it last year. The families of the poorer sort of people universally are the most subject to it. And it is observable that the fever in some places first broke out in the parish workhouses, and from thence spread among the neighbouring people with great malignity. Wherever it has appeared it has given very apparent and fatal evidence of its infectious nature[1]."

Parliament was summoned to meet in December, 1756, on account of the dearth, which formed the topic of the Speech from the throne. The export of corn (which had reached a million quarters a year not long before) was prohibited, and the use of grain in distilling stopped for two months. The distress was more acute in 1757, and was enhanced by the greed of corn-dealers and millers, who used French bolting-mills to grind the mere husks of wheat, pease, rye and barley together into meal. Short, who practised at Sheffield, says that the fever in October and November, 1757, "was neither so rife nor fatal as in 1741[2]." It raged fiercely in several towns at a

---

[1] Johnstone, u. s. Short says: "a slow, malignant, putrid fever in some parts of Yorkshire, Cheshire, Worcestershire and the low parts of Leicestershire, which carried off very many." In October, 1757, it set in at Sheffield and raged all the winter.

[2] Short, *Increase and Decrease of Mankind in England, etc.* London, 1767, p. 109.

distance, "where it went by the name of the miliary fever," and was mostly among the poor, half-starved in the dearth of 1756–57. It is heard of again in the district of Cleveland in the winter of 1759–60, where it seems to have been mostly a disease of children complicated with sore-throat, and allied more to scarlet fever than to the putrid fever of adults[1]. But at Sunderland, near at hand, there was spotted fever at the same time, and in Newcastle there was dysentery.

The accounts of fever in Ireland in the same period as in England (see chapter II.) are not without value, as showing that the "putrid" or nervous type of fever, contrasting with the ordinary typhus of the country, had been remarked there also. Rutty and Sims describe, during a certain period, the symptoms of the low, putrid fever, sometimes with miliary eruptions, identifying it both by name and in character with the fever then prevalent in England. The most significant thing in Rutty's annals is that there occurred in the midst of the low, putrid fever with miliary pustules in 1746, a more acute fever, ending after five or seven days in a critical sweat, and relapsing. The same fever, not very fatal, reappeared in 1748. Sims brings the history of the nervous or putrid or miliary fever in Ireland (Tyrone) continuously down to the year 1772, as elsewhere related. The remarkable phenomenon of tremors or shakings, which most witness to, was seen by him in perfection in the year 1771:

> The tremulousness of the wrists, he says, extended to all the body, "insomuch that I have seen the bed-curtains dancing for three or four days, to the no small terror of the superstitious attendants, who, on first perceiving it, thought some evil spirit shook the bed. This agitation was so constant a concomitant of the fever as to be almost a distinguishing symptom." These were not the shakings of an ague, for there might be no intermission for days[2].

Perhaps the most surprising testimony to the existence of an "epidemic constitution" of slow, continued nervous fever comes from the island of Barbados. Hillary, who had kept a record of the prevalent diseases at Ripon, continued the same when he settled in Barbados in 1751[3]. There can be no doubt as to

[1] Charles Bisset, *Essay on the Medical Constitution of Great Britain*, 1 Jan. 1758, to Midsummer, 1760. Together with a narrative of the Throat-Distemper and the Miliary Fever which were epidemical in the Duchy of Cleveland in 1760. London, 1762, pp. 265, 270, &c.
[2] James Sims, M.D., *Obs. on Epid. Disorders.* Lond. 1773, p. 181.
[3] W. Hillary, M.D., *Changes of the Air and Concomitant Epid. Disorders in Barbadoes.* 2nd ed., Lond. 1766.

the appearance of this fever in February 1753, its prevalence all over the island for eighteen months, and its disappearance in September 1754, when, as he writes, "It now totally disappeared and left the island, and, I think, has not been seen in it since" (1758). He gives the same account of it as the observers in England and Ireland, except that he does not describe miliary eruptions and describes jaundice in convalescent children. It was insidious in its onset (as in London), the patient often keeping afoot five or six days; the symptoms included pains in the head, vertigo, torpor, lassitude, vigil, delirium, faintings, partial sweats, involuntary evacuations, gulpings, tremors, twitchings, catchings, coma and convulsions. Recovery was marked by copious equable sweats and plentiful spitting. "This slow, nervous fever was certainly infectious, for I observed that many of those who visited, and most of them that attended the sick in their fever were infected by it, and got the disease, and especially those who constantly attended them and performed the necessary offices of the sick." It was last heard of in the remoter parts of the island.

Miliary Fever.

It will have been observed in the foregoing accounts of the predominant fevers of the years (roughly) from 1750 to 1760 that there was often a miliary eruption, but that it was far from constant. The constant things were the lowness, depression, ill-smelling sweats, tremors of the whole body or of the wrist-tendons, and other nervous or ataxic symptoms. But we hear more of a miliary eruption in connexion with that than with any other period of fevers in the history; and this was the time when a controversy arose as to whether there was in reality a distinctive kind of fever marked by miliary eruption. Some of the school of Boerhaave contended that the phenomenon of miliary vesicles was due solely to the heating and sweating treatment of the alexipharmac physicians. De Haën and others answered that miliary fever was a natural form, independent of the mode of treatment. The Boerhaavian contention may be admitted as good for such miliary fevers as were described under that name in 1710 by Sir David Hamilton[1]; nearly the

---

[1] *Tractatus duplex de Praxeos Regulis et de Febre Miliari*, Lond. 1710. Engl. transl. of the latter, Lond. 1737.

whole of his sixteen cases appear to have been made miliary by treatment, in so far as they became miliary at all. What this physician did was to foretell the approach of miliary symptoms in various maladies (about one-half of the cases being of lying-in women, and the rest various), and then to prescribe Gascoign's powder, Goa stone, Gutteta powder, Venice treacle or other diaphoretics, along with diluents and the application of blisters; the miliaria appeared about the breast, neck, and clefts of the fingers in due course (tenth to fourteenth day).

So far as his clinical cases are concerned, the late appearance of miliary vesicles, lasting a few days, is sufficiently explained by the powerful drenches administered; and it can hardly be doubted that much of what was called miliary fever was of that factitious kind. But even in Hamilton's essay we find indications of a real miliary type of fever; thus he mentions a class of cases which look to be the same as those described by Johnstone, Rutty, Sims and others forty years after—cases with wakefulness, depression, tremblings of the tongue and hands, convulsive movements and delirium. He mentions also a complication of this with sore-throat in 1704, which destroyed many.

As to the association of miliary eruption with the low putrid fever so characteristic of the sixth decade of the 18th century, it is asserted by too many and in too various circumstances for any doubt as to its reality. There is nothing to show that the alexipharmac treatment was the one always used; and it is not certain that some in Ireland and elsewhere who had miliary eruption received any medical treatment at all. Again, miliary vesicles, not always with perspiration, were commonly found in the relapsing fever of Irish emigrants in London during the great famine of Ireland in 1846–47, by which time the powerful drenches of the alexipharmac treatment had been long disused[1]. The controversy as to the reality of miliary fever was one of the kind usual in medicine: certain physicians, of whom Hamilton in 1710 was an obvious instance, took up an untenable position; they were answered according to the weakness of their argument; and that has been held in later times to be an answer to all who alleged the existence of a type of fever marked by miliary eruptions. There can be no question as to a low, "putrid" kind of fever in which miliary eruptions were usual;

[1] Ormerod, *Clin. Obs. on Continued Fever.* London, 1848.

C. II.

9

but offensive sweats were perhaps more usual, whence the name of putrid in a literal sense, different from the theoretical sense of Willis; more constant also were the starting of tendons, the tremors and shakings, together with very varied hysteric symptoms, from which the fevers received the name of nervous. Dr John Fordyce in his 'History of a Miliary Fever' (1758) really describes under that name the symptoms of the low, nervous, putrid fever, often attended with miliary vesicles, which had been the common type in England in the years immediately preceding, and was a common type for some time after, although less is heard of the miliary eruptions in the later history[1].

About the last quarter of the 18th century medical writers were inclined to drop the names of nervous and putrid as distinctive of certain fevers. Pringle, in his edition of 1775, says he had been careful to avoid the terms nervous, bilious, putrid and malignant, which conveyed either no clear idea or a false one. Armstrong, another army physician, writing in 1773, says: "Nervous, putrid, bilious, petechial or miliary, they are all of the malignant family; and in this great town [London] these are almost the only fevers that have for many years prevailed, and do so still, to the great destruction of mankind. For inflammatory fevers...have for many years been remarkably rare[2]." Dr John Moore becomes sarcastic over the variety of names given to continued fever, some such generic name as Cullen's "typhus," then newly introduced, being what he desired[3].

Haygarth, writing of the Chester fevers in 1772, said that the miliary fever had been "supposed" endemic there for more than thirty years past, but he thought it probable that the eruption had generally, or always, been fabricated "by close, warm rooms, too many bed-cloaths, hot medicines and diet." He had seen only one case in the epidemic that year, and he believed its rarity at that time was due to the treatment by fresh air and by

[1] *Historia Febris Miliaris, et de Hemicrania Dissertatio.* Auctore Joanne Fordyce, M.D., Londini, 1758. Symptoms at p. 16. In an Appendix Dr Balguy makes the following curious division of the miliary vesicles: the white in malignant continued fever, the dull red in remittent fever, the "almost efflorescent" in intermittent. Fordyce makes them to appear as early as the third day, and to begin to disappear in four or six days in favourable cases.

[2] London, 1773, p. 9. See also Sir W. Fordyce's essay of the same year.

[3] John Moore, M.D., *Medical Sketches*, Lond. 1786. Part II. "On Fevers." Referring to the "putrid" fever in particular, he says that certain unbelievers, of whom he was probably one, "assert that mankind are tenacious of opinions, when once adopted, in proportion as they are extraordinary, disagreeable and incredible." Dr Moore is best known as the author of *Zeluco*.

"such regimen and medicines as are cooling and check putre-faction[1]." We shall see later that Percival, for Manchester, contents himself with saying that miliary fevers, which were formerly very frequent in that town and neighbourhood, now [1772] rarely occur[2]. In Scotland as late as 1782 the type was still nervous or low, and hardly ever inflammatory[3].

Mortalities in London from fever and all causes.

Year	Fever deaths	All deaths	Year	Fever deaths	All deaths
1741	7528	32169	1756	3579	20872
1742	5108	27483	1757	2564	21313
1743	3837	25700	1758	2471	17576
1744	2670	20606	1759	2314	19604
1745	2690	21296	1760	2136	19830
1746	4167	28157	1761	2475	21063
1747	4779	25494	1762	3742	26326
1748	3981	23069	1763	3414	26148
1749	4458	25516	1764	3942	23202
1750	4294	23727	1765	3921	23230
1751	3219	21028	1766	3738	23911
1752	2070	20485	1767	3765	22612
1753	2292	19276	1768	3596	23639
1754	2964	22696	1769	3430	21847
1755	3042	21917	1770	3214	22434

It is singular to observe that in the five successive years in this period with lowest fever-deaths and deaths from all causes, the years 1757–61 England was at war on the Continent. A similar low fever-mortality corresponded with the wars under Marlborough and Wellington.

The era of agricultural prosperity in England, which had its only considerable interruptions in the years 1727–29 and 1740–42, may be said to have met with a more serious check from the bad harvest of 1756. There was a recurrence of agrarian troubles in 1764–67, partly through actual scarcity caused by the extreme drought of 1764, partly through the pulling down of cottages and the discouragement of country villages, which Goldsmith has pathetically described in his poem of the time. Short says that the country in 1765 was in general very healthy but for children's diseases. "In some parts the putrid fever roamed about from place to place in the highest degree of putrefaction, so as several dead bodies were obliged to be buried the same day as they died." The price of provisions was excessive, meal riots broke out, and the export of corn was

[1] Haygarth, *Phil. Trans.* LXIV. 73. [2] Percival, *ibid.* LXIV. 59.
[3] Hutchinson, u. s.

stopped, Parliament having been summoned for the occasion in November, 1766[1]. In 1769, at the time of the formation of Chatham's ministry, the same train of incidents recurred,—bread-riots, flour-mills wrecked, corn and bread seized by the populace and sold at low prices, collisions with the military, the gaols full of prisoners[2]. The long period of cheapness, having lasted half a century, was coming to an end. Moralists and economists had much to say as to the meaning of the national distress which began to be felt in the sixties. Want of industry, want of frugality, want of sobriety, want of principle, said one, had brought trouble on the working class. "The tumults that have lately arisen in many counties of England are no other than the murmurs of the people, which have been heard for some years, bursting forth at last into riot and confusion." The English, it seems, had returned to their old medieval taste for the best food they could get; they would not give up the finest bread, although the Irish lived on potatoes, and the French on turnips and cabbage: "The ploughman, the shepherd, the hedger and ditcher, all eat as white bread as is commonly made in London, which occasions a greater consumption of wheat." Women must have tea and snuff, though children go naked and starved. Another writes: "The poorest people will have the finest or none." The enclosures had made a want of tillage. "What must become of our poor, destitute of work for want of tillage?" The country had for the most part been sickly, labourers scarce, and the farmers not able to get their usual quantity threshed out. The profligacy of the poor, profane swearing, etc., are remarked upon[3].

In the last thirty years of the 18th century the accounts of

---

[1] *Annual Register*, 1766, p. 220. The King's Speech on 11 Nov. was chiefly occupied with the dearth. The use of wheat for distilling was prohibited by an order of Council of 16 Sept. 1766. *Gent. Magaz.* p. 399. To show the hardships of the rural population at this time, Mr Gladstone, in a speech at Hawarden in 1891, read the following words copied from a stone set up in the park of Hawarden to commemorate the rebuilding of a mill: "Trust in God for bread, and to the king for protection and justice. This mill was built in the year 1767. Wheat was within this year at 9*s*., and barley at 5*s*. 6*d*. a bushel. Luxury was at a great height, and charity extensive, but the poor were starved, riotous, and hanged."

[2] Lecky, III. 115.

[3] *Gent. Magaz.*, series of letters by various hands in 1766. See also a long essay in the *Annual Register* for 1767 (then edited by Edmund Burke), "On the Causes and Consequences of the present High Price of Provisions," p. 165. The evidence of a rise in the standard of living, in the matter of dress and luxuries as well as of food, is equally clear from Scotland in the articles written by the parish ministers for the 'Statistical Account.'

fever in England became more detailed as to its circumstances, and more numerically precise. I shall accordingly bring together all that I can find relevant to fever in London, Liverpool, Newcastle and Chester, and thereafter in those towns, such as Manchester, Leeds, and others in the North, which were specially touched in their public health by the movement known as the Industrial Revolution.

Typhus Fever in London, 1770–1800.

In the London bills of mortality the item of fevers diminishes steadily during the latter part of the 18th century, the deaths from all causes diminish, the births come nearer to the number of the deaths, and in three years of the last decade they exceed them. This statistical result is doubtless roughly correct; but the bills were becoming more and more inadequate to the whole metropolitan area; and even for the original parishes which they included they have not the same value for fever in the later period as they had for plague at their beginning[1]. On the other hand, from about the year 1770 we begin to have more exact medical accounts of fever in London, which are not indeed numerically exhaustive, but good as samples of what was going on. Whatever improvement there was in the prevalence of typhus fever touched the richer classes. The Paving Act of 1766 is credited with having improved the health of the City, and there were many new streets and squares being built in the west end that were, of course, free from typhus. It is to these desirable residential quarters that the eulogies of Sir John Pringle[2], Dr John Moore[3] and others apply. The slums of London were as yet unimproved, and but little known to the physicians. Lettsom, who was one of the first of his class to visit among the poor in their homes, has much to say of typhus fever; but he is emphatic that it was nearly all an infection of the poor. "In the airy parts of this city," he writes in 1773, "and in large, open streets, fevers of a putrid tendency rarely

---

[1] For a judicious estimate of the value of the Parish Clerks' bills of mortality see the elaborate paper by Dr William Ogle, *Journ. Statist. Soc.* LV. (1892), 437.

[2] *Diseases of the Army.* New ed. 1775, pp. 334–5. Pringle admitted, however, that "in some of the lowest, moistest and closest parts of the town, and among the poorer people, spotted fevers and dysenteries are still to be seen, which are seldom heard of among those of better rank living in more airy situations."

[3] *Medical Sketches,* Lond. 1786, p. 464.

arise....In my practice I have attentively observed that at least forty-eight out of fifty of these fevers have existed in narrow courts and alleys." The same is remarked by Currie for Liverpool, by Clark for Newcastle, by Percival and Ferriar for Manchester, by Haygarth for Chester, and by Heysham for Carlisle.

The quarters of the rich had gradually become detached from those of the poor. I have shown this more especially for Chester, where the old walls made a clear division; but it was general in the second half of the 18th century[1].

Medical practice lay mostly among the richer classes; the physicians knew little of the state of health in the cellars and tenement-houses of large towns. Those physicians who did know how much typhus fever there was in these purlieus had to enter a caveat against the incredulity of the rest. Dr Currie of Liverpool, whose facts I shall give in their place, protested that he was not exaggerating; a protest the more necessary that a contemporary of his own, Mr Moss, a middle-class practitioner, who wrote a book specially on the medical aspects of Liverpool, declares that fever is "rare" in that city, while Currie was treating from his dispensary a steady average of three thousand cases of typhus every year. In the same years, in February, 1779, a physician to the army, Dr John Hunter, who had commenced practice in Mayfair, found on visiting in the homes of the poorer classes in the west of London cases of fever for which he had no other name than the gaol or hospital fever of his military experience; it was so much a novelty to him, apart from campaigns or transport ships, that he gave an account of his discovery of domestic typhus to the College of Physicians[2]. At length he found so many cases steadily winter after winter that he had them sent to the infirmary of the Marylebone Work-house. The practitioners who knew most of the sicknesses of the poor were such as Robert Levett, Dr Samuel Johnson's

---

[1] Lecky, *History of England in the Eighteenth Century*, II. 636, generalizes the facts as follows: "The wealthy employer ceased to live among his people; the quarters of the rich and of the poor became more distant, and every great city soon presented those sharp divisions of classes and districts in which the political observer discovers one of the most dangerous symptoms of revolution."

[2] "This disease, as it appears in jails and hospitals, has been well described by Sir John Pringle; and other authors have given accounts of it on board of ships, especially crowded transports and prison-ships, but I do not find that its originating in the families of the poor in great cities during the winter has been taken notice of." *Med. Trans. Coll. Phys.* III. 345.

dependant, who lived with the doctor in the house in Gough Square. Levett had been a waiter in a Paris coffee-house frequented by the medical fraternity, and had acquired a taste for and perhaps some knowledge of the healing art. He made his modest living by the small fees or articles of food and drink which his poor patients gave him. He had only to issue from the back of Gough Square by the courts and alleys behind Fleet Street, and he would find in the region between Chancery Lane and Shoe Lane hundreds of families seldom visited by a physician or by a qualified surgeon-apothecary. The good Levett was only one of a class. There had always been such humble medical attendants of the poor in London. An Act of the third year of Henry VIII. was directed against them at the instance of the privileged practitioners; but the regular faculty is said to have proved in the sequel both greedy and incompetent, and after thirty years there came another Act, couched in terms that the bluff king himself might have indited (31–32 Henry VIII.), which asserts those qualities of the profession in so many words, and establishes the right of any subject of the king to practise minor surgery and the medicine of simples upon his or her neighbours. That Act is still part of the law of England, and under it Levett exercised a statutory right, perhaps without knowing it[1]. There were many other regions of courts and alleys all round the City on both sides of the water, which must have been medically served by such as Levett, if served at all. It was there that typhus was found and at length clinically described by competent physicians, among the earliest of whom was Lettsom.

The General Dispensary in Aldersgate Street having been started in 1770 with one physician, Lettsom was chosen additional physician in 1773, and threw himself into the work with great zeal[2]. In the first twelvemonth he saw many cases of fever, as in the following table:

[1] He has been immortalised by Johnson's verses:

"Well tried through many a varying year
See Levett to the grave descend,
Officious, innocent, sincere,
Of every friendless name the friend.
In misery's darkest cavern known
His ready help was ever nigh;" etc.

[2] John Coakley Lettsom, M.D., *Medical Memoirs of the General Dispensary in London, April* 1773 *to March* 1774. London, 1774.

Lettsom's practice in Fevers at the Aldersgate Dispensary.

1773   1774

Febris	April	May	June	July	Aug.	Sept.	Oct.	Nov.	Dec.	Jan.	Feb.	March	Total in 12 months	Died
hectica	2	2	4	13	4	2	3	4	9	12	18	13	86	3
inflammatoria	—	—	—	—	—	—	1	1	1	—	2		5	—
intermittens	3	1	7	1	1	1	1	—	2	1	2	2	22	
nervosa	4	3	4	14	7	11	4	5	1	1	5	4	65	3
putrida	14	19	14	25	14	21	34	22	11	6	7	5	192	8
remittens	6	10	5	4	3	6	7	3	12	13	10	3	82	—
simplex vel diarium	—	2	1	6	2	5	4	5	—	—	—	4	29	—

The nervous, putrid and remittent fevers, belonging to the same group, make up the bulk of the fevers. The hectic fevers were almost all of children. The fatal cases of fever were fourteen, the fatal cases in all diseases for the year having been forty-four. What these putrid, nervous and remittent fevers were, will now appear from some of Lettsom's descriptions. Fevers with symptoms of putrescency were marked by nausea, bitter taste, and frequent vomiting, by laboured breathing and deep sighing, offensive breath, sweats offensive and sometimes tinged with blood, almost constant delirium, the tongue dry, the tongue, teeth and lips covered with black or brown tenacious foulness, thrush and ulceration in the mouth and throat, the urine with a dark sediment, the stools excessively nauseous and foetid, and blackish or bloody, the eyes horny or glassy, with the whites often tinged of a deep blood colour, spots on the skin like flea-bites, or larger haemorrhagic vibices, bleeding from the gums, nose or old ulcers, hiccup near death, often a cough through the fever. Lettsom's treatment consisted in good liquors, Peruvian bark, and above all fresh, or "cold" air: "When it is considered that putrid fevers originate in close unventilated places, the introduction of fresh air seems so natural a remedy that I have often admired its aid should have been so long neglected[1]." Accordingly he persuaded the poor people to open their windows, and dragged the sick out of doors as soon as it was safe to do so; the effects, he says, were wonderful. His fifty-one cases are most valuable illustrations of the perennial fever in the crowded parts of London:

[1] Nothing could be clearer than Dr John Arbuthnot's reasoning and advice on this matter half a century before.

Case 1 is of a man aged forty who had occasion to visit a miserable crowded workhouse in Spitalfields. He was instantly seized with such a nausea and debility as induced him to keep his room as soon as he got home. At the end of a week Lettsom found him in "the true jail-fever, or, what is the same, a true workhouse-fever." He had involuntary stools and leaping of the tendons, and took more wine in a week than he had done for many years.

Cases 2 to 12 were of several families in one house in a court in Long Lane, Aldersgate Street, who had been infected by a discharged prisoner from Newgate. Other cases follow, where the infection was caught from visiting the sick. In Case 17, Lettsom applied blisters "owing to the importunity of the friends," but without advantage. Case 30, on 26th October, 1773, was of a family of six persons near Christ Church, Lambeth, father, mother, boy of seventeen, child of two (slight attack) and two maids. Other localities were courts off Whitecross Street, Jewin Street, Little Moorfields, Chiswell Street, and St Martin's-le-Grand. Case 43 was of a woman, aged thirty, in Bunhill Row; she attended a relation who died of a putrid fever, and was herself attacked; her eyes were bloodshot, her skin marbled and interspersed with a general deep-coloured eruption, her cheeks and nose mortified. Cases 44–47 were of people in a "very helpless situation" in Gloucester Court, Whitecross Street.

The year 1773, to which these experiences in a small part of London relate, was one of high febrile mortality, according to the Bills. Two years after, Dr William Grant was moved to write an 'Essay on the Pestilential Fever of Sydenham, commonly called Gaol, Hospital, Ship and Camp Fever[1],' which, as he said in his preface, "I often see in this city: and though so common and fatal, appears not at present to be generally understood." It was, he says, "an indigenous plant, frequent in this city, being produced by close confinement; but it often passes unnoticed, because unknown." The deaths by "fever" in the London Bills were as follows until the end of the century:

Deaths from Fever and from all causes in London.

Year	Fever deaths	All deaths	Year	Fever deaths	All deaths
1771	2273	21780	1786	2981	20454
1772	3207	26053	1787	2887	19349
1773	3608	21656	1788	2769	19697
1774	2607	20884	1789	2380	20749
1775	2244	20514	1790	2185	18038
1776	1893	19048	1791	2013	18760
1777	2760	23334	1792	2236	20213
1778	2647	20399	1793	2426	21749
1779	2336	20420	1794	1935	19241
1780	2316	20517	1795	1947	21179
1781	2249	20719	1796	1547	19288
1782	2552	17918	1797	1526	17014
1783	2313	19029	1798	1754	18155
1784	1973	17828	1799	1784	18134
1785	2310	18919	1800	2712	23068

[1] London, 1775.

There were higher figures in the years immediately before 1771, the years to which the generalities of Fordyce and Armstrong relate. There is a decline in the fever-mortality towards the end of the century; but it is just from the years 1799–1800 that we have an account by Willan of the prevalence and conditions of London typhus, than which nothing can well be imagined worse. The intermediate glimpses we get of typhus in London in the writings of Dr Hunter, physician, and of Dr James Sims, show that the disease was perennial.

"In the month of February, 1779," says Hunter[1], "I met with two examples of fever in the lodgings of some poor people whom I visited that resembled in their symptoms the distemper which is called the jail or hospital fever. It appeared singular that this disease should show itself after three months of cold weather. Being therefore desirous of learning the circumstances upon which this depended I neglected no opportunity of attending to similar cases. I soon found a sufficient number of them for the purpose of further information. It appeared that the fever began in all in the same way and originated from the same causes. A poor family, consisting of the husband, the wife, and one or more children, were lodged in a small apartment not exceeding twelve or fourteen feet in length, and as much in breadth. The support of them depended on the industry and daily labour of the husband, who with difficulty could earn enough to purchase food necessary for their existence, without being able to provide sufficient clothing or fuel against the inclemencies of the season. In order therefore to defend themselves against the cold of the winter, their small apartment was closely shut up, and the air excluded by every possible means. They did not remain long in this situation before the air became so vitiated as to affect their health and produce a fever in some one of the miserable family. The fever was not violent at first, but generally crept on gradually...soon after the first a second was seized with the fever, and in a few days more the whole family perhaps were attacked, one after another, with the same distemper. I have oftener than once seen four of a family ill at one time and sometimes all lying on the same bed. The fever appeared sooner or later as the winter was more or less inclement, as the family was greater or smaller, as they were worse or better provided with clothes for their persons and beds, and with fuel, and as their apartment was more or less confined. The slow approach of the fever, the great loss of strength, the quickness of the pulse with little hardness or fulness, the tremors of the hands, and the petechiae or brown spots upon the skin, to which may be added the infectious nature of the distemper, left no doubt of its being the same with what is usually called the jail or hospital-fever."

Dr James Sims, who had seen much of Irish typhus in Tyrone in his earlier years, and had removed to London, wrote of typhus among the poor there in 1786, ten years before the more systematic and more circumstantial descriptions by Willan[1].

[1] *Med. Trans. of the Coll. Phys. Lond.* III. (1785), 345: "Observations on the Disease commonly called the Jail or Hospital Fever." By John Hunter, M.D., physician to the army.

[2] James Sims, M.D., "Scarlatina anginosa as it appeared in London in 1786," *Mem. Med. Soc. Lond.* I. 414. Willan, who saw the same epidemic of scarlatinal sore-throat in London in 1786, believed that the angina was also "connected with a

This fever was exceedingly mortal, several medical men, he had reason to believe, falling sacrifices to it. Sims never saw the cases till the 7th or 8th day, when they were desipient, insensible, with pulse scarcely to be felt and not to be counted, all having petechiae. None had scarlet rash or sore-throat. They sank and died quietly; the strongest cordials did not produce the smallest effect, and blisters in many did not even raise the skin[1].

It is in the year 1796 that we begin to have the full and accurate records by Willan of the prevailing diseases of London month by month as he saw them at the Carey Street Dispensary, situated in the crowded quarter between Holborn and the Strand[2]. His first reference to typhus is as follows :

"In September, also, fevers usually appear which from their commence-ment exhibit symptoms of malignancy; being attended with a brown dry tongue, violent pain of the head, delirium, or coma, deep-seated pains of the limbs, petechial spots and haemorrhagy. These fevers become highly contagious, especially when they occur in close, confined situations, and in houses where little attention is paid to ventilation or cleanliness. The disease is extended by infection during the months of October and November, but its progress is generally stopped by the frosts of December."

Willan says little more of fever in London until September, 1798, when these contagious malignant fevers became more numerous, both in the city and adjacent villages, than had been known for many years before; also the fever was more fatal than usual, one in five or six dying, whereas one in seven was formerly a very unfavourable death-rate, and one in twenty not unknown. Haemorrhages, aphthae, diarrhoea, starting of the tendons, picking the bedclothes, violent delirium, ending in deafness, stupor, hiccough and involuntary evacuations, were the usual accompaniments of this fever. In the corresponding months of 1799 he recurs to the symptoms of this "malignant contagious fever," and depicts typhus as clearly as may be. In September, 1799, it was "attended with a dull pain of the head, great debility or sense of lassitude and pains referred to the bones, tremblings,

different species of contagion, namely, that of the typhus or malignant fever originating in the habitations of the poor, where no attention is paid to cleanliness and ventilation." *Cutaneous Diseases*, 1808, p. 333.

[1] The rumour of London fevers seems to have reached Barker, who kept an epidemiological record at Coleshill. Referring to the winter of 1788-89, he says: "At this time there were dreadful fevers in London, fatal to many, and a very infectious one in Coventry, of which many among the poor died, most of them being delirious, and many phrenetical."

[2] Robert Willan, M.D., *Reports on the Diseases of London, particularly during the years* 1796-97-98-99 *and* 1800. London, 1801.

restlessness with slight delirium, a querulous tone of voice, a small and frequent pulse, heat of the skin, thirst and a fur upon the tongue, first of a dirty white colour, but turning in the latter stage of the disease to a yellowish brown. In this form the fever continued thirteen days without any dangerous symptoms, and then suddenly disappeared, leaving the patient, for some time after, languid and dispirited. All the individuals of a family were successively affected with the same train of symptoms; many of them so slightly as not to be much confined to their beds." In October and November he describes the symptoms of the disease in a more dangerous form. By this fever, he was informed, some houses of the poor had been almost depopulated, the infection having extended to every inmate. "The rumour of a plague was totally devoid of foundation."

He then describes the state of the dwellings where such fevers occurred—the unwashed bed-linen, the numbers in one bed, the rooms encumbered with furniture or utensils of trade, the want of light and air in the cellars and garrets and in the passages thereto, the excremental effluvia from the vault at the bottom of the staircase. It cannot be wondered at, he concludes, that contagious diseases should be thereby formed, and attain their highest degree of virulence; and he estimates that "hundreds, perhaps thousands" of labourers in and near London, heads of families and in the prime of life, perished annually from such fevers. He denies that his account is exaggerated, and appeals for the truth of it to medical practitioners whose "situation or humanity has led them to be acquainted with" the localities[1].

Typhus in Liverpool, Newcastle and Chester in the last quarter of the 18th century.

Liverpool, in the last quarter of the 18th century, came next in size to London, having a population (in 1790) of 56,000 to the capital's estimated 800,000. According to a medical author,

[1] He names specially some streets of St Giles's parish, the courts and alleys adjoining Liquorpond Street, Hog-Island, Turnmill Street, Saffron Hill, Old Street, Whitecross Street, Golden Lane, the two Bricklanes, Rosemary Lane, Petticoat Lane, Lower East Smithfield, some parts of Upper Westminster, and several streets of Southwark, Rotherhithe, etc. "I recollect a house in Wood's Close, Clerkenwell, wherein the fomites of fever were thus preserved for a series of years; at length an accidental fire cleared away the nuisance. A house, notorious for dirt and infection, near Clare-market, afforded a farther proof of negligence: it was obstinately tenanted till the wall and floors, giving way in the night, crushed to death the miserable inhabitants."

whose experiences lay among the middle classes, it was everything that could be wished in the way of healthfulness and
prosperity; but it had a dark side as well. About 7,000 of the
people lived in cellars underground, and nearly 9,000 in back
houses, in small confined courts with a narrow passage to the
street. "Among the inhabitants of the cellars," says Currie[1],
"and of these back houses, the typhus is constantly present; and
the number of persons under this disease that apply for medical
assistance to the charitable institutions, the public will be
astonished to hear, exceeds three thousand annually...In sixteen
years' practice I have found the contagious fever of Liverpool
remarkably uniform among the poor. Seldom extending itself
in any considerable degree among the other classes of the
community, it has been supposed that Liverpool was little
subject to fever; but this will be shewn from authentic documents to be a great and pernicious error." At the Dispensary
in the year 1780 the cases of typhus averaged 160 per month,
the numbers being as remarkably steady from month to month
as from year to year. In the ten years from 1 January, 1787, to
31 December, 1796, 31,243 cases of fever were entered on the
books of the Dispensary, an average of 3124 per annum[2].

Of 213,305 cases of all diseases at the Dispensary in seventeen years, 1780 to 1796, 48,367, nearly one-fourth, were labouring under typhus. Supposing that these were all the cases of
typhus in Liverpool, and that 1 in 15 died, we should have some
150 deaths from typhus in a year. Supposing also that typhus
was relatively as common at that time in London, it will follow
that nearly all the deaths under "fever" in the bills of mortality
might well have been from typhus fever; for London in its
several densely populated out-parishes was the fever-quarter of
Liverpool a dozen times over[3].

---

[1] *Medical Reports on the Effects of Water, Cold and Warm, as a Remedy in Fever and other Diseases.* 2nd ed., 1798. It need hardly be explained that Dr Currie was competent on fevers, his use of the clinical thermometer marking him as a man of precision. He is best known to the laity as the biographer of Robert Burns and the generous helper of the poet's widow and family.

[2] "If it be supposed," says Currie, "that some cases may be denominated typhus by mistake, let it be considered how many cases of this disease do not appear in the books of the Dispensary, though occurring among the poor, being attended by the surgeons and apothecaries of the Benefit Clubs to which they belong."

[3] Moss (*A Familiar Medical Survey of Liverpool,* 1784), who had not the same means of knowing the prevalence of typhus in Liverpool as Currie, declares that "there has been but one instance of a *truly* malignant fever happening in the town for many years; it was in the autumn of 1781. and appeared in Chorley Street, which is one of the narrowest and most populous streets in the town, and nine died of it in

The Newcastle Dispensary was opened in October, 1777, by the exertions of Dr John Clark, who was in correspondence with Lettsom in London[1]. Dr Clark had been in the East India Company's service, and had seen much of ship-fever and of the fevers of the East. During a visit to his home in Roxburghshire in the summer of 1770, between his voyages, he attended several persons in continued fever. When he settled at Newcastle he saw the worst kinds of contagious fever, in workhouses and "in the sordid and crowded habitations of the indigent." Putrid fever, or typhus, was by far the most common disease attended from the new dispensary, although less than at Liverpool, the operations of the charity being on a much smaller scale. It was seldom out of Newcastle a whole year; and in some years, as 1778, 1779, 1783, 1786 and 1787 it was unusually rife in particular districts, often attacking whole families. Scarlet fever was epidemic and very fatal in 1778 and 1779, while dysentery attacked great numbers of the poor in the autumns of 1783 and 1785. The following Table shows the principal diseases attended from the Dispensary during the first twenty-three months of its working, 1 Oct. 1777, to 1 Sept. 1779:

Newcastle Dispensary 1777–79.

	Cases visited	Cured	Too far advanced	Dead
Putrid fever	391	357	9	16
Ulcerated sore-throat	146	125	11	9
Dysentery	72	55	5	4
Smallpox	45	29	5	6

From 1 Oct. 1777, to 1 Sept. 1789, the cases of typhus visited were 1920, of which 121 were fatal. During the winter of 1790 and the spring and summer of 1791 it was prevalent amongst the poor, and was frequently introduced into genteel families and sometimes even into those of the first distinction. That outbreak was supposed to have been generated in the Gateshead poorhouse. For some time its ravages were confined chiefly to the low, ill-aired, narrow street called Pipewell Gate. In Sep-

one week; it was only of short duration, and did not spread in any other part of the town." He admits that the habitations of the poorer class were confined, being chiefly in cellars; yet the diet of the *sober* and *industrious* is wholesome and sufficient, the comfortable artizans being ship-carpenters; coopers, ropers and the like.

[1] John Clark, M.D., *Observations on the Diseases which prevail in Long Voyages,* &c. 2nd ed., Lond. 1792; *Account of the Newcastle Dispensary from its Commencement in 1777 to March 1789,* Newcastle, 1789; and subsequent Annual Reports.

tember it made its appearance in Newcastle; at first the
contagion was easily traced from Pipewell Gate, and afterwards
from one house to another.   In that outbreak, 188 poor persons
were visited from the Newcastle Dispensary, the Gateshead
poor having been attended by the parochial surgeon.   Clark's
ten cases recorded of the epidemic were all of people in good
circumstances.   The Dispensary Tables show cases of typhus
every year down to 1850, the largest totals being in 1793 (374,
18 deaths), 1801 (435, 20 deaths), and 1819 (368, 14 deaths); and
these, we may take it, were but a small fraction of all the cases
in Newcastle.

Perhaps the most unexpected revelation of typhus is at
Chester, from the time when Haygarth began to write upon its
public health in 1772.   Chester was then one of the most
desirable places of residence in England.   Boswell wrote to
Johnson, " Chester pleases me more than any town I ever saw."
The old city within the walls was occupied by a superior class
of residents, including the cathedral clergy, county families,
retired officers and Anglo-Indians, professional men, merchants
and tradesmen.   It had the best theatre out of London.
Squares, crescents and broad streets were replacing most of the
old buildings.   The six parishes that lay entirely within the
walls had a population, in 1774, of 3502, and an annual average
death-rate (in the ten years 1764 to 1773) of 1 in 58 or 17·2 per
1000, the central parish of St Peter having a rate of 1 in 62, and
the cathedral parish 1 in 87.   It passed as one of the healthiest
cities in the kingdom, being far before Shrewsbury and Nottingham, to say nothing of the large towns where the burials
exceeded the baptisms.   But its moderate death-rate over all,
1 in 42 living, would have been much lower but for the four
poor suburban parishes, with a population of 11,211, which had
a death-rate of 1 in 35.   Haygarth gives a deplorable account
of them.   The houses were small, close, crowded and dirty, ill
supplied with water, undrained, and built on ground that
received the sewage from within the walls.   The people were
ill-fed and they seldom changed or washed their clothes; when
they went abroad they were noisome and offensive to the smell.
Many of them worked on the large farms around Chester, others
at shipbuilding and shipping (Chester had then a considerable
foreign trade), others at the mills and markets, others at a
nail-factory, while others were employed by the tradesmen

within the walls. Fever seems to have been perennial among them, the deaths from typhus having been 23 in 1772, 33 in 1773 and 35 in 1774. "In these poor habitations," says Haygarth, "when one person is seized with a fever, others of the family are generally affected with the same fever in a greater or less degree." It became rifer than usual in August, 1773, and attacked 285, proving fatal to 28, or to one in ten. It had the common symptoms of malignant fevers produced by human effluvia, and particularly affected the head with pain, giddiness and delirium. It attacked in general the lowest, few of the middle rank, and none (or only one) of the highest rank [1].

Chester had no manufactures. Its population had grown rapidly of late, as that of Liverpool had grown, the poorer classes being the prolific part of the community; but it had no share in the industrial revolution, it did not employ its women and children in factories, and it was in some respects better than Leeds, Warrington, Manchester, or Carlisle. It is a good illustration of a town growing rapidly without manufactures, and of a community divided by the old walls into two quite distinct sections, a rich and a poor. Such had been the drift of things in England apart from the industrial revolution; but it is the latter which furnishes the best illustrations of a poor prolific populace, of a growing struggle, and of the attendant typhus fever.

Fever in the Northern Manufacturing Towns, 1770–1800.

The prosperity of the first two-thirds of the 18th century had been attended with a very small increase of population. From 1700 to 1750 the numbers in England are estimated to have grown no more than from about six millions to six millions and a half. The fecundity of many rural parishes was swallowed up by emigration to the American and West Indian colonies, by the army and navy, and by the great waste of life in London and some other towns. The increase was nearly all north of the Trent, while the old weaving towns of the south-west had actually declined. Gloucestershire, Somerset and Wilts were the most crowded counties in 1700. During the next fifty

[1] Haygarth, *Phil. Trans.* LXIV. 67; Hemingway, *History of Chester*, I. 344 *seq.*

years, the greatest increase was as in the following rough estimate[1]:

	1700	1750	Increase per cent.
Lancashire	166,200	297,400	78
West Riding of Yorks.	236,700	361,500	52
Warwickshire	96,600	140,000	45
Durham	95,500	135,000	41
Staffordshire	117,200	160,000	36
Gloucestershire	155,200	207,800	34

In the counties where population had increased most, much of the increase was still rural or semi-rural. Defoe describes how the land near Halifax was divided into lots of from two to six or seven acres, hardly a house out of speaking distance from another, at every house a tenter, and on almost every tenter a piece of cloth, or kersey or shalloon. Every clothier kept one horse at least, to carry his manufactures to the market, and nearly every one kept a cow, or two or more, for his family. The houses were full of lusty fellows, some at the dye-vat, some at the looms, others dressing the cloths, the women and children carding or spinning, being all employed from the youngest to the oldest: not a beggar to be seen, nor an idle person[2]. We have no accounts of the health of this population, except Nettleton's statistics of smallpox in and around Halifax in 1721 and 1722, given elsewhere, and the "epidemic constitutions" recorded by Wintringham at York during the same period, and by Hillary at Ripon.

Before the earliest of the inventions of spinning by machinery, the weavers were gathering to the towns of Yorkshire, Lancashire and other counties north of the Trent. The spinning-jenny of Hargreaves was wrecked by a Blackburn mob in 1768, and a mob wrecked the cotton-mill built by Arkwright at Chorley eleven years later. This was decidedly a time of movement from the country to the towns, a movement which preceded the spinning ingenuity of the sixties and may have been stimulated by the earlier use of the fly-shuttle in weaving.

[1] Arnold Toynbee, *Lectures on the Industrial Revolution of the 18th Century, etc.* London, 1884.

[2] Toynbee (u. s.) says of the time before the mills were built: "The manufacturing population still lived to a very great extent in the country. The artisan often had his small piece of land, which supplied him with wholesome food and healthy recreation. His wages and employments too were more regular. He was not subject to the uncertainties and knew nothing of the fearful sufferings which his descendants were to endure from commercial fluctuations, especially before the introduction of free trade."

Much of the country round Manchester, though it doubtless retained those farm-houses, hedgerows, and field paths which come into the idyllic opening of 'Mary Barton' more than half a century later, was "crowded with houses and inhabitants," as Percival says: so populous were the environs of Manchester that every house in the township had been found by a late survey to contain an average of six persons. The proportion of deaths was less than in 1757; but that was chiefly due to the accession of new settlers from the country, which raised the ratios of marriages and births[1]. Manchester had increased from a population of about 8000 in 1717 to one of 19,839 (inclusive of Salford) in 1757. When the inhabitants were next counted in 1773, they were found to be 22,481 in Manchester (5317 families in 3402 houses) and 4765 in Salford (1099 families in 866 houses). According to Percival, who gives these figures, the death-rate in 1773 was 1 in 28·4, the births exceeding the deaths by forty in a year. The poor, he says, were now better lodged, and some of the most dangerous malignant distempers were less violent and less mortal. Manchester, however, was still an unhealthy place compared with the country, especially to young children. Thus, the thirty-one townships in the parish of Manchester contained, exclusive of the city, 13,786 inhabitants (2525 families in 2371 houses), and of these only 1 in 56 died annually (compared with 1 in 28 in the city)—the births being to the deaths as 401 to 246 in the year 1772.

Again, the bleak upland parish of Darwen with a population in the year 1774 of 1850 souls mostly occupied in the cotton manufacture, had, during the seven years before, more than twice as many baptisms as burials (508 to 233), the birth-rate (1 in 25·5) being high and the death-rate (1 in 56) low.

Leeds had a population of some six or seven thousand at the time of the Civil Wars, and lost 1325 in nine months of the year 1645 from plague, all of them the poorer class. A generation or two later, in the time of Thoresby's 'Diary,' it was a centre of the cloth trade; and it appears to have grown steadily throughout the 18th century. In 1775 it had a population of 17,117. We hear from Lucas of an epidemic typhus in it previous to 1779[2]. Eighty persons had died of that fever in one year, and

[1] Percival, "Population of Manchester." *Phil. Trans.* LXIV. 54.
[2] James Lucas, "Remarks on Febrile Contagion." *London Medical Journal,* X. 260.

many who struggled through the disease died afterwards of lingering complaints.   In two courts or yards (such as might have been the Lantern Yard which Silas Marner found pulled down when he revisited Leeds) forty persons were affected with the fever; some families had received ten shillings a week from the assessment for the poor.   As early as 1779 Lucas proposed a house of reception for contagious fever, a proposal which was carried into effect in 1804, after a whole generation of typhus and at a time when there was little fever in Leeds or elsewhere. The infectious fevers, being chiefly confined to the poor, often prevailed, says this writer, for a length of time without exciting much alarm, or without their fatality being attended to ; but, he adds about the year 1790, "should a few of the higher rank receive the infection, then the disease is described in most exaggerated terms."

Carlisle was a good instance of the increase of urban population and the breeding of typhus.   In seventeen years, from 1763 to 1780, the inhabitants had increased from 4158 to 6229, many of the immigrants being Scots and Irish with their families.   The chief industry was the making of calico, in which the women and children were employed as well as the men. When Dr Heysham surveyed the town and suburbs for his census of 1779, he had "opportunity of seeing many scenes of poverty and filth and nastiness[1]"; and in the bill of mortality for that year he confesses himself astonished that there should be so little fever.

The great outburst of typhus at Carlisle began in the end of March, 1781, with no very obvious special provocation[2].   Upwards of 600 had typhus to February 7th, 1782, at which date 12 or 15 were still suffering from it.   The deaths were less than 1 in 10 of all attacked : viz. 2 in May, 4 in June, 8 in July, 8 in August, 7 in September, 9 in October, 8 in November, 6 in December, and 3 in January, 1782, a total of 55.   Of this total of fatal cases, 3 were boys, 4 bachelors, and 15 husbands : 3 girls, 2 maids, 22 wives, and 6 widows.   Two-thirds of all the deaths were of married people; Heysham saw no case in a child under three years.   It affected about a tenth part of the inhabit-

---

[1] In Appendix to Hutchinson's *Cumberland,* 1794.   Reprinted in Appendix to Joshua Milne's *Valuation of Annuities,* Lond. 1815.

[2] John Heysham, M.D., *Account of the Jail Fever, or Typhus Carcerum, as it appeared at Carlisle in* 1781. London, 1782.

ants of Carlisle (6299), and raged most among the lower class
who lived in narrow, close, confined lanes and in small crowded
apartments, of which there were a great many in Carlisle,
generally going through all the inmates of a house where it had
once begun.   On seeking to trace the origin of the epidemic, he
found that it began in the end of March, 1781, in a house in
Richard-gate, which contained about half-a-dozen very poor
families.   Every window that could be spared was shut up, to
save the window-tax.   The surgeon who attended some of these
poor wretches told Dr Heysham that the smell was so offensive
that it was with difficulty he could stay in the house.   One
of the typhus patients in this house was a weaver, who, on his
recovery, went to the large workshop where he worked, and
there, it was supposed, gave the infection (in his clothes) to his
fellow workmen, by whom new centres of infection were made
in various other houses.   In August, a young man just recovered
from the fever went to his mother's in the small village of
Rockliffe, four or five miles from Carlisle, to get back his
strength in the country air; his mother soon took the fever and
died, and a neighbour woman who came to her in her sickness
likewise caught it and died.   These were all the cases known in
the village, and they show the enormously greater fatality of
typhus in those not inured to its atmosphere and conditions.

The state of population and health at Warrington was
peculiar, and is given fully in another chapter.   There could
be no more striking instance of the growth of what the foreign
writers call the proletariat; an old market-town, with a small
sail-cloth industry from Elizabethan times, it became a busy
weaving town owing to the demand for sail-cloth during the war
with the American colonies.   The whole population of some
9000 men, women and children, were wage-earners; the women
were all the while unusually prolific, and the sacrifice of infant
life was enormous, especially by smallpox.   We have no
particular accounts of fevers; but in the bill of mortality for
1773, the year of a disastrous smallpox epidemic, there were
25 deaths from fever, of which 10 were of "worm fever," or the
remittent of children[1].

By the year 1790, when Ferriar's accounts of fever in
Manchester begin, the industrial revolution had been accomplished, mills were everywhere, and the characteristic hardships

[1] Aikin, *Phil. Trans.* LXIV. 473.

and maladies of a prolific working class in a time of slack trade were already much the same as we find them pictured with fidelity and pathos in the pages of Mrs Gaskell half a century after.

But, so as not to exaggerate the ill health of the working class in Manchester at the end of the 18th century, let us compare the births with the deaths according to the doubtless imperfect registers[1]:

Manchester, Births and Deaths, 1770–91.

Year	Births	Deaths	Year	Births	Deaths
1770	1050	988	1781	1591	1370
1771	1169	993	1782	1678	984
1772	1127	904	1783	1615	1496
1773	1168	923	1784	1958	1175
1774	1245	958	1785	1942	1734
1775	1359	835	1786	2319	1282
1776	1241	1220	1787	2256	1761
1777	1513	864	1788	2391	1637
1778	1449	975	1789	2487	1788
1779	1464	1288	1790	2756	1940
1780	1566	993	1791	2960	2286

The mean lodging-houses in the outskirts of the town, says Ferriar, in 1790[2], were the principal nurseries of febrile contagion: some of these were old houses with very small rooms, into each of which four or more people were crowded to eat, sleep, and frequently to work. They commonly bore marks of a long accumulation of filth, and some of them had been scarcely free from infection for many years past. As soon as one poor creature dies or is driven out of his cell he is replaced by another, generally from the country, who soon feels in his turn the consequences of breathing infected air. There was hardly any ventilation possible, many of these old houses being in dark narrow courts or blind alleys. In other parts of the town the lodging-houses were new, and not yet thoroughly dirty; but in these there was a long garret under the tiles, in which eight or ten people often lodged, the beds almost touching. Again, many lived in cellars, sleeping on the damp floor with few or no bedclothes; the cellars of Manchester, however, were better ventilated than those of Edinburgh, and

[1] John Aikin, M.D., *The Country from 30 to 40 miles round Manchester.* Lond. 1795, p. 584.

[2] John Ferriar, M.D., *Medical Histories and Reflections.* 4 vols., 1810–13, I. 172

freer from fever. These cellar-tenants were subject to the constant action of depressing passions of the mind. "I have seen patients," says Ferriar, "in agonies of despair on finding themselves overwhelmed with filth and abandoned by everyone who could do them any service, and after such emotions I have seldom found them recover." Addressing the Literary and Philosophical Society of Manchester previous to 1792, he pointed out in an *argumentum ad hominem* that "the situation of the poor at present is extremely dangerous, and often destructive to the middle and higher ranks of society[1]." And again, "the poor are indeed the first sufferers, but the mischief does not always rest with them. By secret avenues it reaches the most opulent, and severely revenges their neglect or insensibility to the wretchedness surrounding them[2]."

In an address to the Committee of Police in Manchester, he instances the following cases:

A family of the name of Turner in a dark cellar behind Jackson's Row: they have been almost constantly patients of the Infirmary for three years past on account of disorders owing to their miserable dwelling. There are other instances of the same kind in Bootle Street.

In Blakely Street, under No. 4, is a range of cellars let out to lodgers, which threatens to become a nursery of disease. They consist of four rooms communicating with each other, of which the two centre rooms are completely dark; the fourth is very ill-lighted and chiefly ventilated through the others. They contain four or five beds in each, and are already extraordinarily dirty.

In a nest of lodging-houses in Brook's entry near the bottom of Long-mill-gate, a very dangerous fever constantly subsists, and has subsisted for a considerable number of years. He had known nine patients confined in fevers at the same time in one of those houses and crammed into three small dirty rooms without the regular attendance of any friend or of a nurse. Four of these poor creatures died, absolutely from want of the common offices of humanity and from neglect in the administration of their medicines. Another set of lodging-houses constantly infected is known by the name of the Five Houses, in Newton Street[3].

The fever in Manchester was not always malignant typhus: sometimes it had the symptoms and low rate of mortality that suggest relapsing fever. Thus, in the winter epidemic of 1789–90, very prevalent in Manchester and Salford, out of Ferriar's first ninety patients only two died; in some the skin had a remarkable, pungent heat, in others there were profuse watery sweats; women were commonly affected with hysterical symptoms during convalescence, which was often tedious[4]. A certain

---

[1] Ferriar, I. 261.   [2] *Ibid.* I. 234.   [3] *Ibid.* II. 213–20.
[4] *Ibid.* I. 153–6; and II. 57.

number of these cases would run into "a formed typhus," with petechiae and all the other signs of malignity; and in some seasons, as in the distressful year 1794, typhus was the usual form. Two fatal cases in children, examined after death, had peritonitis; "in the one no marks of the disease were discernible within the cavity of the [intestinal] tube;" in the other, the patient was covered with petechiae[1]. These cases of localized inflammation in typhus he compares with Pringle's cases of spotted fever complicated with abscess of the brain.

The years 1792 and 1793 passed, says Ferriar, without any extraordinary increase of fever patients, although the noxious influences were always present. But in the summer and autumn of 1794 "the usual epidemic fever" became very prevalent among the poor in some quarters of the town, particularly after a bilious colic had raged among all ranks of people. This was a time when work was slack; many workmen enlisted and left their families. In November and December 1794, as many as 156 sent applications to the Infirmary in a week to be visited in fever at their homes.

This was a memorable time of scarcity and distress all over the country, the beginning of a twenty-years' period of so-called "war-prices," when farmers' profits were so large that they could afford to double or treble their rents to the landlords. The history of epidemics comes at this point into close contact with the economic history, which I shall touch on in the sequel, after giving a few more particulars of typhus in England and Scotland generally, previous to the outbreak of the war with France in 1793.

Typhus in England and Scotland generally, in the end of the 18th century.

The introduction of machinery and the building of mills brought typhus fever to places much less crowded than Leeds, or Manchester, or Carlisle.

Dr David Campbell of Lancaster saw much of typhus in that town, and in mill villages near it, in the years 1782, 1783, and 1784. In Lancaster town he saw about 500 cases, of which 168 were in men, with 20 deaths, 236 in women, with 11 deaths,

---

[1] Ferriar, I. 166–8.

and 94 in children under fourteen, with 3 deaths. At Backbarrow cotton mill, twenty miles from Lancaster, there were 180 cases, of which 38 were in men, with 5 deaths, 11 in women, with 2 deaths, and 131 in children under fourteen, with no deaths[1] At this mill there was an extremely offensive smell in the rooms, which came from the privy; the doors of the latter, "for indispensable reasons in the economy of these works, where so many children are employed, always communicate with the workrooms." Every care had been taken to keep the air sweet, but without effect. The offensive smell was in all the cotton mills from the same cause; and in the Radcliffe mill belonging to Mr Peel, the typhus was ascribed to that source, the nuisance having been at length got rid of. Both at Backbarrow and Radcliffe the houses of the workpeople were new, airy and comfortable. In the same years typhus raged with uncommon severity at Ulverston and in various parts of Lancashire, where cotton-mills had been set up[2].

The typhus of Liverpool and Newcastle was reproduced in Whitehaven and Cockermouth on a scale proportionate to their size. Whitehaven, the port of the Cumberland coal-field, was the Newcastle of the west coast, and had a large trade with Ireland. Many of the labourers lived in cellars. Brownrigg's experiences of typhus fever in it went back to near the middle of the 18th century. The Whitehaven Dispensary was opened in 1783, the occasion for it being thus explained :—

"Previous to the establishment of dispensaries Whitehaven and Cockermouth were infested by nervous and putrid fever. Many of their respectable inhabitants became its victims; and among the lower class of people it prevailed with deplorable malignancy. The present period happily exhibits a different picture. Notwithstanding our connection with the metropolis of Ireland, and other commercial places, contagion rarely appears; or, when accidentally introduced, is readily suppressed[3]."

The following is the abstract of "contagious fever cases" from the records of the Whitehaven Dispensary from 30 June, 1783, to 9 June, 1800[4]:

[1] This is perhaps the first numerical evidence of the slight fatality of typhus in children. A more elaborate proof of the same was given long after by Geary for Limerick. An early age-table for Whitehaven is given under Smallpox, *infra.*

[2] David Campbell, M.D., *Observations on the Typhus or Low Contagious Fever.* Lancaster, 1785.

[3] Joshua Dixon, M.D., *Annual Reports of the Whitehaven Dispensary,* 1795 *to* 1805. Details for 1773-4 in his note in *Memoirs of Lettsom,* III. 353.

[4] Dixon, *Literary Life of Dr Brownrigg,* pp. 238-9.

Year	Cured	Dead	Total		Year	Cured	Dead	Total
1783	75	1	76		1792	17	2	19
1784	401	9	410		1793	7	3	10
1785	350	20	370		1794	13	1	14
1786	91	6	97		1795	28	2	30
1787	21	1	22		1796	48	1	49
1788	53	7	60		1797	35	2	37
1789	103	2	105		1798	12	1	13
1790	288	21	309		1799	11	1	12
1791	74	6	79		Total	1627	85	1712

The year 1790 is indicated as an unhealthy one, by the excess of burials over christenings, also at Macclesfield, where there were 316 christenings to 380 burials, the proportion being usually the other way[1].

Dr John Alderson of Hull wrote in 1788 an essay on the contagion of fever, in which there are no authentic details for Hull: "The calamity itself is the constant complaint of every neighbourhood, and almost every newspaper presents us with an example of the direful consequences of infection"—the reference being to gaols more particularly[2]. Whatever was the reason, there was undoubtedly a great deal of typhus in England in the eighties of the eighteenth century. Oxfordshire, Gloucestershire, Worcestershire, Wiltshire and Buckinghamshire experienced much typhus from 1782 to 1785, although we have few particulars. "The remembrance of its ravages at Gloucester, Worcester and Marlborough," says Dr Wall of Oxford, "is still fresh in every mind, where its virulence proved so peculiarly fatal to the medical world." At Aylesbury, Dr Kennedy survived an attack of the "contagious fever," to write an account (1785) of the epidemic, which he traced to the gaol (the date, be it observed, is subsequent to Howard's visitations)[3]. At Maidstone, also, in 1785, the gaol fever was the subject of a special account[4].

At Worcester in 1783 the younger Dr Johnstone caught typhus while visiting the gaol, which was thereafter rebuilt at great expense. A prisoner took it to Droitwich where 14 died[5].

Dr Wall gives clinical details of fifteen cases of typhus treated by him in private practice at Oxford in 1785; one of his patients was an apothecary whose business had exposed him very much to the influence of contagion, as he was much

[1] Aikin, *Country round Manchester.* Lond. 1795, p. 616.
[2] *Nature and Origin of the Contagion of Fevers.* Hull, 1788.
[3] *Account of a Contagious Fever at Aylesbury.* Aylesbury, 1785.
[4] Thomas Day, *Some Considerations...on the Contagion in Maidstone Jail,* 1785.
[5] See Barnes, in *Mem. Lit. Phil. Soc. Manchester,* II. 85. Dr Samuel Parr wrote his epitaph in the Cathedral. Also Johnstone sen. to Lettsom, *Memoirs,* III. 241.

employed amongst the poor in the suburbs of the town and neighbouring villages and in the House of Industry[1]." In the year 1783–85, much of the epidemic fever was of the nature of ague, as described in another chapter. It is not always easy to separate it from typhus; but there is no doubt that both were prevalent together. Thus in the parish of Painswick, Gloucestershire, in the spring of 1785 there occurred both "a contagious fever" and an "epidemic ague," the latter having left a good many persons dropsical and cachectic[2]. This had been part of an epidemical fever which had raged for some time in the county of Gloucestershire, and is said to have lately carried off a great number of poor. At Norton, within five miles of Gloucester, there lived in two adjoining tenements two families: in one a man and his wife and three children, in the other a man and his wife, of whom only one remained alive on the 1st of March, 1785[3].

The extraordinary failure of the harvest in Scotland in 1782 produced much distress, and with it fever, in the winter following. The Glasgow and Edinburgh municipalities imported grain for the public benefit. Various traces of the scarcity and fever appear in the Statistical Account written a few years after. Thus, in Holywood parish, Dumfriesshire, some fevers were wont to appear in February and March among people of low circumstances living in a narrow valley; and the unusual mortality in the dear year 1782 was owing to an infectious fever in the same cottages. In the regular bills of mortality of Torthorwald parish, Dumfriesshire, the deaths from "fever" fall in the dear years, 1782–3, 1785, &c. In Dunscore parish, in the same county, the burials of 1782 rose to the most unusual figure of 30 (the baptisms being 17), "owing to a malignant fever[4]."

[1] Martin Wall, M.D., *Clin. Obs. on the Use of Opium in Low Fevers and in the Synochus.* Oxford, 1786.

[2] J. C. Jenner, in *Lond. Med. Journal,* VII. 163.

[3] *Gent. Magaz.* 1785, I. 231, March 1.

[4] This is the period and the district to which Robert Burns refers, under date of 21 June, 1783, in a letter to his cousin, James Burness, of Montrose: "I shall only trouble you with a few particulars relative to the wretched state of this country. Our markets are exceedingly high, oatmeal 17*d.* and 18*d.* per boll, and not to be got even at that price. We have, indeed, been pretty well supplied with quantities of white peas from England and elsewhere; but that resource is likely to fail us, and what will become of us then, particularly the very poorest sort, heaven only knows." The lately flourishing silk and carpet weaving had declined during the American War, and the seasons had been adverse to farmers. The lines in Burns' poem, "Death and Dr Hornbook":
> 'This while ye hae been mony a gate
>   At mony a house.'
>   'Ay, Ay,' quoth he, and shook his head.—
are explained by a note, "An epidemical fever was then raging in the country."

But Scotland was now past the danger of actual famine from even a total failure of the harvest. Some farmers were ruined, and many more were unable to pay the year's rent; but the very poorest were enabled to find food, one source being "the importation of white pease from America." From Delting, in Shetland, one of the poorest parishes, the report is: "There is reason to believe that none died from mere want; but there is no doubt that many, from the unwholesome food, contracted diseases that brought them to their graves."

The following relating to the parishes of Keithhall and Kinkell, Aberdeenshire, in the scarcity following the lost harvest of 1782, is a curiously detailed glimpse of the time:

"Several families who would not allow their poverty to be known lived on two diets of meal a day. One family wanted food from Friday night till Sunday at dinner. On the last Friday of December, 1782, the country people could get no meal in Aberdeen, as the citizens were afraid of a famine; and a poor man, in this district, could find none in the country the day after. But the distress of this family being discovered, they were supplied. Next day the [Kirk] session bought at a sale a considerable quantity of bere, which was made into meal. This served the poor people until the importation at Aberdeen became regular, and every man of humanity rejoiced that the danger of famine was removed [1]."

We hear most of fevers in the Highland parishes, with their subdivisions of holdings and an excess of population. Thus of Gairloch, Ross-shire, it is said: "Fevers are frequent, sometimes they are of a favourable kind, at other times they continue long and carry off great numbers"—the poor in this parish, upon the Kirk Session roll, numbering 84 in the year 1792, and the aggregate money paid to the whole number averaging £6. 7s. in a year, whereas the fertile parish of Ellon, Aberdeenshire, with 40 on the poor's roll, paid them £43 per annum.

Again, of the fishing village of Eyemouth, it is said: "The only complaints that prove mortal in this place are different kinds of fevers and consumptions; and these are mostly confined to the poorest class of people, and ascribed to their scanty diet." And of another fishing parish, in Banffshire, Fordyce, including Portsoy, it is said: "The most prevalent distemper is a fever, and that for the most part not universal, but confined to particular districts. It is sometimes thought to arise from infection and communication with other parts of the country; at other times from local situations and circumstances of the people's houses and habits of living in particular districts [2]."

[1] Account by Rev. Geo. Skene Keith, *Statist. Act.* 11. 544.   [2] Also Banff, *ibid.* XX. 347.

The beginning of the great French war was the occasion of a considerable increase of fever; although no records make it appear so fatal a time as the years 1783–86. The commercial distress and want of work which began in the autumn of 1792, were intensified by the bad harvests of 1794 and 1795, which followed two harvests also deficient. This was the period of distress and of epidemic fever to which Wordsworth referred in the passage in the first book of the 'Excursion,' where he is relating the story of Margaret's ruined cottage[1].

There is little medical writing upon the epidemic fever of 1794–95; and, in the very district of Wordsworth's story, the records of the Whitehaven Dispensary bear no traces of a great concourse of patients. There is reason to think that the fever, if slow and weakening, was seldom fatal, that it was *typhus mitior*, and that it was sometimes, perhaps often, relapsing. One glimpse we get of it in the family of the afterwards celebrated Dr Edward Jenner of Berkeley, in the winter of 1794–95. He thus writes to a friend about the visitation of "grim-visaged typhus:"

"You shall hear the history of our calamities. First fell Henry's [his nephew and assistant] wife and sister. From the early use of bark, they both appeared to recover; but the former, after going about her ordinary business for some days, had a dreadful relapse which nearly destroyed her. It was during my attendance on this case that the venomed arrow wounded me...Like Mrs Jenner's fever, at an early period there was a clear inter-

[1]
"Not twenty years ago, but you I think
Can scarcely bear it now in mind, there came
Two blighting seasons, when the fields were left
With half a harvest. It pleased heaven to add
A worse affliction in the plague of war, &c."

Trotter, *Medicina Nautica*, I. 182, 1797, gives these real cases:—"During the short time that I attended the dispensary at Newcastle, just at the beginning of the [French] war, I was sent for to a poor man in a miserable and low part of the town called Sandgate. He was ill with what is called a spotted fever." Six children were standing round his bed, the oldest not more than nine. They had been ill first, then his wife, who was recovered and had gone out to pawn the last article they had to buy meal for the children. The man worked on the quay at 1s. 2d. per diem. Again, "When I practised as a surgeon and apothecary at the end of the late [American] war in a small town in Northumberland, with an extensive country business, some similar scenes came under my view. Two servants of two opulent farmers applied to me for relief. The first had seven children, who took the fever one by one till the whole became sick. His wages were 1s. per diem. His master, a rich man, thought himself charitable by allowing them to pull turnips from his field for food. The other servant was a shepherd; but his herding, as the saying is, was a poor one. The first and second of six children were able to work a little, till they got a fever in a severe winter, and down they fell, one after another, the father and mother at last." They wanted to sell the cow; but some charitable ladies raised a small subscription, by which means the comforts of wine and diet came within their reach; their master, for his part, sent them the carcase of a sheep, which had been found dead in a furrow, with a request that the skin should be returned.

mission for four days...On the eighth day after the first seizure it again set in, in good earnest, and continued one-and-twenty days...Dr Parry was with me from Bath five times, Dr Hicks and Dr Ludlow as many, and my friend George was never absent from my bedside...But, to return to that mansion of melancholy, Henry's. His infant girl has now the fever; a servant maid in the house is dying with it; and to complete this tragical narrative, about five days ago fell poor Henry himself. · His symptoms at present are such as one might expect: violent pain in the head, vertigo, debility, transient shiverings....His pulse this evening is sunk from 125 to 100. The stench from the poor girl is so great as to fill the house with putrid vapour; and I shall remove him this morning by means of a sedan-chair to a cottage near my own house[1]."

This is a tolerably clear picture of a short-period fever with relapses, or of relapsing fever strictly so-called; the stench, also, of one patient is characteristic. Barker, of Coleshill or Birmingham, has much to say under the same year 1794, of a slow, tedious fever, marked by " sluggish action and comatose symptoms," and much subject to relapses; but he does not give the duration of the first or subsequent paroxysms, as Jenner does, or the usual length of the clear intervals, his most definite case being of a young woman who died in twenty-four hours from a relapse which came on about three weeks after the fever had left her[2].

It was the access of fever in 1794–5, and the alarm that it caused among the richer classes, that led to the opening of the Manchester House of Recovery in 1796. In certain streets in the neighbourhood chosen for the hospital, Portland Street, Silver Street and others in the same block, the cases of contagious fever for nearly three years before the hospital was opened are given by Ferriar as follows:

    Sept. 1793 to Sept. 1794, cases of fever, 400
    Sept. 1794 to Sept. 1795,   „   „   „   389
    Sept. 1795 to May 1796,   „   „   „   267

The cases began to be sent to the hospital on the 27th May, 1796, and an attempt was made to extinguish contagion in the houses, by white-washing, disinfecting and the like; so that in the same group of streets there were only 25 cases of fever from 13 July, 1794 to 13 March, 1797. Meanwhile the admissions to the hospital were few until the dearth of 1799–1802. One of the manufacturing towns which is known to have shared in the epidemic fever of 1794–96 was Ashton-under-Lyne, where upwards of three hundred cases (with few deaths)

[1] Jenner to Shrapnell, Baron's *Life of Jenner*, I. 106–7.
[2] John Barker, *Epidemicks*, pp. 201–6.

occurred in less than three months at the end of 1795. This epidemic must have been somewhat special to Ashton, for it produced much alarm in neighbouring places and caused Ashton to be avoided from fear of infection.

Shortly after 1796, Ferriar made an inquiry into an epidemic of fever at a village within a mile of Manchester; the houses were many of them new, built for the convenience of a large cotton mill; but even the new houses were offensive, with cellars occupied by lodgers, and almost every house overcrowded. This was the first fever in the village, and it was traced to a family who had come from Manchester with infected clothes. Stockport about the same time erected a House of Recovery, having "the same general causes of fever which render the disease so common in Manchester"; and Ferriar adds: "I believe there is not a town in the kingdom containing four thousand inhabitants which would not be greatly benefited by similar establishments."

The bad harvest of 1794 raised the price of wheat to 55s. 7d. on 1 January, 1795, and the prospect of another short harvest to 77s. 2d. on 1 July. A famine being threatened, the Government caused neutral ships bound to French ports with corn to be seized, and brought into English ports, the owners receiving an ample profit. Agents were also sent to the Baltic to buy corn. By these means the price of wheat, which had risen in August to 108s. 4d., fell in October to 76s. 9d. Parliament met on the 29th October, and various measures were taken[1]. In the spring

---

[1] The dearth of 1794–95 called forth one notable piece, the 'Thoughts and Details on Scarcity,' drawn up by Mr Burke, from his experience in Buckinghamshire, originally for the use of Mr Pitt, in November, 1795. Burke takes an optimist line, and preaches the economic doctrine of *laissez faire:* "After all," he asks, "have we not reason to be thankful to the Giver of all good? In our history, and when 'the labourer of England is said to have been once happy,' we find constantly, after certain intervals, a period of real famine; by which a melancholy havock was made among the human race. The price of provisions fluctuated dreadfully, demonstrating a deficiency very different from the worst failures of the present moment. Never, since I have known England, have I known more than a comparative scarcity. The price of wheat, taking a number of years together, has had no very considerable fluctuation, nor has it risen exceedingly within this twelvemonth. Even now, I do not know of one man, woman, or child, that has perished from famine; fewer, if any, I believe, than in years of plenty, when such a thing may happen by accident. This is owing to a care and superintendence of the poor, far greater than any I remember...Not only very few (I have observed that I know of none though I live in a place [Beaconsfield] as poor as most) have actually died of want, but we have seen no traces of those dreadful exterminating epidemicks, which, in consequence of scanty and unwholesome food, in former times not unfrequently wasted whole nations. Let us be saved from too much wisdom of our own, and we shall do tolerably well." The last sentence is his favourite principle of "a wise and salutary neglect" on the part of Government.

of 1796, the climax of distress was reached, wheat being at 100s. per quarter. The harvest of 1796 was abundant and wheat fell to 57s. 3d. The harvests of 1797 and 1798 were not equally good, but they were not altogether bad, and the price of wheat kept about 50s. for nearly three years, which were years of comparative comfort between the dearth of 1794–96 and the dearth of 1799–1802.

Fevers in the Dearth of 1799–1802.

Although Willan chooses the end of the year 1799 to enlarge upon the London fever, he does not connect it with the dearth that was already beginning to be felt (soup kitchens having been opened in various parts of London). The price of wheat, which had been steadily about 50s. in 1797 and 1798, rose in May, 1799 to 61s. 8d., after a hard winter which had probably injured the autumn-sown corn. The harvest turned out ill, and the price of wheat rose in December, 1799, to 94s. 2d. Bounties were offered on imported foreign grain, but in June, 1800, the price was 134s. 5d., falling in August to 96s. 2d. on the crops promising well. The latter end of harvest proved wet, much of the grain being lost, so that the price per quarter of wheat rose to 133s. in December. There was much suffering, and some rioting. Parliament met on the 11th November, 1800, on account of the dearth, the opinions of the members being much divided as to the causes of the high prices. In March, 1801, wheat was at 156s. 2d. per quarter, beef from 10d. to 10½d. per pound, mutton 11d. to 12d. per pound. It is to this year, when the quartern loaf was at one-and-eightpence, that a comparison by Arthur Young belongs, showing the great change in the purchasing power of wages[1]. By the end of summer, 1801,

---

[1] A labourer at Bury St Edmunds, receiving a weekly wage of five shillings, was able to buy therewith at the old prices:

		Cost of same in 1801		
		£	s.	d.
	A bushel of wheat	0	16	0
	A bushel of malt	0	9	0
5s.	A pound of butter	0	1	0
	A pound of cheese	0	0	4
	Tobacco, one penny	0	0	1
		£1	6	5
Weekly wage in 1801, 9s.				
Parish bonus 6s.			15	0
		0	11	5 deficiency

wheat rose to 180s., and the quartern loaf was for four weeks at 1s. 10½d.

Whatever statistics were then kept of fever-cases, show a decided rise in the years 1800 and 1801 :

Year	Manchester House of Recovery (fever-cases)	Glasgow Royal Infirmary (fever-cases)	Newcastle Dispensary (fever-cases)	London Bills of Mortality (fever-deaths)
1796	371	43	201	1547
1797	339	83	65	1526
1798	398	45	67	1754
1799	364	128	—	1784
1800	747	104	—	2712
1801	1070	63	425	2908
1802	601	104	—	2201
1803	256	85	352	2326
1804	184	97	255	1702
1805	268	99	74	1307

The London Fever Hospital was not opened until February, 1802, a small house in Gray's Inn Lane containing sixteen beds. It came at the end of the epidemic, and was in small request during the next fifteen years. The same epidemic at Leeds was the occasion of opening a House of Recovery there in 1804, twenty-five years after Lucas had first called for it. The state of affairs in Leeds, which at length moved the richer classes to that step, is thus described by Whitaker[1]:

"In the years 1801 and 1802 an alarming epidemic fever spread in Leeds and the neighbourhood. The contagion extended so rapidly and proved so fatal that some hundreds were affected at the same time, and two medical gentlemen, with several nurses, fell victims to the disease...In 1802 whole streets were infected house by house; in one court, of crowded population, typhus raged for four months successively."

One of the Leeds physicians, Dr Thorp, seized the occasion to urge the need of a fever hospital, in a pamphlet written in 1802, in which he said :

"In a visit made a few days ago to those abodes of misery, I saw in one particular district upwards of twenty-five families ill in contagious fever. In some houses two, in others six or seven [families] were confined, many of whom appeared to be in extreme danger." The superintendent of the sick poor stated to Dr Thorp "that sixty families in epidemic fever are under his care at this time. New applications are making daily. In some families three, in others six or seven, are in the disease. Forty persons in fever have applied to him for medical aid within the present week[2]."

[1] *Loidis and Elmete*, 1816, p. 85.
[2] Thorp, Tract of 1802, cited by Hunter, *Ed. Med. Surg. Journ.* April, 1819, p. 239.

The wonder is that, with the enormous prices of food, things were not worse. At the time when provisions were dearest, work was slack in several industries. A commercial report of 1 April, 1801, speaks of the trade of Birmingham as very distressed, a large proportion of the men being out of work; the ribbon trade of Coventry was deplorable, and the woollen trade of Yorkshire still worse. Evidence of epidemic typhus in various parts of England came out in connexion with the reports on influenza in 1803. Holywell, in Flintshire, with a large cotton-making industry, had not been free from a bad kind of typhus for two years previous to the influenza of 1803[1]. In Bristol there was a good deal of fever in 1802–3, which found its way, through domestic servants, into good houses in Clifton, "and proved fatal in some instances[2]." It is probable that these are only samples, the writings on epidemics being singularly defective at this period. The following, dated 10th April, 1802, by a surgeon at Earlsoham, near Framlingham, Suffolk, gives us a glimpse of malignant contagious fever in a farm-house:

"The most prevailing epidemics for the last twelve months have been typhus maligna and mitior, scarlatina anginosa, measles, and mumps. Many of the former have proved alarmingly fatal in several of our villages, whilst those of the second class of typhoid fevers have put on the appearance of the low nervous kind attended with great prostration of strength, depression of spirits, loss of appetite, etc., which frequently continue many weeks before a compleat recovery ensues." Five cases, of "the most malignant kind of typhus," occurred in a farmer's family: one of the sons, aged eighteen, died in a few days with delirium, and black sordes of the mouth, tongue and throat; then the father, two daughters, and another son, took the infection but all escaped with their lives. Of four persons who nursed them, one caught the fever, and died. Four persons in a neighbouring family, who visited them, took infection, of whom two died[3].

There was perhaps nothing very unusual in such instances of country fevers at the beginning of the century. The incident is exactly in the manner of one that figures prominently in a story of Scottish life and customs at the same period, which long passed current as a faithful picture and as enforcing a much-needed moral[4].

---

[1] Currie, *Med. Phys. Journ.* X. 213.   [2] Beddoes.
[3] Goodwin, *Med. Phys. Journ.* IX. 509. Cf. Gervis, *Med. Chir. Trans.* II. 236.
[4] Elizabeth Hamilton, *The Cottagers of Glenburnie*, Edin. 1808: "The only precaution which the good people, who came to see him [the farmer] appeared now to think necessary, was carefully to shut the door, which usually stood open...The prejudice against fresh air appeared to be universal...The doctor did not think it probable that he would live above three days; but said, the only chance he had was in removing him from that close box in which he was shut up, and admitting as much air as possible into the apartment...While the farmer yet hovered on the brink of death, his wife and Robert, his second son, were both taken ill...Peter MacGlashan

Comparative immunity from Fevers during the War and high prices of 1803–15.

From 1803 to 1816 there was comparatively little fever in this country. This was notably the case in London, but it was also true of all the larger towns where fever-hospitals had been established, and it was as true of Ireland as of England. This was, indeed, a time of great prosperity, which reached to all classes, the permanent rise of wages having more than balanced the increased cost of the necessaries of life. The following prices of wheat will show that a dear loaf did not necessarily mean distress while the war-expenditure lasted:

Prices of wheat (from Tooke).

	s.	d.			s.	d.			s.	d.
1802	57	1	1810 June		113	5	1817 Sept.		77	7
1803	52	3	Dec.		94	7	1818 Dec.		78	10
1804 Lady Day	49	6	1811 June		86	11	1819 Aug.		75	
Dec.	86	2	Nov.		101	6	1820		72	
1805 Aug.	98	4	1812 Aug.		155		1821 July		51	
Dec.	74	5	Nov.		113	6	Dec.		50	
1806	73	5	1813 Aug.		112		1822		42	
1807 Nov.	66		Dec.		73	6	1823 Feb.		40	8
1808 May	73	6	1814 July		66	5	June		62	5
Dec.	92		1815 Dec.		53	7	Oct.		46	5
1809 March	95		1816 May		74		Dec.		50	8
July	86	6	Dec.		103		1824		65	
Dec.	102	6	1817 June		111	6				

The only years in the period from 1803 to 1816 in which there was some slight increase of fever were about 1811–12. There was undoubtedly some distress in the manufacturing districts at that time, owing to the much talked-of Orders in Council, which had the effect of closing American markets to British manufactures[1].

had taken to his bed on going home and was now dangerously ill of the fever....All the village indeed offered their services; and Mrs Mason, though she blamed the thoughtless custom of crowding into a sick room, could not but admire the kindness and good nature with which all the neighbours seemed to participate in the distress of this afflicted family."

[1] Charlotte Brontë's story of *Shirley* falls in this period and turns upon the industrial crisis in Yorkshire; but it is on the whole a happy idyllic picture. Harriet Martineau wrote in *Household Words*, vol. I. 1850, Nos. 9–12, a story entitled "The Sickness and Health of the People of Bleaburn," a Yorkshire village supposed to have been Osmotherly. It is, in substance, an account of a terrible epidemic of fever in the year 1811, the story opening with the news of the victory of Albuera and the rejoicings thereon. It appears to have been constructed very closely from the real events of the plague of 1665–66 in the village of Eyam, in the North Peak of Derbyshire, and had probably a very slender foundation in any facts of fever in Yorkshire or elsewhere in the year 1811. "Ten or eleven corpses," says the novelist, "were actually lying unburied, infecting half-a-dozen cottages from this cause." Cf. infra, Leyburn, p. 167.

The small amount of fever in London between the year 1803 and the beginning of the epidemic of 1817–19 rests on the testimony of Bateman[1], who in 1804 took up Willan's task of keeping a systematic record of the cases at the Carey Street Dispensary. He has only two special entries relating to typhus: one in the autumn of 1811, when some cases occurred in the uncleanly parts of Clerkenwell and St Luke's ("but I have not learned that it has existed in any other districts of London"); the other in October and November 1813, when there was more typhus among the Irish in some of the filthy courts of Saffron Hill, near Hatton Garden, than for several years past, the infection having spread rapidly and fatally in several houses. The best evidence of this lull in typhus in London is the almost empty state of the new fever-hospital:

Year	Admissions		Year	Admissions
1802	164		1810	52
1803	176		1811	43
1804	80		1812	61
1805	66		1813	85
1806	93		1814	59
1807	63		1815	80
1808	69		1816	118
1809	29		1817	760

Until it was removed to Pancras Road, in September, 1816, the London fever-hospital had only sixteen beds. But Bateman says that no one was refused admission, and that for several years the house was frequently empty three or four weeks together. Also at the Dispensary, in Carey Street, he had an opportunity during the period 1804–1816,

"Of observing the entire freedom from fevers enjoyed by the inhabitants of the numerous crowded courts and alleys within the extensive district comprehended in our visits from that charity." And again, writing in the winter of 1814–15, Bateman says: "To those who recollect the numerous cases of typhoid fevers [this term did not then mean enteric] which called for the relief of dispensaries twelve or fourteen years ago, and the contagion of which was often with great difficulty eradicated from the apartments where it raged, and even seized the same individuals again and again when they escaped its fatal influences, the great freedom from these fevers which now exists, even in the most close and filthy alleys in London, is the ground of some surprise." And once more, in the summer of 1816, just as the new epidemic period was about to begin, he says: "The extraordinary disappearance of contagious fever from every part of this crowded metropolis during the long period comprehended by these Reports [since 1804], cannot fail to have attracted the attention of the reader."

[1] T. Bateman, M.D., *Reports on the Diseases of London...from 1804 to 1816.* Lond. 1819.

11—2

Bateman concluded, not without reason, that this immunity of London from fever was due to the high degree of well-being among the poorer classes in times of plenty; and although he made out that the poor of Dublin, Cork and some Scotch towns did not profit by times of plenty so much as those in London, yet his reason for the abeyance of fever from 1804 to 1816 applied to England, Ireland and Scotland at large, and was doubtless the true reason.

The following figures from Manchester[1], Leeds[2] and Glasgow[3] hospitals, as well as the Irish statistics elsewhere given, are closely parallel with those of London:

Manchester House of Recovery.

Year	Cases	Deaths	Year	Cases	Deaths
1796–7	371	40	1807–8	208	15
1797–8	339	16	1808–9	260	21
1798–9	398	27	1809–10	278	30
1799–1800	364	41	1810–11	172	15
1800–1	747	63	1811–12	140	18
1801–2	1070	84	1812–13	126	13
1802–3	601	53	1813–14	226	17
1803–4	256	33	1814–15	379	29
1804–5	184	34	1815–16	185	14
1805–6	268	29	1816–17	172	6
1806–7	311	33			

Leeds House of Recovery.

Year	Cases	Deaths	Year	Cases	Deaths
1804 (2 mo.)	10	0	1812	80	12
1805	66	6	1813	137	11
1806	75	2	1814	79	4
1807	35	1	1815	146	15
1808	80	3	1816	121	13
1809	93	8	1817	178	8
1810	75	14	1818 (10 mo.)	254	20
1811	92	4			

Glasgow Royal Infirmary (Fever Wards).

Year	Cases	Year	Cases
1795	18	1807	25
1796	43	1808	27
1797	83	1809	76
1798	45	1810	82
1799	128	1811	45
1800	104	1812	16
1801	63	1813	35
1802	104	1814	90
1803	85	1815	230
1804	97	1816	399
1805	99	1817	714
1806	75	1818	1371

[1] Parl. Committee's Report on Contag. Fev. 1818, p. 33. Table by P. M. Roget.
[2] Adam Hunter, *Ed. Med. Surg. Journ.*, April, 1819.
[3] Cleland, *Glasgow and Clydesdale Statist. Soc. Transactions*, Pt. I. Nov. 2, 1836.

Even such fever as there was in Britain from 1804 to 1817 was not all certainly typhus. The high death-rates at the Manchester fever-hospital in 1804 and 1805 (1 death in 7·5 cases and 1 death in 5·25 cases) may mean a certain proportion of enteric cases in those years. "From 1804 to 1805," says Ferriar, "many cases were admitted of a most lingering and dangerous kind....Many deaths took place from sudden changes in the state of the fever, contrary to the usual course of the disease, and only imputable to the peculiar character of the epidemic. Similar cases occurred at that time in private practice." Next year, 1806, there was an epidemic among the troops at Deal, described under the name of "remittent fever," which Murchison claims to have been enteric[1]. In September, 1808, says Bateman, several were admitted into the London House of Recovery, with malignant symptoms; "and some severe and even fatal instances occurred in individuals in respectable rank in life." He still uses the name of typhus; but he is aware that the cases of continued fever, especially in the summer and autumn of 1810, had often symptoms pointing to a bowel-fever rather than to a head-fever[2].

The years 1807 and 1808 appear to have been the most generally unwholesome during this period of comparative immunity from fever; they were marked by the occurrence of dysenteries, agues, and infantile remittents, as well as of fevers of the "typhus" kind. The chief account comes from Nottingham[3]. The cases of "typhus" there were very tedious, but not violent, nor attended with any unfavourable symptoms, only one case having petechiae, and all having diarrhoea. The following

[1] Sutton, *Account of a Remittent Fever among the Troops in this Climate.* Canterbury, 1806.

[2] In the first three months of 1811 a singular fever occurred among working people in part of a suburb of Paisley, one practitioner having 32 cases in 13 families. It was marked by rigors at the onset, pain in the back, headache, dry skin, loaded very red tongue, quick fluttering pulse, watchfulness, delirium-like fatuity, abdominal pain in many, foetid stools, great prostration, gradual recovery after fifteen or sixteen days without manifest crisis, and relapses in some. In this fever Murchison discovers enteric or typhoid. Its limitation to a part of one of the suburbs of Paisley is, of course, in the manner of enteric fever; on the other hand, only one of those 32 cases died, which is a rate of fatality perhaps not unparalleled in typhoid but much more often matched in typhus or relapsing fever of young and old together; while the length of the fever, fifteen or sixteen days or sometimes more, is too great for the abortive kind of enteric and too little for enteric fever completing both its first and second stages. James Muir, *Edin. Med. and Surg. Journ.* VIII. 134. Murchison, *Continued Fevers,* p. 428.

[3] James Clarke, M.D., "Medical Report for Nottingham from March 1807 to March 1808," *Edin. Med. and Surg. Journ.* IV. 422. His account of the unwholesome state of the weavers' houses is as bad as any of those already given.

table of admissions for various kinds of fever (as classified by
Cullen) at the Nottingham General Hospital, 25 March, 1807,
to 25 March, 1808, shows the preponderance of "synochus" and
next to it, of infantile remittent :

Admitted to the Nottingham General Hospital, 1807.

Intermittent fever	7
Synocha	10
Typhus	27
Febris nervosa	26
Synochus	155
Febris infantum remittens	88
Dysentery	5

The state of war in the Peninsula was favourable to
epidemic or spreading diseases, and there is a good deal to show
that such diseases did exist among the British troops[1]. But
there is only one good instance of England getting a taste of
that experience of war-typhus which the Continent had to
endure for many years. This was on the return of the remnant
of the army after the defeat at Corunna on 16 January, 1809.
The troops were crowded pell-mell on board transports, which
had a very rough passage home. Dysentery broke out among
them, and was the most urgent malady when they landed at
Plymouth in a state of filth and rags. Typhus fever followed,
but in the first three weeks at Plymouth, to the 18th of February,
it was not of a malignant type, only 8 dying of it in the Old
Cumberland Square Hospital; in the next three weeks, 28 died
of it there. Up to the 27th of March, 1809, the sick at Plymouth
from the Corunna army numbered 2432, of whom 241 died.
Of 4 medical officers, 3 took the contagion, of 29 orderlies,
25 took it. The fever was in some cases followed by a relapse,
which was more often fatal than the original attack[2]. This
was a typical instance of typhus bred from dysentery or other
incidents of campaigning, a contagion more dangerous to others
than to those who had engendered it. "Within a few yards of
the spot where I now write," says Dr James Johnson, of Spring
Gardens, London, "the greater part of a family fell sacrifices
to the effects of fomites that lurked in a blanket purchased
from one of these soldiers after their return from Corunna[3]." In

[1] McGrigor, "Med. Hist. of British Armies in Peninsula," *Med. Chir. Trans.* VI.
381.

[2] Richard Hooper, "Account of the Sick landed from Corunna," *Edin. Med. and
Surg. Journ.* V. (1809), p. 398. See also Sir James McGrigor, *ibid.* VI. 19.

[3] James Johnson, *Influence of Tropical Climates*, p. 20.

August, 1813, an Irish regiment passing through Leyburn, a small market-town of the West Riding of Yorkshire, in an airy situation, was obliged to leave behind a soldier ill of typhus, who died of the fever after a few days. The infection appeared soon after in the cottages adjoining, and remained in that end of the town for several months, choosing the clean and respectable houses. In a farmer's family, a son, aged twenty-nine, died of it, while another son and two daughters had a narrow escape. The disease appeared also in the village of Wensby, a mile distant, and in other villages. Few lives were lost[1].

These were, perhaps, not altogether solitary instances in Britain of typhus spread abroad by the movements of troops during the great French war. Let us multiply such instances by hundreds, and we shall vaguely realize the meaning of the statement that the period of the Napoleonic wars, and more particularly the period from the renewal of the war in 1803 until its close in 1815, was one of the worst times of epidemic typhus in the history of modern Europe. It was precisely in those years that England, Scotland and Ireland enjoyed a most remarkable degree of freedom from contagious fever.

The Distress and Epidemic Fever (Relapsing) following the Peace of 1815 and the fall of wages.

The long period of comparative immunity from typhus near the beginning of the 19th century was first broken, both in Great Britain and in Ireland, by the very severe winter of 1814–15; but it was not until the great depression of trade following the peace of 1815 (which made a difference of forty millions sterling a year in the public expenditure) and the bad harvest of 1816 that typhus fever and relapsing fever became truly epidemic, chiefly in Ireland but also in Scotland and England. The lesson of the history is unmistakable: with all the inducements to typhus from neglect of sanitation in the midst of rapidly increasing numbers, there was surprisingly little of the disease so long as trade was brisk and the means of subsistence abundant. The reckoning came in the thirty years following the Peace.

[1] J. Terry, in *Ed. Med. and Surg. Journ.*, Jan. 1820, p. 247.

In London, says Bateman[1], the epidemic began in the autumn of 1816, before the influence of scarcity was acutely felt, in the courts about Saffron Hill, the same locality in which he mentioned fever in the winter of 1813–14 among the poor Irish. But this means little more than that the Irish, whether in Ireland or out of it, are the first to feel the effects of scarcity in producing fever. At the very same time that it began among them in Saffron Hill, it began among some young people at a silk factory in Spitalfields. In March, 1817, there was a good deal more of it in Saffron Hill, as well as among the silk-weavers in Essex Street, Whitechapel, in Old Street, in Clerkenwell, and in Shadwell workhouse. Many poor-houses, and especially those of Whitechapel, St Luke's, St Sepulchre's and St George's, Southwark, were getting crowded in 1817 with half-starved persons, among whom fever was rife in the summer and autumn. There was also much of it in the homes of working people in the eastern, north-eastern and Southwark parishes, with more occasional infected households in Shoe Lane, Clare Market, Somers Town and St Giles's in the Fields ("in the filthy streets between Dyot Street and the end of Oxford Street")[1]. The hospitals and dispensaries were fully occupied with fever, and the new House of Recovery in Pancras Road, with accommodation for seventy patients, was soon full. At the Guardian Asylum for young women, more than half of the forty inmates were seized with the fever in one week. The cases were on the whole milder than in ordinary years; of 678 admitted to the House of Recovery in 1817, fifty died or 1 in 13·5. In two-thirds of these patients the fever lasted two weeks or to the beginning of the third week; of the remaining third, a few lost the fever on the 7th, 8th or 9th day, a larger number on the 12th to the 14th day, while a considerable number kept it to the end of the third week or beginning of the fourth. Of the whole 678, only 75 had a free perspiration, and in only 19 of these was the perspiration critical so as to end the fever abruptly. The fever relapsed in 54 of the 678, a proportion of relapsing cases which seemed to Bateman to be "remarkably great[2]." In most

---

[1] Bateman, *Account of the Contagious Fever of this Country.* Lond. 1818.
[2] The following from the "Observations on Prevailing Diseases," Oct.—Nov., 1818 (perhaps by Dr Copland), in the *London Medical Repository*, x. 525, shows that the relapses in the earlier part of this epidemic had been commonly remarked in London: "Fevers are still prevalent...Relapses have been noticed as of frequent occurrence in the instances of the late epidemic. To what are these to be attributed?

the symptoms continued without break throughout the illness. Besides other febrile symptoms, there were pains in the limbs and back, aching of the bones, and soreness of the flesh, as if the patients had been beaten. There was a certain proportion of severe complicated cases of typhus. Bateman held that the differences in type depended on the differences of constitution, giving the following reason for and illustration of his opinion :

"Thus, in the instance of a man and his wife who were brought to the House of Recovery together, the former was affected with the mildest symptoms of fever, which scarcely confined him to bed, and terminated in a speedy convalescence; while his wife was lying in a state of stupor, covered with *petechiae* and *vibices*; in a word, exhibiting the most formidable symptoms of the worst form of typhus. Yet these extreme degrees of the disease manifestly originated from the same cause; and it would be equally unphilosophical to account them different kinds of fever and give them distinct generic appellations as in the case of the benign and confluent smallpox, which are generated in like manner from one contagion." Besides this woman, only eight others had petechiae.

The House of Commons Committee were unable to find out with numerical precision how much more prevalent the fever was in 1817–18 than in the years preceding[1]. To their surprise they found that in six of the general hospitals of London, which admitted cases of fever, "no register is kept in the hospital to distinguish the different varieties of disease." The apothecary of St Luke's Workhouse told them that he attended, on an average of common years, about 150 cases of fever; in the last year [1817] the number rose to 600 ; and they were assured by several besides Bateman, that the great decrease of the deaths from "fever" in the London bills of mortality during a space of fourteen years at the beginning of the century (1803–17), was not a mere apparent decrease, from the growing inadequacy of the bills, but was a real decrease.

The epidemic which began in 1817 continued in London throughout the years 1818 and 1819, chiefly in the densely populated poorer quarters of the town. Two instances of the London slums of the time came to light before the House

Are we to ascribe them to the influence of the atmosphere, to anything in the nature of the disorders themselves, or to the vigorous plans of treatment which are adopted for their removal? These relapses are more common in hospital than in private practice...It has recently become the fashion to consider the state of recovery from fever as one which will do better without than with the interposition of the cinchona bark. Has the prevalence of this negative practice anything to do with the admitted fact of frequent relapse?"

[1] *Report of the Select Committee of the House of Commons on Contagious Fever*, Parl. Papers, 1818.

of Commons Committee on Mendicity and Vagrancy in 1815–16: firstly, Calmel's Buildings, a small court near Portman Square, consisting of twenty-four houses, in which lived seven hundred Irish in distress and profligacy, neglected by the parish and shunned by everyone from dread of contagion; and, secondly, George Yard, Whitechapel, consisting of forty houses, in which lived two thousand persons in a similar state of wretchedness. The dwellings of the poorer classes in London at this period, before the alleys and courts began to disappear, were described thus generally by Dr Clutterbuck[1]:

"The houses the poor occupy are often large, and every room has its family, from the cellar to the garret. Thirty or forty individuals are thus often collected under the same roof; the different apartments must be approached by a common stair, which is rarely washed or cleansed; there are often no windows or openings of any kind backwards; and the *privies* are not unfrequently within the walls, and emit a loathsome stench that is diffused over the whole house. The houses are generally situated in long and narrow alleys, with lofty buildings on each side; or in a small and confined court, which has but a single opening, and that perhaps a low gateway: such a court is in fact little other than a well. These places are at the same time the receptacles of all kinds of filth, which is only removed by the scavenger at distant and uncertain intervals, and always so imperfectly as to leave the place highly offensive and disgusting."

In England, generally, this epidemic of 1817–19 is somewhat casually reported. One writes from Witney, Oxfordshire, "on the prevailing epidemic," which began there in July, 1818, among poor persons, in crowded, filthy and ill-ventilated situations. At first it was like the ordinary contagious fever of this country, "a disease familiar to common observation"; but afterwards it showed choleraic and pneumonic complications. Sometimes the parotid and submaxillary glands were inflamed; petechiae were absent[2]. The type of fever at Ipswich in the spring of 1817 was contagious (e.g. six cases in one family) and sthenic, or of strong reaction, admitting of bloodletting, according to the teaching which Armstrong, Clutterbuck and others had been reviving for fevers[3]. Those instances, one from Oxfordshire the other from Suffolk, must stand for many. Hancock says that the fever of 1817–19 "visited almost every town and village of the United Kingdom[4]." Prichard says that

[1] *On the Epidemic Fever at present prevailing.* Lond. 1819, p. 40.
[2] J. B. Sheppard, "Remarks on the prevailing Epidemic." *Edin. Med. Surg. Journ.*, July 1819, p. 346. Also for Taplow, Roberts, *Lond. Med. Repos.* XIV. 186.
[3] W. Hamilton, M.D., *Med. and Phys. Journ.*, June 1817, p. 451.
[4] *Laws and Phenomena of Pestilence,* Lond. 1821, p. 39. Christison says: "All great towns, with the exception it is said of Birmingham."

it began in Ireland, "where the distress was most urgent, and afterwards prevailed through most parts of Britain," some of the more opulent also being involved in the calamity. As to its prevalence in the manufacturing towns of Yorkshire we have ample testimony. The Leeds House of Recovery, which had not been fully occupied at any time since its opening in 1804, received 178 cases in 1817, and 254 in the first ten months of 1818. Of the latter, 66 came from low lodging-houses, of whom upwards of 50 were strangers. Of 50 admitted in January, 1818, 20 came from four or five lodging-houses in March Lane, and from another locality equally bad—Boot and Shoe Yard; while the rest of the 50 in that month came from houses and streets in the same vicinity. March Lane was one of the worst seats of the great Leeds plague in 1645. By the month of April, 1820, the epidemic had decreased a good deal in Leeds, the cases becoming at the same time more anomalous[1].

The following is one of the Rochdale cases:

June 2, 1818, Alice Eccles, a delicate young woman living in a crowded and filthy court from which fever had not been absent for nearly a year, was bled to ten ounces, purged, and recovered. On September 20th the same woman returned, desiring to be bled again. She was labouring under her former complaint; "since her last illness she had been repeatedly exposed to contagion, or rather, she had been living in an atmosphere thoroughly saturated with infectious effluvia, the house in which she resided, and generally the room in which she slept, having had one or more cases of fever in them," and the windows kept closed[2].

At Halifax in the summer of 1818, typhus (or relapsing fever) had increased so much that fever-wards were added to the Dispensary. It had been alarmingly fatal in a high-lying village near Settle. It was prevalent in Ripon, Huddersfield and Wakefield; and had been brought from Leeds to Atley. A Bradford physician visited 27 cases of fever in one day at a neighbouring village. Throughout Yorkshire, it was confined to the lower orders, and was not very fatal[3]. At Carlisle it began about July, 1817, and became somewhat frequent in the winter and spring following; of 457 cases treated from the Dispensary 46 died, or 1 in 10[4]. At Newcastle, a mild typhus (typhus mitior) broke out in the autumn of 1816, not in the poorer quarters, but mostly among the domestics of good

[1] Adam Hunter, *Edin. Med. Surg. Journ.*, Apr. 1819, p. 234, and Apr. 1820.
[2] Wood, "Cases of Typhus." *Edin. Med. Surg. Journ.*, April, 1819.
[3] Adam Hunter, u. s.
[4] T. Barnes, *Edin. Med. Surg. Journ.*, April, 1819.

houses in elevated situations. There was much privation at Newcastle, as elsewhere, at this time, among the poor. Murchison takes this fever of the autumn of 1816 at Newcastle to have been enteric or typhoid; but it is described as a simple continued fever, with vertigo, headache, and bloodshot eyes, lasting from five or six days to four or five weeks, ending usually without a marked crisis, and causing few deaths[1]. The epidemic continued in Newcastle for three years, the admissions to the Fever Hospital from 4 Sept. 1818, to 4 March, 1819, having been 160, with 12 deaths. Dr McWhirter wrote, in April, 1819, that he saw on his rounds as dispensary physician "too many of the obvious causes of fever," including the filth and wretchedness of the poor inhabitants : "one rather wonders that so many escape it than that some are its victims[2]."

Thus far there has been little besides Bateman's essay to indicate the nature or type of the fever in England. In Ireland it was to a large extent relapsing fever, and, as we shall see, it was so also in Scotland. Bateman found less than a tenth part of the cases at the London Fever Hospital to have relapses, which was an unusually large proportion, in his experience. Elsewhere in England the tendency to relapse was either wanting or the relapses were described or accounted for in other ways; to understand this it has to be kept in mind that the epidemic was the occasion of a great revival of blood-letting, a practice which had fallen into disuse in fevers since the last half of the 18th century, and was something of a novelty in 1817. The fever of that year was undoubtedly abrupt in its onset, strong, "inflammatory," with full bounding pulse, beating carotids, hot and dry skin, intense headache, suffused eyes, and the like symptoms, which seemed to call for depletion. The common practice was to bleed *ad deliquium*, which meant to ten, or fourteen, or twenty ounces, at the outset of the fever. There was hardly one of the writers upon the epidemic, unless it were Bateman, an advocate of the cordial and supporting regimen, who did not consider the stages or duration of the fever as artificially determined by the blood-letting, and not as belonging to the natural history.

In order to show how much the treatment by blood-letting dominated the view of the fever itself, of its type, its stages,

[1] H. Edmonston, *ibid.* XIV. (1818), p. 71.
[2] T. McWhirter, *ibid.* April, 1819, p. 317.

or duration, I shall take the Bristol essay of Prichard, who adopted phlebotomy, as he says, at first tentatively and with some fear and trembling, but at length practised it vigorously, having found it to answer well[1]. The epidemic of fever in Bristol began about June, 1817, and lasted fully two years. The first cases brought to St Peter's Hospital, which was the general workhouse of the city, were of wretched vagrants found ill by the wayside or abandoned in hovels. About the same time forty-two felons in the Bristol Newgate, "one of the most loathsome dungeons in Britain, perhaps I might say in Europe," were infected, of whom only one died, and he of a relapse. From June, 1817, to the end of 1819, there were 591 cases in the poor's house, 647 in the General Infirmary, and 975 treated from the Dispensary, making 2213 cases, of which a record was kept. But there were also many cases in private practice among the domestics, children, and others in good houses, such as those on Redcliff Hill. The cases in the poor's house were classified by Prichard as follows:

	1817	1818	1819
Simple Fever	22	45	40
with cephalic symptoms	24	27	25
„ pneumonic symptoms	7	10	16
„ gastric symptoms	3	11	5
„ enteric symptoms	3	4	5
„ hepatic symptoms	5	3	3
exhausted and moribund	1	6	4
not characterised	30	44	2
	95	150	105
Of these there died	20	16	11

The "genuine form," or ground-type, according to Prichard, was "simple fever," of which the cases with cephalic symptoms were merely the more protracted or more serious. "The pneumonic, hepatic, gastric, enteric and rheumatic forms may be regarded as varieties"—the gastric and hepatic being cases mostly in summer with jaundice, the enteric in autumn and winter with diarrhoea and dysentery. Nearly all these patients were bled within four or five days from the commencement of the disease: "in a very large proportion of the cases the fever was immediately cut short"; when it did not end thus abruptly,

[1] J. C. Prichard, M.D., *History of the Epidemic Fever which prevailed in Bristol,* 1817–19. Lond. 1820.

its symptoms declined gradually, and the attack was over within eight or ten days. After the blooding "sleep very frequently followed, and a partial or sometimes a complete remission of the symptoms." Only one case of relapse is mentioned, No. 118, of the year 1818, and that was a relapse in a very prolonged case: the patient was admitted on 6 October, had a relapse on 18 November, and was discharged on 23 December. Prichard has not one word in his text to suggest relapsing fever; the bulk of his cases were simple continued fever, with or without cephalic or other local symptoms, ending in four, six, eight or ten days, while some were cases of *typhus gravior*. The fever was undoubtedly contagious: it spread through whole families, and in St Peter's Hospital itself it attacked seventy of the ordinary pauper inmates, including a good many lunatics.

The Epidemic of 1817–19 in Scotland : Relapsing Fever.

Let us now turn to the epidemic in Scotland, where the relapsing type was as marked as in Ireland, if not more so. The destitution in the Scots towns in the autumn of 1816, and following years, was fully as great as anywhere in the kingdom, although the peasantry of Scotland were not famine-stricken, as those of Ireland were. The state of the poorer classes in Edinburgh was graphically set forth in an essay by Dr Yule, in 1818[1], and in an article in *Blackwood's Magazine* the year after. Vigorous efforts to relieve the distress were made by the richer classes, and a special fever-hospital was opened at Queensbery House, the admissions to which, together with the fever-cases at the Royal Infirmary, were as follows :[2]

Year	Admitted	Died	Ratio of deaths
1817	511	33	1 in 15$\frac{14}{33}$
1818	1572	75	1 in 21
1819	1027	30	1 in 34
(to 1 Dec.)			

Of this epidemic several accounts were published at the time, including one by Welsh, superintendent of the fever hospital, which is dominated, like the Bristol account of Prichard, by the idea that blood-letting cut short the fever[3]. Christison,

[1] *Obs. on the Cure and Prevention of the Contagious Fever now in Edinburgh.* Edin. 1818.
[2] *Edin. Med. Surg. Journ.* XVI. 146.
[3] Benj. Welsh, *Efficacy of Bloodletting in the Epidemic Fever of Edinburgh.* Edin. 1819.

who had experience of the relapsing form in his own person[1], describes also two other forms mixed with the cases of relapsing fever: a mild typhus, the *typhus mitior* (*typhus gravior* being exceedingly rare in that epidemic), and a form which began like the inflammatory relapsing *synocha*, and gradually after a week put on the characters of mild typhus.

The admissions for fever to the Glasgow Infirmary, which was then the only charity that received fever cases, had been at a somewhat low level since the last epidemic in 1799–1801. They began to rise again with the distress of 1816 :—

Admissions for Fever, Glasgow Infirmary.

Year	Cases	Year	Cases
1814	90	1819	630
1815	230	1820	289
1816	399	1821	234
1817	714	1822	229
1818	1371	1823	269

At the height of the epidemic in 1818 an additional fever hospital was opened at Spring Gardens, to which 1929 cases were admitted in that and the following year. Great efforts were made in Glasgow to "stamp out" the contagion by disinfectants and removal to hospital[2]; but the course of the epidemic seemed to follow the economic conditions more than anything else.

The outbreak at Aberdeen was later than in the south of Scotland, having begun in August, 1818. The infection was said to have been brought to the city by a woman who found a lodging in Sinclair's Close. A group of houses in the close, covering an area of seventy by fifty feet and containing one

[1] *Life of Sir Robert Christison,* Edin. 1885, I. 142 :—"I had been scarcely three weeks at my post in the fever hospital when I was attacked suddenly—so suddenly, that in half-an-hour I was utterly helpless from prostration. I had nearly six days of the primary attack, then a week of comfort, repose and feebleness, and next the secondary attack, or relapse, for three days more. My pulse rose to 160, and continued hard and incompressible even at that rate. My temperature under the tongue was 107° &c." He was bled to 30 oz. and next day to 20 oz. more. Before the end of the epidemic, in August, 1819, he had another attack of relapsing fever, for which he was bled to 24 oz. and a third, after exposure to chill, the same autumn, which last was a simple five-days' fever without relapse, also treated by the abstraction of 24 oz. of blood. In 1832 he had two attacks of the same *synocha* without relapses, and throughout the rest of his life many more: e.g. 16 June, 1861, "I have had something like the relapsing fever of my youth"—a five-days' fever with a relapse on the 18th day; and again, on 19 March, 1868, "Incomprehensible return of mine ancient enemy." These experiences coloured Christison's view of relapsing fever, the so-called relapses being, in his opinion, comparable to the returning paroxysms of ague.

[2] Cleland.

hundred and three inmates, became the first centre of the fever. The scenes described are like those of the Irish epidemics: in one room, a man, his wife, and five children were lying ill on the floor; in another, a man, his wife and six children; in a third, a young girl, whose mother had just died of fever, was left with three infant brothers or sisters. More than three-fourths of the denizens of the close were " confined to bed in fever, and all the others crawling about during the intervals of their relapses." The value of all the furniture and clothing belonging to 103 persons could little exceed £5. There was a horrible stench both within and without the houses (relapsing fever being remarkable for its odour). Yet this close was usually as healthy as any other part of the town. A House of Recovery, with sixty beds, was opened in the Gallowgate, and thirty beds were given up to fever-cases in the Infirmary of the city. Besides those ninety hospital cases at the date of 17 December, 1818, it was estimated that were three hundred more. Begging had been put down, so that the contagion had not spread to the richer classes. Despite these removals to hospital, the epidemic became more general about the New Year, 1819, and of a worse type; two physicians died of it, and some others had a narrow escape. At the outset, the fever had been of the relapsing kind—"subject to relapses for a third and fourth time, more especially when they return too early to their usual labour[1]." At a later period the epidemic seems to have become ordinary typhus, as it did also in Ireland and elsewhere; and it was called typhus in the essay upon it by Dr George Kerr[2].

The extent of this epidemic of 1818–19 over Scotland generally is not known; but the following notice of it in a country parish of Forfarshire was probably a sample of more that might have been given.

Early in the summer of 1818 an epidemic of continued fever appeared in a manufacturing village seven miles from Lintrathen; it attacked at first young and plethoric subjects, and ran through whole families. In August it reached Lintrathen parish, in which one practitioner had forty cases, with no deaths. The fever was of an inflammatory nature; the bulk of the cases fell in October, and were nearly all of young women. They were bled to syncope, which then meant usually to 32 ounces. There was a prejudice

[1] Report signed A. Brebner, provost, printed in Harty, *Historic Sketch of the Contagious Fever in Ireland*, 1817–19. Dublin, 1820, Appendix, p. 110.
[2] *Memoir concerning the Typhus Fever in Aberdeen*, 1818–19. By George Kerr, Aberdeen, 1820.

against blooding among the old people, who said "they had had many fevers, and in their time no such thing was ever allowed." But, according to the doctor, this withholding of the lancet had the effect of protracting their illnesses : "they toasted sick for six weeks, and were often confined to bed for months[1]."

The epidemic of 1817–19 brought into prominence two questions, the one theoretical, the other practical. The theoretical question (not debated at the time) was touching the place or affinities of relapsing fever in the nosology. Christison maintained that it was the inflammatory fever, or *synocha* of Cullen, showing a peculiar tendency to relapse. The fever of the same epidemic period in England was also undoubtedly a fever of strong or inflammatory reaction, corresponding to Cullen's definition of *synocha*, but it relapsed much less frequently than in Ireland and Scotland in the same years. Even in Ireland and Scotland there were always many cases of "relapsing fever" which did not relapse. The law of its relapses was reduced to great simplicity by a physician learned in fevers, Dr John O'Brien, in the Dublin epidemic of 1827. The bulk of that epidemic was a fever of short periods—three, five, seven or nine days, most of the attacks ending on the fifth or seventh night of the fever. The attack being ended in a free perspiration, there might or might not happen, after an interval, a relapse, and again a relapse after that, or even a third. The five-days' fever was more liable to relapse than the seven-days' fever, the seven-days' fever more liable than the nine-days' fever, the fevers of the longest periods not liable at all. In other words, the sooner the patient "got the cool," by a night's sweating, the more liable he was to have one or more relapses[2].

The logical position of relapsing fever was completed by Dr Seaton Reid, of Belfast, when he proposed, in his account of the epidemic in 1846–7, to call it Relapsing Synocha[3]. Other fevers have shown a tendency to relapse in certain circumstances. Three fevers which have many points in common, the sweating sickness, dengue and influenza, are all subject to relapses. It was doubtless of the sweating sickness that Sir Thomas More was thinking when he wrote : "Considering there is, as physicians say, and as we also find, double the peril in the relapse that

---

[1] William Gourlay, "History of the Epidemic Fever as it appeared in a Country Parish in the North of Scotland." *Edin. Med. and Surg. Journ.*, July, 1819, p. 329, dated 20 Nov. 1818.

[2] *Trans. K. and Q. Cal. Phys. Ireland*, v. 527.   [3] *Dub. Q. J. Med. Sc.* VIII. 297.

was in the first sickness." Plague, also, might relapse, or recur in an individual once, twice, three times, or oftener in the same epidemic season. Enteric is an instance of a long-period fever which has at times a tendency to relapses[1]. None of these, however, can dispute the claim of relapsing synocha to be relapsing fever *par excellence*. For whatever reason, the short period fever of times of distress and dearth or famine has shown a peculiar tendency to relapse, and has shown that tendency more in the 19th century than in the 18th, and more among the Irish and Scotch poor than among the English.

The practical question that came to the front in the epidemic fever of 1817–19 was that of isolation hospitals for the sick. It was thus stated by Dr Millar, of Glasgow, in a letter of advice to the authorities of Aberdeen :

"It is only by a universal, or nearly universal sweep of the sick into Fever Hospitals, joined to a universal or nearly universal purification of their dwellings, that anything is to be hoped for in the way of suppressing our epidemic. So far as this grand object is concerned, all the rest is folly: it is worse than folly[2]."

This was the well-meant but somewhat fanatical application of a trite and commonplace notion. It was well understood by reflective persons at that time, who were quite sound on the contagiousness of fever, that the whole question of segregating the poor in fever hospitals was beset with difficulties, not merely of expense but also of expediency. A Select Committee of the House of Commons sat upon it in 1818, and published their report, with the minutes of evidence, on the 20th May. So much had been said in Parliament by Peel and others, and said so truly, of the spreading of fever all over Ireland by whole families turned adrift in beggary, that the Select Committee were full of ideas of contagion, and of the great opportunity of suppressing fever by destroying its germs or seeds. But they had soon occasion to learn that a fever may be potentially contagious, yet not contagious in all circumstances, and that segregation in fever hospitals had a rival in dispersion through general hospitals. Half-a-dozen London physicians of position, answering respectively for Guy's, St Thomas's, the London, St Bartholomew's, St George's, the Westminster and the

---

[1] A succession of thirty-one cases of relapsing typhoid at Charing Cross Hospital in 1877–78 were made the subject of an able essay by J. Pearson Irvine, M.D., *Relapse of Typhoid Fever*, London, 1880.

[2] Cited in Aberdeen Report, 17 Dec. 1818, in Harty, App. p. 110.

Middlesex Hospitals, declared that they mixed their cases of contagious fever in the ordinary wards among the other patients; and when asked by the astonished Committee whether the fever did not spread, they answered one after another with singular unanimity, "Never," which under cross-examination, became in one or two instances, "hardly ever," as, for example, in the evidence for St Thomas's Hospital, where a sister and a nurse had caught fever and died.   The point of this London evidence was that the great safeguard against febrile contagion was free dilution with air, and that the great provocation of a contagious principle was to "concentrate" the cases of fever[1].   The Bristol experience in the same epidemic, although it did not come before the Select Committee, was wholly in agreement with medical opinion in London.   The fever-cases there were received either into St Peter's Hospital, which was the city poor-house, or into the General Infirmary.   The former was an old irregular building, badly ventilated, in which the contagion spread freely to the ordinary inmates and became very virulent.   Contrasting with the apartments of the old poor's house, the wards of the Bristol General Infirmary were spacious, lofty, well-ventilated:

"Here the patients labouring under fever were dispersed among invalids of almost every other description; so that, whatever effluvia emanated from infected bodies became immediately diluted in the mass of air free from such pollution. Here, accordingly, no instance occurred of the propagation of fever. None of the nurses were attacked, nor were patients lying in the adjacent beds in any instance infected, though cases of the worst description, some of them exhibiting all the symptoms of typhus gravior, were placed promiscuously among the other patients, scarcely two feet of space intervening between the beds[2]."

The same practice was kept up in the Edinburgh Infirmary until 1858 or longer; Christison, who gives a diagram of an ordinary ward with four fever-beds in it, declared in 1850 that there had been no spread of fever for fifteen years before, except on one occasion, when the rules of the house were neglected[3].   The bold policy of dispersing fever-patients among the healthy was begun by Pringle and Donald Monro during the campaigns of 1742–48 and 1761–63 in the Netherlands and North Germany.   They found that concentration raised the contagion to high degrees of virulence and that dispersion

[1] *Report of Select Committee*, u. s. p. 6, and minutes of evidence.
[2] Prichard, pp. 74, 88.
[3] Christison, *Month. J. Med. Sc.* x.; Bennett, *Princip. and Pract. of Med.* 944–5.

weakened it to the point of non-existence, Monro's success at Paderborn in 1761 having been of the most signal kind[1].

The Select Committee of 1818 were more influenced by what they were told of the good effects of the earliest Houses of Recovery, at Waterford, Manchester and other places in the end of the last century. For several years after their opening they were little needed, the epidemic which gave the immediate impulse to their establishment having subsided in due time both in the towns provided with Houses of Recovery and in the innumerable places where no such provision had been made. The recommendations of the Committee do not appear to have been carried out; for the London Fever Hospital, in Pancras Road, which had been enlarged to seventy beds when the epidemic began in 1817, remained the only special fever hospital in London until the establishment of the hospitals of the Metropolitan Asylums Board in 1870[2].

The confusion of commerce, depression of trade and lack of employment which followed the Peace of Paris, and gave occasion to the British and Irish epidemic fevers of 1817–19, gradually righted themselves. The price of wheat, which would have been still higher after the four-months drought of 1818, but for large imports, gradually fell, and was about 50s. in 1821, and 40s. in the winter of 1822–23. After that, it rose somewhat again, and the third decade of the century, in the middle of which occurred the great speculative crash of 1825, was on the whole a hard time for the working classes. The history of fever has few illustrations between the epidemic of 1817–19 and that of 1826–27, excepting the great famine-fever of Connemara and other parts of the West of Ireland

---

[1] See above, p. 110–11.

[2] A complementary measure, namely, notification of contagious sickness to the authorities, was put in practice at Leeds in 1804 on the opening of the House of Recovery there. The Leeds House of Recovery, with fifty beds, was opened on 1 November, 1804, the epidemic of fever being then about over. One of its officers was an inspector, whose duty was "to detect the first appearance of infection, to cause the removal of the patient to the House of Recovery, and to superintend the fumigating and whitewashing of the apartment from which he is removed. So great is the solicitude of the physicians to promote early removal that rewards are offered to such as shall first give information of an infectious fever in their neighbourhoods." It was claimed that this had been a great success, Leeds having been for twelve years previous to the epidemic of 1817 nearly exempted from two of the most infectious and fatal diseases, namely, typhus and scarlet fever. (It happened, however, that the whole of England, Scotland and even Ireland were exempted to the same remarkable, and of course gratifying degree.) Whitaker, *Loidis and Elmete*, 1816, p. 85.

in 1822, elsewhere described, which coincided with a somewhat prosperous time in England and called forth a princely charity[1].

The Relapsing Fever of 1827–28.

The epidemic of relapsing fever which was at a height in Dublin in 1826, did not culminate in Edinburgh, Glasgow. and other towns of Scotland until 1828. It was a somewhat close repetition of the epidemic of 1817–19, except that it was chiefly an affair of the towns, owing to depression of trade and want of work following the great crash of commercial credit in 1825–26. In Glasgow, the admissions for fever to the Royal Infirmary began to rise in 1825[2]:

Glasgow: Admissions for Fever.

Year		Year	
1824	523	1828	1511*
1825	897	1829	865
1826	926	1830	729
1827	1084*		

* Some of these were treated at the extra fever-hospital in Spring Gardens.

At Edinburgh the cases of fever treated in hospital were fewer in ordinary years than at Glasgow, but they rose to a higher point in the epidemic years[3]:

Edinburgh: Admissions for Fever.

Year		Year	
1824	177	1828	2013
1825	341	1829	771
1826 (nine months)	456	1830	346
1827	1875		

[1] A strange epidemic of the early summer of 1824 in a semi-charitable girls' school at Cowan Bridge, between Leeds and Kendal, which is the subject of a moving chapter in 'Jane Eyre,' was inquired into by Mrs Gaskell, the biographer of Charlotte Brontë. Forty girls were attacked with fever. A woman who was sent to nurse the sick, saw when she entered the school-room from twelve to fifteen girls lying about, some resting their heads on the table, others on the ground; all heavy-eyed and flushed, indifferent and weary, with pains in every limb, the atmosphere of the room having a peculiar odour. The symptoms, so far as known, and the circumstances of the school, point more to relapsing fever than to typhus, which is the name given to it by Charlotte Brontë. None died of the fever (it is otherwise in the tale), but one girl died at home of its after-effects. Dr Batty, of Kirby, who was called in, did not consider the type of fever to be alarming or dangerous. The dietary of the school had undoubtedly been most meagre for growing girls, and its discipline severe. The house was old and unsuited for the purposes of a boarding-school.

[2] Cowan, *Journ. Statist. Soc.* III. (1840) p. 271; *Glas. Med. Journ.* III. 437.

[3] From the table by Christison, *Edin. Med. Journ.*, Jan. 1858, p. 581.

Christison gives the following account of the epidemic in Edinburgh in 1827–28:

"Like that of 1817–19, it arose in Edinburgh during a protracted period of want of work and low wages among the labouring classes and tradespeople; it prevailed only among the working classes and unemployed poor—in the Fountainbridge and West Port districts, the Grassmarket 'closes,' the Cowgate and the narrow 'wynds' descending on either side of the long sloping back of the High Street and Canongate." The fever had the same three types as in 1817–19—many cases of inflammatory, or relapsing, or synocha, a few of low fever (typhus), and some between the two—militant or inflammatory for a week, then becoming low, and running the continuous course of typhus..."The inflammatory fever presented the same extreme violence of reaction as in the former epidemic—the same tendency to abrupt cessation, with profuse sweating—the same liability to return abruptly a few days afterwards—and the same disposition to depart finally in a few days more, and again abruptly with free perspiration. The cases of typhus were more frequently severe than in 1818–19. Icteric synocha occurred also oftener, although far from frequently[1]."

The epidemic of relapsing fever in 1826–28, which made a great impression in the towns of Ireland and Scotland, has left few traces in specially English records. But it is clear that there was some increase of fever about the same time in London; and it becomes a matter of interest, as well as of no little difficulty, to ascertain the type or types of the same. It was just after this quasi-epidemic in London that Dr Burne published his essay on fevers, the preface bearing the date of 28th February, 1828[2]. The materials of this essay came from Guy's Hospital, and they were both clinical and anatomical. The author seeks to find a common name for all varieties of continued fever, the name that he chooses being "Adynamic Fever." "By far the greater number of cases," he says, "are of the first or second degree only of severity, and not dangerous." These were cases of "simple continued fever," or fever of short duration, with flushed face, suffused eyes and other signs of the "inflammatory" type, or of synocha. Although Burne does not give the exact proportion of cases with relapse, as Bateman had done for the London epidemic of 1817–18, yet he makes it clear that relapses did occur, and he discusses the phenomenon in a manner which makes his testimony interesting: "Convalescents are more liable to a relapse after the adynamic fever than after any other disease; and this may be accounted for by the very enfeebled and exhausted state in which the powers

[1] *Life of Christison,* "Autobiography."
[2] John Burne, M.D., *Pract. Treatise on the Typhus or Adynamic Fever.* London, 1828.

of the system are left." His relapses were obviously a return of the original fever, beginning again suddenly in the midst of convalescence with flushing of the face, headache, dry tongue, and scanty urine, and with a great access of febrile heat in the night, a disturbance of the system which generally continued for several days, while in some it went off sooner with a diarrhoea. He assigned three principal causes for the relapse —overloading the enfeebled but craving stomach, walking out in the open air too soon, and giving way to emotion[1].

The references to relapse apply almost certainly to fevers of the shorter periods (synocha or "inflammatory" fever), and not to those cases of enteric fever which did undoubtedly occur in the practice of Guy's Hospital in the same seasons.

Typhoid or Enteric Fever in London, 1826.

The identification of enteric fever and relapsing fever respectively, or the separation of each from typhus, became actual in Britain at one and the same time. I have already said all that seems necessary as to the earlier appearances of relapsing fever on the stage of epidemiological history. This will be the fitting point in the chronology, the third decade of the 19th century, to bring in the question of enteric or typhoid fever. As to its identification, or recognition as a distinct species, that was not really completed, to the satisfaction of everyone, until the elaborate analysis of the symptoms respectively of typhus and enteric fevers by Sir William Jenner in 1849–51[2]. But, for ten years before that, the co-existence with maculated typhus of a different long-period fever, having abdominal symptoms and abdominal lesion, had been recognised,

[1] To show the effect of emotion in causing a relapse, he gives an instance, almost the only concrete illustration in all his book: An Irishwoman, Ann McCarthy, aged 26, was admitted to Guy's Hospital on 20 June, 1827, with "adynamic fever of the second degree," having been already ill for two weeks: the course of her fever was favourable and she was "soon convalescent." While still in the ward mending her strength, she lent her bonnet to another female patient to go out with; finding that her kindness had been abused by the woman forgetting to return the bonnet, she became exceedingly angry, relapsed into the fever on the 10th of July, was wildly delirious for several days, and died on the 19th of July. At this time it was the practice at Guy's to examine the bodies after death; but permission was refused in the case in question, so that Burne was unable to say "whether the bowels were affected." The case, therefore, may have been one of relapsing enteric fever. A similar ambiguity is discussed by Hughes Bennett in his *Principles and Practice of Physic* (p. 923), and decided in favour of relapsing fever proper, or relapsing synocha.
[2] Sir William Jenner, M.D., *Lectures and Essays on Fevers and Diphtheria,* 1849 to 1879. London, 1893.

and the characteristic ulceration or sloughing of the lymph-follicles of the ileum, with sphacelation of the mesenteric lymph-glands, had been clearly described by several London physicians and depicted in coloured plates, in the years 1826 and 1827, during an unusual prevalence of such cases in London. The authentic history of enteric fever in Britain really begins with these writings by physicians of St George's and Guy's Hospitals. But, as it is improbable that the type of fever was absolutely new in the years 1825 and 1826, it may be asked whether the enteric type cannot be discovered in the old accounts of British fevers, and if so, whether we may assume in the past as much enteric fever relatively to spotted typhus, relapsing fever, or simple continued fever, as in the period after 1850.

Having adverted to this point from time to time in the preceding history as it arose, for example in connexion with Willis's fever of 1661, Strother's fever of 1727–29, the Rouen fever of 1750, and other instances both in children (remittent or convulsive or comatose fever of children) and in adults, I shall not recapitulate farther back than the beginning of the 19th century.

There was a certain amount of post-mortem observation in the 18th century, especially in camp sicknesses, by Pringle and others; but there is no trace of intestinal ulceration among their fatal fevers. It was found, however, in the epidemic of 1806 among the troops at Deal, and it is probable that Ferriar's cases at Manchester about 1804, and Bateman's cases of continued fever in London from 1804 to 1816, were in some part enteric, although the anatomical test is wanting. That was a period when there was singularly little of the old London fever in the houses of the poorer class. Then came the remarkable "constitution" of relapsing or simple continued fever, from about 1816 to 1828, the relapsing character of which was far more obvious in Ireland and Scotland, than in London, Bristol, or elsewhere in England, but was not altogether unobserved in London, whether in 1817–19 or in 1827–28. The relapsing type disappeared after that for fifteen or twenty years, and was replaced by typhus more maculated than had been seen for many years. But, before the relapsing or simple continued fever disappeared for a time, enteric fever was seen in London in company with it.

The chief season of enteric fever in London was the autumn of 1826, following a long period of great drought and heat. The remarkable weather of that season was the same in England, Ireland and Scotland, and is thus described for the last by Christison :

"The spring and summer seasons of that year were remarkable for the extraordinary drought and heat which prevailed for many continuous months. No such seasons could be recollected by anybody, and assuredly there has been nothing similar in this country since....The fine weather set in with the beginning of March, and continued, with scarcely a check, well into the autumn....The drought prevailed and the heat increased till the middle of June, when a thunderstorm with heavy rain cooled the air for a day or two. But the heat then became greater than ever, and there was continuous sunshine and no rain till after the middle of July, when again there was thunder and rain, after which sun, heat and drought ruled the season once more." The shade temperature at Edinburgh was 84° Fahr., at 3 p.m. on three successive days of July[1]. The two summers preceding had also been exceptional, that of 1824 having been hot and moist, that of 1825 hot and dry, with dysentery in Dublin.

In August, 1826, Dr Cornwallis Hewett, of St George's Hospital, published ten fatal cases of enteric fever, four of which had occurred in his own practice, six in the practice of his colleagues[2]. The first was admitted on 23 April, 1825, the latest on 3 July, 1826. While his paper was under hand, he had read in the *Medico-chirurgical Review* for July, 1826, some extracts from Bretonneau's paper on "Dothiénentérite" (enteric fever), and he pronounced the London cases to be the same as those recently observed at Tours. Several other cases occurred at St George's Hospital in the autumn of 1826, three of them reported by Dr Chambers[3]. At the very same time, there was a run of enteric cases at Guy's Hospital. Dr Bright says: "Fever occurred with considerable frequency among the patients who presented themselves for admission into Guy's Hospital, during the months of October, November and December, 1826. On the whole, the disease was not severe." The more comprehensive account of these cases was given by Burne, early in 1828, from which it appears that the bulk of them were fevers of the shorter period, that there were relapsing cases among them, and that some were cases of enteric fever, verified by post-mortem

[1] Christison, *Life*, u. s. I. 341.
[2] "Cases showing the frequency of the occurrence of Follicular Ulceration in the Mucous Membrane of the Intestine during the progress of Idiopathic Fever, with Dissections, and Observations on its Pathology." *Lond. Med. and Physical Journ.*, Aug. 1826, p. 97.
[3] *Ibid.* p. 351.

examination[1]. It was the enteric cases that attracted the notice of Dr Bright, who says nothing of the relapsing cases, or of cases of simple continued fever. The fact that the intestinal mucous membrane may become diseased during fever was, he says, "long known in particular cases, but never suspected to be so general till brought into view by the French physicians, and which has lately been illustrated in this country with great beauty [this does not mean in plates] by the pens of my able and assiduous friends Dr Chambers and Dr Hewett." He gives ten fatal cases, with coloured plates of the intestinal or mesenteric lesion in some of them, the earliest coloured plate having been made from a case admitted on 13 October, 1825, and the most typical plate of the sloughing Peyer's follicles from a case admitted on 25 November, 1826. He gives also eleven cases of recovery, to show the benefit of treating the diarrhoea by calomel[2]. Nearly all the cases occurred in the end of the year, either of 1825 or 1826; and Burne confirms this when he says that the cases with enteric lesion were found at Guy's Hospital only in autumn. Some two years after, in 1830, Drs Tweedie and Southwood Smith, physicians to the London Fever Hospital, described cases of fever with ulcerated intestine and sphacelated mesenteric glands. After that, the interest shifted to typhus, which reappeared in London of an unusually maculated type; so that the years 1826–30 make a somewhat distinct period in which the new fever, with enteric lesion, was an engrossing medical topic. It is tolerably certain that it was the unusual seasons of 1825 and 1826 which brought enteric fever into prominence; while, as soon as it became frequent, it could hardly have escaped the systematic apparatus of clinical case-taking and post-mortem examination, with preservation and drawing of specimens, for which Guy's Hospital was already noted under the influence of Bright and his colleagues, and in which the staff of St George's Hospital would appear to have been not less competent. Although Dr Hewett, in 1826, identified his cases with the *dothiénentérite* of Bretonneau, yet neither he nor Dr Bright took the abdominal ulcerations or sloughs as distinctive of a new kind of fever. They regarded them rather as a new complication of "idiopathic" typhus fever, a "complication" which appealed to them more on the side

[1] Burne, u. s.
[2] Richard Bright, M.D., *Reports of Medical Cases.* Part I., 1827.

of treatment than of systematic nosology; hence the writings of both physicians are occupied mainly with the benefit of calomel in relieving the congestion of the bowels and in checking the diarrhoea.

It is undoubted that cases of enteric fever in 1826–27 were relatively more numerous in London than in Dublin and Edinburgh, where the epidemic fever was almost wholly of the relapsing type. In Edinburgh, at least, the comparative in-frequency of enteric fever for years after it had been recognized in Paris, Tours and other French cities, and had been found in London as a common autumnal type, can be proved beyond cavil. Writing long after of the first epidemic of relapsing fever in Edinburgh, Christison said :

"Of enteric typhus (typhoid fever) we saw nothing then [1817–20], nor for many years afterwards. If it might have been overlooked during life, it could not have been missed after death. For our dissections were many, and, to meet the bias of the day for finding a local anatomical cause for all fevers [the doctrine of Broussais], every important organ in the body was habitually looked to. Nevertheless we were constantly met with the want of morbid appearances anywhere, unless slight signs of vascular congestion in various membranous textures be considered such[1]."

These vascular congestions were, indeed, scanned closely for traces of ulceration, after Bright's plates of 1828, and any little irregularity on the surface of a congested Peyer's patch was liberally construed in that sense, as in Craigie's reports subsequently. But in the Edinburgh epidemic of 1827–29, the anatomical signs of enteric fever were wanting until the end of it. Writing in 1827, Alison said that he had dissected 26 cases dead of the epidemic fever, without finding intestinal ulceration in one of them. Christison, however, says that a very few cases of enteric fever were dissected in Edinburgh in 1829[2].

In Dublin, also, the anatomical mark of enteric fever was missed in 1826–27, in the few dissections that were made during the epidemic[3]. An opinion in a widely different sense was given on that point by Stokes twelve years after the event, to which I refer in a note[4].

[1] *Life of Sir Robert Christison*, I. 144. Also in *Trans. Soc. Sc. Assn.* 1863, p. 104.
[2] *Edin. Med. Journ.*, Jan. 1858, p. 588. Cf. *infra*, under Dysentery, 1828.
[3] Reid, *Trans. K. and Q. Coll. of Phys. in Ireland*, v.; O'Brien, *ibid.*
[4] Writing in 1839, Dr Stokes, of Dublin, made the following remarkable assertion (*Dub. Journ. Med. and Chem. Sc.* XV. p. 3, note): "In the epidemic of 1826 and 1827 we observed the follicular ulceration (dothienenteritis of the French) in the greater number of cases." As the epidemic of 1826–27 was almost wholly one of relapsing

Return of Spotted Typhus after 1831: "Change of Type."
Distress of the Working Class.

A fever with relapses, and a fever with sloughing of the follicles and lymph glands of the intestine, were not the only novelties in the first thirty or forty years of the 19th century. Relapsing fever and enteric or typhoid fever were each clearly separated, at a later date, from typhus fever. But what was the "typhus fever" from which they were at length separated? It was a fever which came prominently into notice after the "constitution" of 1826–29 was ended—a fever with a mottled, measly, or rubeoloid rash, and with variou. . ... spots, on account of which it was described by Dr Roupell in 1831, in a lecture before the College of Physicians of London, as a "new fever[1]." It was a new fever only in the sense in which each new febrile "constitution," whether it were an influenza, an epidemic ague, or a malignant typhus, was apt to be called popularly "the new fever," in the 16th and 17th centuries. There were, of course, erudite men at the College of Physicians in 1831 who knew that a fever with a mottled rash, with vibices and petechiae, and with all other symptoms of typhus gravior, had often occurred in England, Scotland and Ireland in former times. The "spotted fever" was perhaps the most familiar name of typhus in the 17th century. The mottled rash, like that of measles, was described for the fever of Cork by Rogers in the beginning of the 18th century, and for various other English and Irish epidemics by Huxham, O'Connell, Rutty and others. But undoubtedly the maculated typhus was somewhat new to the generation who saw it about 1830 and following years, the continued fevers which had prevailed in England, Scotland and

---

fever, the statement is at least puzzling. It was made twelve years after the epidemic, at a time when the discrepancies between British and French observers, as to the occurrence of ulceration of the ileum in continued fever, were much discussed. Dr Lombard, of Geneva, having visited Glasgow, Dublin and other places, and confirmed the fact that the characteristic lesion of enteric fever was at that time only occasional, went on to say that Irish typhus was a species of disease by itself, a *morbus miseriae*. Whereupon the editor of the 'Dublin Journal of Medical Science' (XII. 503, in a review of Cowan's Glasgow Statistics) gave the following truly Irish reply: "Had Dr Lombard made more inquiries, he would have found that Ireland is not so sunk in misery and debasement but that she can produce occasionally a fever which, in abdominal ulcerations, can compete with the sporadic diseases of her wealthier and more enlightened neighbours." It may have been in the same patriotic spirit that Stokes declared "the greater number of cases" in the epidemic of 1826 and 1827 to have had follicular ulceration.

[1] G. L. Roupell, M.D., *Some Account of a Fever prevalent in* 1831. Lond. 1837.

Ireland since 1816 having been for the most part the simple continued, or synocha, with or without the relapsing character, and to some extent enteric fever[1].

It was from 1830 to 1834 that a change in the reigning type of fever began to be remarked in London, Dublin, Edinburgh and Glasgow, the new type becoming more and more evident as fevers became more prevalent in the 'thirties' and 'forties.' Typhus at length became so much a spotted fever that the question arose whether it should not be classed among the exanthemata. In 1840, Dr Charles West, having observed "the alteration in character which fever has undergone within the last few years," went over the history (but more the foreign than the English) with a view " to illustrate the question whether typhus ought not to be classed among the exanthematous fevers[2]:" of course he found many old descriptions of a mottled rash or other spots, but saw no reason to make spotted typhus one of the exanthemata. Dr Kilgour, of Aberdeen, who treated more than a thousand cases in his fever-ward at the infirmary there from 1838 to 1840, wrote in 1841, "I am perfectly satisfied that this fever, call it by what name we will, is truly an exanthematous fever[3]." Previous to 1835, the spots of fever-cases in the Glasgow Infirmary had hardly been remarked; but after that date all cases were classed either as spotted or not, the spotted cases being three-fourths of the whole. Besides being spotted, the fever of the new constitution was insidious in its approach and low in its reaction, very unlike the sthenic, militant, inflammatory synocha of the generation before. The blood-letting which had been all but universally used in the fever from 1816 to 1828, and had seemed to answer well, was continued for a time in the fever of the 'thirties.' But it was soon found to be injurious: the patients in the new fever were apt to faint when only a few ounces of blood (four or six) had been drawn, whereas in the other fever (whether relapsing or

[1] In addition to what has been said on this point already, for particular epidemics, I shall give a statement for ordinary years by Dr Carrick, of Bristol, in his ' Medical Topography' of that city: *Trans. Prov. Med. Assocn.* II. (1834), p. 176. "Continued fever is common enough, but nine-tenths of the cases are of a simple character, terminating for the most part within seven days, and unaccompanied with anything more serious than slight catarrhal or rheumatic disorder. Typhus gravior is rare—much more so than might be expected."

[2] Charles West, M.D., "Historical Notices designed to illustrate the question whether Typhus ought to be classed among the Exanthematous Fevers." *Edin. Med. and Surg. Journ.* 1840, April, p. 279.

[3] Alexander Kilgour, M.D., *ibid.* Oct. 1841, p. 381.

simple continued) they had often lost thirty ounces before deliquium was reached. It was found, on the other hand, that fever-cases in the 'thirties' needed wine and other cordial regimen. There was nothing new in these revolutions, whether of the fevers themselves, or of the opinions as to their treatment. Sydenham's method of taking his cue for treatment from the "constitution" of the season, which was the method of Hippocrates, appeared to be once more the best suited to the circumstances.

It is not easy to make out what were the circumstances of the time that led to the supersession of simple continued fever (or relapsing fever in Ireland and Scotland), by spotted fever or typhus gravior in all parts of the kingdom. Sydenham would have looked, among other things, to the weather and the character of seasons; but from 1830 onwards there was no season so notable as the dry and hot summer of 1826, although the end of the year 1836 was remarkably wet. The period of typhus gravior was a time of much sickness of other kinds—the Asiatic cholera of 1831–32, the influenza of 1831, 1833. and 1836–37, and the general unhealthiness of the year 1837. This was also the decade when the "condition-of-England question" was a common topic, a time of strikes and of much distress among the working classes, as shown in the reports of the Poor Law Commission.

In Glasgow there was a considerable prevalence of fevers year after year from the relapsing-fever epidemic of 1827–29, according to the following table of admissions for fever to the Royal Infirmary and the special fever-hospitals[1]:

Admissions for Fever, Glasgow.

Year	Fever cases		Year	Fever cases
1827	1084		1833	1288
1828	1511		1834	2003
1829	865		1835	1359
1830	729		1836	3125
1831	1657		1837	5387[3]
1832	1589) [2]1148}		1838	2047
			1839	1529

The worst year of the series for fever was 1837, and the worst month of that year was May, when the fever-deaths were

[1] Cowan, "Vital Statistics of Glasgow," *Journ. Statist. Soc.* III.
[2] Cases at Mile-End Fever Hospital.
[3] Including 906 male fever-patients at Albion Street temporary hospital.

1 in 3·22 of the mortality from all causes. That great access of fever in Glasgow followed immediately upon the great strike of the cotton-spinners, on 8th April, 1837, by which eight thousand persons, mostly women, were thrown out of work[1]. The death-rate in Glasgow was in those years as high as anywhere in the kingdom, and was higher in the nine years from 1831 than in the nine years preceding. The population of Glasgow, says Cowan, had increased on the industrial side, out of proportion to its middle and wealthiest class[2]; and to that he would attribute the higher death-rates in the second peri·d (right-hand side), of the following table :

Glasgow Death-rates.

	1822—1830			1831—1839	
Year	Death-rate over all. One in	Death-rate under five. One in	Year	Death-rate over all. One in	Death-rate under five. One in
1822	44·4	101	1831	33·8	79
1823	36·4	78	1832	21·67	63
1824	37·0	81	1833	35·7	77
1825	36·3	81	1834	36·3	81
1826	40·6	105	1835	32·6	67
1827	37·0	84	1836	28·9	62
1828	33·0	79	1837	24·6	65
1829	37·9	100	1838	37·9	83
1830	41·5	97	1839	36·1	72

The high death-rates in some of the years in the second column were owing to special causes—Asiatic cholera in 1832, smallpox of children in 1835 and 1836, and to influenza, as well as to typhus, in 1831, 1833 and 1837. As to the fever which prevailed from 1831 to 1836, as it was not relapsing in type, so it was not associated with scarcity.

"The increase of fever in Glasgow," says Cowan, "during the seven years prior to 1837, had taken place, not in years of famine or distress, but during a period of unexampled prosperity, when every individual able and willing to work was secure of steady and remunerating employment. From the close of 1836, one of those periodical depressions in trade, arising from the state of our monetary system, had visited this city, and deprived a large proportion of the population of the means of subsistence[3]."

It was then that the cases of typhus trebled in number.

[1] *Blackwood's Magazine*, March, 1838, p. 289.
[2] In 1819 the Irish in Glasgow had been estimated at 1 in 9·67: in 1831 the Irish part of the population had risen to 1 in 5·69. Dr Cowan, however, said of them: "From ample opportunities of observation, they appear to me to exhibit much less of that squalid misery and habitual addiction to the use of ardent spirits than the Scotch of the same grade."
[3] Robert Cowan, M.D., "Statistics of Fever in Glasgow for 1837." *Lancet*, April 10, 1839.

The epidemic of fever reached its height in Dundee about the same time as in Glasgow, and in both towns sooner than anywhere else in Scotland or England. One reason of this was the labour-troubles culminating in strikes. In the twelvemonth from 15 June, 1836, to 12 June, 1837, more than three-fourths of all the admissions to the Dundee Infirmary on the medical side were for fever (700 cases). After the wet autumn of 1836 there were a good many cases of dysentery, of which 22 were treated in the infirmary, with two deaths[1].

At Edinburgh, as at Glasgow, there had been an unusual amount of fever in 1831 and 1832, and a steady prevalence of it thereafter. The epidemic of 1836–39 was for the most part typhus of the winter seasons, declining each spring and disappearing each summer, except in the   of 1836, when many cases came in June, July and August from airy parts of the town[2]. The climax of the epidemic was in 1838, a year later than in Glasgow and Dundee, according to the admissions to the fever-wards of the infirmary[3]:

Admissions for Fever, Edinburgh Infirmary.

Year	Cases	Year	Cases
1831	758	1836	652
1832	1394	1837	1224
1833	878	1838	2244
1834	690	1839	1235
1835	826	1840	782

At Aberdeen the epidemic appears to have been later even than at Edinburgh, if the following admissions to one of the two fever-wards (Dr Kilgour's) may be taken as a fair measure of it[4]:

Admissions for Fever, Aberdeen.

Year	Cases	Deaths
1838 (March to December)	189	26
1839	286	29
1840	534	53

In all these large towns of Scotland, the fever was purely typhus. The various observers all describe the fever as of the spotted kind, the proportion of cases with spots varying somewhat.

[1] James Arrott, M.D., *Edin. Med. and Surg. Journ.*, Jan. 1839, p. 121.
[2] Craigie *ibid.* April, 1837.
[3] Christison, *Monthly Journ. Med. Sc.* x. 1850, p. 262.   [4] Kilgour, u. s.

Thus, at Glasgow Infirmary, from 1835 to 1839, there were 4202 cases with eruption, 1270 without eruption, and 143 doubtful. And, that the cases without eruption were not cases of enteric or typhoid, is probable from the record kept of the fatalities in Dr Anderson's fever-wards[1]:

In 1885 cases with eruption,   275 deaths, or 14·58 per cent.
  ,,   324 cases without eruption,   11 deaths, or 3·33 per cent.
  ,,   143 cases doubtful,   7 deaths, or 4·89 per cent.

At Aberdeen, Kilgour counted 59 cases spotted in a total of 189 in 1838, 96 in a total of 286 in 1839, and 278 in a total of 534 in 1840, all the cases, whether spotted or not, being of the same fever, which he considered an exanthematous malady as a whole. Of 169 cases tabulated by Craigie at Edinburgh, from 28 June, 1836, to 12 February, 1837, there were 79 with an eruption, which was usually the mottled or rubeoloid rash.

The fatalities were relatively more in Edinburgh than in Dundee, comparing two periods which were not the same. Of 700 cases at Dundee, from June, 1836, to June, 1837, only 50 died, or 1 in 14, notwithstanding a good many complications from chest complaints and bowel complaints[2]. At Edinburgh during fifteen months of 1838–39, there died 276 in 2037 cases, or 1 in 7·3; of those cases, 1075 were in females, with 116 deaths, or 1 in 9, and 962 males, with 160 deaths, or 1 in 6[3]. The most common age for the fever at Dundee was from twenty to forty years (416 out of 700 cases, with 26 deaths, or 1 in 16), while the most fatal age, as usual, was from forty to sixty years, at which one person died of three attacked. At Aberdeen, in the last year of the epidemic, the years of life from ten to twenty had more cases (233 in a total of 657) than any other decade of life. The average stay of a patient in the Aberdeen fever-wards was 18·67 days. The great preponderance of deaths in adolescents or adults was clearly shown in the Glasgow fever-statistics, 1835–39.

Deaths from typhus fever	Under ten years	Over ten years	Fever-deaths per cent. of deaths from all causes
4788	752	4036	11·57

The corresponding epidemic of typhus in England had the fortune to be recorded in great part under the new system of Registration, which came into force on the 1st of July, 1837. At the beginning of registration of the causes of death, and until a good many years after, no distinction was made in the published tables between typhus fever and enteric fever. But we happen to know that the epidemic of 1837–38 was in London

---

[1] Cowan, *Journ. Statist. Soc.* III. 1841.
[2] Arrott, u. s.   [3] Craigie, u. s.

almost wholly typhus, just as it was in the large towns of
Scotland. Of sixty cases in 1837–38, of which notes were kept
by West, under Latham at St Bartholomew's Hospital, none
that died and were examined post-mortem had ulcerations,
although some had congestion, of Peyer's patches, the cases
being all reckoned typhus exanthematicus[1]. Sir Thomas Watson,
who was then physician to the Middlesex Hospital, says of the
ulceration of Peyer's patches in continued fever:

"Since attention has been drawn to the subject, the patches of glands,
and the whole tract of mucous membrane, from the stomach to the rectum,
have been diligently explored, and the result seems to be that, at certain
times and places (in other words, in certain epidemics), the ulceration of the
inner surface of the intestine is far less common at some than at others. It was
comparatively rare in an epidemic of which I witnessed some part in
Edinburgh [1827–29]. Then I came to London; and for several years I
never saw a body opened after death by continued fever without finding
ulcers of the bowels. More recently, however, and especially during the
present epidemic (1838), I have looked for them carefully, in many cases
that have proved fatal in the Middlesex Hospital, and have discovered
neither ulceration nor any other apparent change in the follicles of the
intestines." And elsewhere he confirms the purely typhus character of the
epidemic of 1838: "Our wards at the Middlesex are full of it, and scarcely
a case presents itself without these spots. We speak of it familiarly as the
spotted fever; or, from the resemblance which the rash bears to that of
measles, as the *rubeoloid* fever[2]."

From which it would appear that not even the ordinary
average number of endemic cases of enteric fever, such as might
have been expected at a hospital in the west end of London,
were forthcoming in the epidemic of 1837–38, so purely was the
type of fever typhus.

The deaths from this epidemic in London, from the 1st of
July, 1837, to the 31st of December, 1838, were as follows[3]:

1837		1838			
3rd Quarter	4th Quarter	1st Quarter	2nd Quarter	3rd Quarter	4th Quarter
826	1107	1285	1176	829	788

—a total of 6011 deaths from fever, nearly all typhus, in eighteen
months. The worst London parishes were Whitechapel and St
Pancras, in which latter the fever-hospital was situated. The
high mortality from fever, which had begun before the 1st of
July, 1837, continued into the year 1839, when the deaths in
London (probably including some enteric) were 1819.

[1] *Edin. Med. and Surg. Journ.* July, 1838.
[2] *Principles and Practice of Physic,* 3rd ed. 1848, II. 742, 732.
[3] *First Report of the Registrar-General,* London, 1839.

Over all England and Wales, including London, the last six months of 1837 produced 9047 deaths from "typhus," and the twelve months of 1838, 18,775 deaths, the winter of 1837–38 having been the most fatal period. After London, the large towns most affected by the epidemic in the latter half of 1837 were as follows :

	Deaths from typhus in six months		Deaths from typhus in six months
Liverpool	524	Dudley	54
Manchester and Salford	274	Abergavenny	53
		Wolverhampton	45
Birmingham	75	Newcastle	44
Bolton	75	Wigan	43
Sunderland	72	Chorley	41
Leeds	71	Swansea	36
Sheffield	68	Halifax	33
Bradford	65	Macclesfield	33
Stockport	63	Norwich	27

In each of the next two years the number of deaths from typhus in the four largest towns was as follows :

	Typhus deaths in 1838	Typhus deaths in 1839
Manchester and Salford	627	416
Liverpool	573	358
Leeds	245	150
Birmingham	123	141

From nearly all the registration districts of England and Wales, deaths from fever were returned in 1837–39, so that the contagion must have been very widely spread in town and country[1]. In London the epidemic declined greatly in 1839, but in many parts of England the deaths registered as "typhus" were hardly less numerous than in 1838, and in some country divisions they were more, as if the contagion had taken longer to reach the villages[2]. One village epidemic in North Devon in the latter half of the year 1839 had been observed by Dr W. Budd, afterwards of Bristol :

[1] The district registrars had hardly organised their work in the first two or three years of registration. Some gave much more complete returns than others. There was a reluctance to register births, and the marriages were not all registered. But the totals of deaths came out very nearly as the actuaries had expected.

[2] The Third Report of the Registrar-General gives the mortality in all parts of England from typhus in 1839 (as well as from scarlatina) in an elaborate table of the registration districts and sub-districts.

The first case in the village (North Tawton, 1100 to 1200 inhabitants) was of a young woman in a poor and crowded cottage, who sickened on 11 July, 1839; her mother, brother, and sister sickened in succession, her father and a young infant escaping the infection. In another cottage, four out of six were ill of fever, in another, three persons had it, and so on, the whole number of cases treated by Dr Budd in the village until the beginning of November being about eighty. It was carried from North Tawton to neighbouring hamlets: thus, a sawyer who lodged next door to the first infected cottage sickened of the fever and, on 2 August, returned to his home in the hamlet of Morchard. As he lay there, he was visited by a friend, who assisted to raise him in bed: "While thus employed, the friend was quite overpowered by the smell from the sick man's body," and on the tenth day thereafter sickened of fever, which spread to two of his children and to a brother who came from a distance to see him. Another sawyer who lodged with the former left North Tawton ill a week after him (9 August) for his home, also at Morchard, where he died after a period not stated; ten days after his death his two children took the fever, his widow escaping it. In a third instance, a widow L—— left North Tawton on 21 August to visit her brother, a farmer in the hamlet of Chaffcombe, seven miles distant. Two days after her arrival she fell ill of fever and recovered slowly. In the same farmhouse the mistress caught it a month or two later and died on 4 November; the farmer himself took to bed with the fever on the day his wife died, and came safe through the attack. Three weeks after, an apprentice on the farm sickened, then a lad (the fifth in order) in the end of December, then the farmer's sister, then another apprentice, then a serving-man, then a maidservant, and lastly the daughter of the widow L—— from North Tawton, who had been the first case in the house months before. This farmhouse at Chaffcombe sent off two distinct offshoots of contagion. The lad, who was fifth in the above series, was sent home ill to his mother's cottage, between Bow and North Tawton, in the end of December. His mother sickened on 24 January, 1840, and died on 2 February. Next door to her lived a married daughter, whose whole household were attacked. Another married daughter, who came from a distance to visit the sick, took the infection on her return home, and so started a new focus. From the same farm at Chaffcombe, the maid, who was ninth in order in the above series, was sent home to her father's cottage in the hamlet of Loosebeare, four miles away; her father caught the fever from her, and a farmer K——, who lived across the road, having visited this man several times in his illness, took the fever next, other cases following under farmer K's. roof, and thereafter throughout the whole hamlet of Loosebeare[1].

---

[1] W. Budd, M.D., *Lancet*, 27 Dec. 1856, and 2 July, 1859. Dr Budd, who had been studying in Paris and seeing much typhoid fever, but little or no typhus, in the service of Louis at La Pitié hospital, took the whole of these cases for enteric or typhoid, and insisted, in his later life, on the ground of his North Tawton experiences in 1839, that typhoid fever spread by contagion. He published numerous papers on this theme (*Lancet*, 27 Dec. 1856, another series in the same journal from 2 July to Nov. 1859, *Brit. Med. Journ.* Nov.-Dec. 1861 and, finally, a volume of reprints with additions, *Typhoid Fever, its Nature, Mode of Spreading and Prevention*, London, 1873). But he published no clinical cases nor post-mortem notes, to make good his 1839 diagnosis, on which the whole matter turned, contenting himself with an assurance that he knew typhoid well from studying it under Louis (who, at that time, believed that the typhus of armies, gaols, &c. and of the British writers, was the same as the fever which he, and others after him, named typhoid). He also made the following six statements, as if he were making affidavit: (1) that the great majority of the cases had early diarrhoea, (2) that three had profuse intestinal haemorrhage, (3) that more or less of tympanitis was almost universal in the epidemic, (4) that in nearly every case he found the rose-coloured lenticular spots, (5) that one case, which was the only one examined post-mortem, had the characteristic ulceration of the intestine,

This was doubtless the way the epidemic spread in all the country districts of England, the unwholesome state of labourers' cottages, as revealed in the reports of the Poor Law Commission, favouring it.   In the chapter on the fevers of Ireland we shall find that the contagion of typhus and relapsing fever was dispersed in the same way, but to a much greater extent, owing to the amount of vagrancy.

In the manufacturing towns of the North of England the fever continued at a somewhat steady epidemic level for several years.   The pathetic scenes of typhus among the poor of Manchester in Mrs Gaskell's famous tale of *Mary Barton* belong to the early part of the year 1839; but they might have been drawn from almost any months of the two or three years following, according to the passage cited below from the same work[1].

and (6) that one fatal case had the symptoms of perforation of the gut. This summary manner, asking in effect to be taken on trust, is not usually accepted from innovators, none of the great discoverers having resorted to it.   Hitherto, however, no one has thought proper to question Budd's diagnosis of the epidemic fever in his North Tawton practice, nor even to remark upon his strange error of treating the epidemic of 1838-39 all over Britain as purely one of typhoid (*Lancet*, 27 Dec. 1856).   But everyone knew that typhoid fever did not spread in the way that he described (doubtless correctly for the above cases).   After the publication of his book in 1873 an attempt was made by an influential layman in the *Times* (9 Nov. 1874) to popularize Budd's fallacies or paradoxes on the contagiousness of typhoid.   "How," it was asked, after a summary of the North Tawton epidemic in 1839, "could a disease whose characters are so severely demonstrable, have ever been imagined to be non-contagious? How could such a doctrine be followed, as it has been, to the destruction of human life?"

1 "For three years past trade had been getting worse and worse, and the price of provisions higher and higher.   This disparity between the amount of the earnings of the working classes and the price of their food occasioned, in more cases than could well be imagined, disease and death.   Whole families went through a gradual starvation.   They only wanted a Dante to record their sufferings.   And yet even his words would fall short of the awful truth; they could only present an outline of the tremendous facts of the destitution that surrounded thousands upon thousands in the terrible years 1839, 1840, and 1841.   Even philanthropists who had studied the subject were forced to own themselves perplexed in their endeavour to ascertain the real causes of the misery; the whole matter was of so complicated a nature that it became next to impossible to understand it thoroughly....The most deplorable and enduring evil that arose out of the period of commercial depression to which I refer, was this feeling of alienation between the different classes of society.   It is so impossible to describe, or even faintly to picture, the state of distress which prevailed in the town [Manchester] at that time, that I will not attempt it; and yet I think again that surely, in a Christian land, it was not known even so feebly as words could tell it, or the more happy and fortunate would have thronged with their sympathy and their aid.   In many instances the sufferers wept first, and then they cursed.   Their vindictive feelings exhibited themselves in rabid politics.   And when I hear, as I have heard, of the sufferings and privations of the poor, of provision shops, where ha'porths of tea, sugar, butter, and even flour, were sold to accommodate the indigent—of parents sitting in their clothes by the fireside during the whole night for seven weeks together, in order that their only bed and bedding might be reserved for the use of their large family—of others sleeping upon the cold hearthstone for weeks in succession, without adequate means of providing themselves with food or fuel—and this in the depth of winter—of others being compelled to fast for days together, uncheered by any hope of better fortune, living, moreover, or rather starving, in a crowded garret, or damp

In 1839 the Lancashire deaths from typhus were 1343; in Wales, Monmouth and H·refordshire they were 1548. There is, indeed, little improvement in the statistical returns as late as 1842. The deaths from "typhus" were as follows in all England and Wales:

1838	1839	1840	1841	1842
18,775	15,666	17,177	14,846	16,201

The deaths from the epidemic maladies of infants and children during the same five years were also very high.

	1838	1839	1840	1841	1842
Smallpox	16,268	9,131	10,434	6,368	2,715
Measles	6,514	10,937	9,326	6,894	8,742
Hooping cough	9,107	8,165	6,132	8,099	8,091
Scarlatina	5,802	10,325	19,816	14,161	12,807
Croup	4,463	4,192	4,336	4,177	4,457
Diarrhoea	2,482	2,562	3,469	3,240	5,241

The epidemic of smallpox corresponded closely to the epidemic of fever, the former being fatal chiefly to infants and young children, the latter fatal chiefly to adults. Before the smallpox epidemic had subsided scarlet fever became unusually mortal, especially in 1840, and kept its higher level of deaths for a generation after. The epidemic of fever, although it affected the mortality of the young comparatively little, was indirectly a reason why many of them died of other diseases; for the prostration of the parents, the impoverishment, and all the other troubles associated with an epidemic of typhus, led to inevitable sufferings among the young, which weakened their power of resistance.

The registration returns were not tabulated (except for London) from the end of 1842 to the beginning of 1847, but there is reason to think that the epidemic fever was not active in the interval. It is undoubted that the enormous construction of railroads in England during those years gave employment and wages to multitudes, and ended the distress the sooner. This effect of railroad-making in England was so obvious that Lord George Bentinck desired to relieve the distress in Ireland in 1846–47 by the same means.

Enteric Fever mixed with the prevailing Typhus, 1831–42.

While there is complete agreement among the hospital physicians of the great towns that the fever of 1837–39 was maculated typhus, to the total exclusion of cases with ulceration

cellar, and gradually sinking under the pressure of want and despair into a premature grave; and when this has been confirmed by the evidence of their careworn looks, their excited feelings, and their desolate homes—can I wonder that many of them, in such times of misery and destitution, spoke and acted with ferocious precipitation?" Mrs Gaskell, *Mary Barton.*

of the bowel, as in the experience of Watson at the Middlesex Hospital and of West (under Latham) at St Bartholomew's, yet some allowance should be made, in interpreting the figures of fever mortality in those years throughout England and Wales, for admixture of enteric fever. Budd's statement that the only case which was dissected in the epidemic at North Tawton, Devonshire, in 1839, had the bowel-lesion of enteric fever, if it is to count in the absence of the usual details (place, date, objective description), would mean that at least one case there was not of the prevailing type of contagious epidemic typhus. The coincidence of some such cases is made the more probable by the evidence from Anstruther, Fifeshire, reported by John Goodsir, afterwards Professor of Anatomy at Edinburgh, who was assisting his father in practice there from 1835 to 1839. During that period, which was the time of the typhus epidemic in the larger towns of Scotland, he attended about one hundred cases of fever annually in Anstruther and the neighbourhood; the fever was usually mild, only some sixteen of the cases having proved fatal; of those sixteen he examined ten after death, finding "ulceration" of the Peyer's patches in all, and perforation of the intestine in four of them. These facts he gave orally to Dr John Reid, pathologist to the Edinburgh Infirmary, whose experience of the morbid anatomy of fever was altogether different. Goodsir, having kept the specimens, made them the subject of a paper some years after (1842), in which he described very minutely the stages and degrees of congestion, ulceration, sloughing and perforation in the lymph-follicles of the intestine in fever, placing congestions at one end of the scale and sloughing at the other, as the French pathologists then did[1]. Reid examined, at the Edinburgh Infirmary from October, 1838, to June, 1839, forty-one bodies dead of fever, to see whether the intestinal lesion, which Goodsir had told him of, occurred in them. The distinctness of the Peyer's patches varied a good deal (differences which are known to be in part congenital and in part to depend on age), and in only two instances were they elevated and seemingly "ulcerated."

[1] John Goodsir, "On a Diseased Condition of the Intestinal Glands," *Lond. and Edin. Monthly Journ. of Med. Science*, April, 1842. He does not enter on the question "as to whether the subject of the present paper constitutes a distinct species of disease, or be merely a form of the ordinary continued fever"; but he appears to recognize that a certain district may have a form of fever special to it, as Reid had probably told him.

One of these was the case of an Irishman, from Sligo, aged 25, who had been so constipated that he was purged with colocynth, etc.: "at the lower part of the ileum, the elliptical patches were irregular on the surface, and presented sever l superficial and ill-defined depressions (ulcerations)." The other was the case of a girl, aged 15, who had not suffered from diarrhoea, but had the intestinal patches elevated and superficially "ulcerated[1]." Neither of these cases would probably be reckoned typhoid or enteric fever at the present time on the anatomical evidence only. The early French observers, Chomel, Louis, Andral and others, included in a scale all the appearances of the Peyer's patches in fever that they thought morbid, from mere prominence of the lymphatic tissue and distinctness of the follicular pits, up to extensive sloughing and ulceration of the same, as if they were all the signs of one and the same fever in its various stages of development. But simple prominence or congestion of Peyer's patches may occur in typhus fever, or in relapsing fever; nor would a slight erosion, or "superficial ulceration" raise in all cases a suspicion of enteric fever.

The observations of Home, Reid's predecessor as pathologist to the Edinburgh Infirmary, from 1833 to 1837, were however conclusive that true enteric fever had occurred now and again during the steady prevalence of typhus fever from year to year. In that space he made 101 post-mortem examinations in fever-cases; in 29 the Peyer's patches were distinct, in 7 of those 29 there was "a greater or less degree of ulceration," and in 2 of those 7 there was perforation[2]. Murchison examined the post-mortem register of the Edinburgh Infirmary for the years 1833 to 1838, and found only fifteen cases of fever with ulceration of the bowel. But in the eight months from 1 November, 1846, to June, 1847, there were nineteen dissections with the characteristic lesion of typhoid, the season having been remarkable everywhere for that disease.

In the following series of years the fatal cases of fever in the Edinburgh Infirmary with ulceration were few[3]:

Year	Enteric deaths		Year	Enteric deaths
1854	5		1858	1
1855	2		1859	2
1856	1		1860	1
1857	8		1861	6

It was thought remarkable that the form of continued fever which was most usually found in the great continental cities, in Paris, Berlin, Prague and Vienna, namely that with ulceration of the lymph-follicles of the intestine, should be but occasionally mixed with the old typhus in England, Ireland and Scotland

[1] John Reid, M.D., "Analysis and Details of Forty-seven Inspections after Death," *Edin. Med. and Surg. Journ.*, Oct. 1839, p. 456.
[2] Reid, u. s., from Home's records.
[3] Murchison, *Continued Fevers*, 2nd ed. 1873, p. 444.

in the very same years.   But there was nothing to discredit the British observations, anatomical and clinical; and in 1836 Dr Lombard, of Geneva, having visited various cities in England, Scotland and Ireland bore witness to the matter of fact, strange as it was to him.   Writing to Graves, of Dublin, on 16 June, 1836, he said : "Before I leave Ireland, allow me to express to you my great astonishment at what I have seen in this country respecting your continued fever;" and in a second letter, of 18 July, after his return to Geneva, he added, that in Liverpool, ulceration of the ileum in continued fever was "occasional," that in Manchester he had been told it occurred "by no means always," that in Birmingham the cases of fever were not many, but "always" with intestinal ulceration, and that in London "not a fourth part" of the cases of fever had the latter condition, and these mostly in autumn[1].   This was before the great epidemic of typhus had begun in the English towns.   To the same non-epidemic period (1834) belongs the statement of Carrick, for Bristol, that fever was often observed to be infrequent or altogether absent in the most crowded and dirty parts of the city at times when there were a good many cases "in institutions and dwellings where cleanliness and free air are most carefully attended to," and that ulceration of the bowel was the most common post-mortem appearance[2].

The comparative rarity of enteric fever in the chief towns of Scotland and Ireland continued for a good many years longer, indeed until after the differences between typhus and typhoid were perceived and admitted by all.   Even at the London Fever Hospital, during twenty-four years (1848–71) after Sir William Jenner's diagnostic points were strictly looked to in its wards, much the greater part of the admissions were of typhus; in only two periods, 1850–55 and 1858–61, during both of which there was comparatively little fever of any kind in London, did the admissions for enteric fever slightly exceed those for typhus; on an annual average of the twenty-four years ending 1871, the cases of the former were only about a fifth part of the

---

[1] Lombard, in *Dublin Journal of Med. Sc.* x. (1836), p. 17. He bore witness, also, to the rarity of the bowel-lesion in the Glasgow fevers. This was confirmed by Dr Perry, of that city, *Ibid.* x. 381. See also Julius Staberoh, M.D., " Researches on the Occurrence of Typhus in the Manufacturing Cities of Great Britain," *Ibid.* XIII. 426.

[2] *Trans. Prov. Med. Assoc.* II. (1834), p. 176.

whole. The cases of enteric fever increased decidedly after 1865. Murchison thought that the increase might be accounted for in part by the enlargement of the Fever Hospital, and by the unusually high temperature of certain years, the summers and autumns of 1865, 1866, 1868 and 1870 having been remarkable for their great heat and prolonged drought; but, he adds, "it is not a little remarkable that this increased prevalence of enteric fever in the metropolis has been contemporaneous with the completion of the main drainage scheme[1]."

Still more recently, the relative proportions of typhus and enteric fever have been reversed, so that there have been years with little or no typhus but with a good deal of enteric fever. There are some persons, unacquainted with the history, who cannot imagine that it was ever otherwise than now, who think of the former times of medicine, not as differing in social, economic, and various other respects from their own, but only as being less clever at diagnosis. There are others who realize clearly enough the historical matter of fact, but find it necessary to explain the almost contemporaneous decline of typhus and rise of typhoid by some hypothesis of the latter being "evolved" out of the former. This evolutional doctrine makes the mistake of ascribing to the species of disease the same comparative fixity of characters that belongs to the species of animals and plants. Beside the latter, the species of disease are the creatures of a day. In the nosological field, the origin of species is not analogous to the evolution of a new species of animal or plant out of an old, as in the hypothesis of Darwin, for the reason that every species of disease is evolved directly and, as it were, *pro re nata*, out of a few simple conditions of human life, variously mixed but always there to give occasion to one infective malady or another, which may have a shorter existence, like sweating sickness, or a longer, like plague. Edinburgh experiences offer a ready criticism of the evolutional doctrine. Typhus declined, and typhoid rose; but it was in the old tenement houses of the Canongate, Cowgate, Grassmarket, and High Street that typhus declined, and it was mostly in the new streets across the valley, or in the New Town of Edinburgh, that enteric fever arose, having sometimes no more mysterious an origin than the results of defective or cheap plumber-work,

[1] *Continued Fevers*, 2nd ed. 1873, p. 443.

for example, the leakage of a soil-pipe fermenting, a foot deep, beneath the basement floor. But it was not until a good many years after that that these new experiences became common; and meanwhile Edinburgh and other towns in Scotland saw much of typhus and relapsing fever.

Relapsing Fever in Scotland, 1842–44.

The epidemic of 1836–39 had been typhus of a specially maculated kind. The period or "constitution" of synocha, rising twice to epidemics of relapsing fever, had lasted from near the beginning of the century until 1828 or 1829. Then came the new constitution of low, depressed, spotted fever, which would not stand blood-letting. But in 1842–44 relapsing fever reappeared in Scotland. This reappearance was a blow to two doctrines of the time—first that Ireland was the original breeding-place of all such fevers, and secondly, that a return of the "constitution" of relapsing fever would warrant a return to the practice of blood-letting, which had fallen into disuse during the epidemic of typhus. The epidemic of 1842–44 was at first purely a Scots affair, with some extension to England, but none to Ireland. As to blood-letting, once it had been given over in fevers it was not readily taken up again, notwithstanding the theory that relapsing fever belonged to those sthenic or inflammatory types of sickness in which the lancet was still thought admissible. Moreover, Christison, who remembered the relapsing synocha of 1817–19 and of 1827–28, said of the third epidemic: "The synocha of 1843–44, though so prevalent, by no means presented the same strong phlogistic or sthenic character as in the earlier epidemics of 1817–20 and 1826–29. The pulse was neither so frequent nor so strong; the heat was not so pungent; the glow of the integuments was less lively and less general[1]."

I take conveniently from Murchison the following succinct account of the Scots relapsing fever of 1842–44[2]:

"The next epidemic of fever in 1843 differed from those that preceded it, inasmuch as it did not originate in or implicate Ireland, but was mainly confined to Scotland. There was no increase of fever in the Irish hospitals

[1] Christison, "On the Changes which have taken place in the Constitution of Fevers and Inflammations in Edinburgh during the last forty years." Paper read at Med. Chir. Soc. Edin. 4 March, 1857. *Edin. Med. Journ.* Jan. 1858, p. 577.
[2] *Continued Fevers*, under the head of "Typhus," p. 47.

during this year, whereas the number of admissions into the Glasgow Infirmary rose from 1,194 to 3,467; in the Edinburgh Infirmary from 842 to 2,080; and in the Aberdeen Infirmary from 282 to 1,280. These numbers, too, are far from representing the true extent of the epidemic, for thousands of sick were sent from the hospital doors. The fever was almost exclusively relapsing fever; typhus was comparatively rare. The first cases were observed on the east coast of Fife, in 1841-2 (by H. Goodsir), and not in the crowded localities of large towns. In Dundee, where the proportion of typhus cases was comparatively great, the fever appeared early in the summer of 1842, and raged to a considerable extent during the whole of the autumn, before it showed itself elsewhere. In Glasgow the first cases occurred in September, 1842; but the fever was not generally prevalent until December, from which month the cases rapidly increased until October, 1843, when the epidemic began to decline. The number of cases in Glasgow was estimated at 33,000, or 11½ per cent. of the entire population. In Edinburgh relapsing fever was first observed in February, 1843. It rapidly spread until October, after which it gradually abated, until, by the following April, it had well nigh disappeared. In the month of October, 1843, the number of fever cases admitted into the Edinburgh Infirmary amounted to 638, and during several months, from thirty to fifty cases were daily refused admission. The total number of cases in Edinburgh was calculated by Alison at 9,000. In Aberdeen the epidemic commenced about the same time, and followed the same course as in Edinburgh. At Leith, curiously enough, it did not appear until September, 1843; it then spread rapidly for two months, after which it declined, and by the end of February, 1844, it had almost ceased; but during this brief period it attacked 1,800 persons, or one in every fourteen of the population. The disease was general over Scotland, and was not restricted to the large towns; it prevailed in Greenock, Paisley, Musselburgh, Tranent, Penicuick, Haddington, Dunbar, the Isle of Skye, etc. Although the epidemic was mostly confined to Scotland, the same fever was observed in some of the large towns of England. The number of admissions into the London Fever Hospital rose from 252 in the preceding year to 1,385 in 1843: and the annual report for 1843 makes it evident that a large proportion of these cases were relapsing fever. The rate of mortality of the epidemic was small, not exceeding from two-and-a-half to four per cent. Although this was the same fever as prevailed in 1817-19, even local bleeding was rarely resorted to, and many of the cases were thought to demand stimulants. All accounts agree in stating that the epidemic supervened upon a period of great distress among the Scottish poor, and that it was restricted throughout to the poorest and most wretched of the population."

This epidemic, which was the subject of an altogether unusual amount of writing in Edinburgh[1], partly on the supposition that relapsing fever was a "new disease," proved once for all that one had not to go to Ireland for the engendering or making of a famine-fever. The demonstration came just in time; for the epidemic was hardly over in Scotland, when the series of great potato-famines in Ireland began in 1845, soon to be followed by the disastrous epidemics of dysentery, relapsing

[1] See especially John Rose Cormack, M.D., *Natural History, Pathology and Treatment of the Epidemic Fever at present prevailing in Edinburgh and other towns.* Lond. 1843; and the papers by Wardell, *Lond. Med. Gaz.* N. S. II—V.

fever and typhus from 1846 to 1848. Indeed, so near was the Scots epidemic to the Irish, that in the North of Ireland the first of the relapsing fever, in 1846, was called "the Scotch Fever," on the supposition that it had reached them from its recent focus in the West of Scotland[1]. The Irish and original part of the great epidemic of 1846–48 has been fully described in another chapter; much of the mortality was due to dysentery, and the most prevalent fever was relapsing fever, with a very low rate of fatality among the poorer classes. But in Ireland itself there was also much typhus, very mortal to the richer classes who came in contact with the starving multitudes.

The "Irish Fever" of 1847 in England and Scotland.

The contagion that reached England and Scotland from the scene of famine in Ireland was more apt to produce typhus than relapsing fever. That the Irish contagion was the principal source of the great epidemics in England and Scotland in 1847–48, seems to be proved by every fact in their progress, direction and other circumstances. But it is not so clear that England and Scotland would not have had an unusual amount of typhus in the same years even if the Irish had been kept out by an ideally strict quarantine. What touched Ireland most, touched Scotland and England in a measure. The seasons were bad in all parts of the kingdom; many were out of work in the manufacturing towns; but as soon as the price of provisions fell in 1848, the epidemic in England came to a sudden end.

The epidemic of fever in England in 1847 was almost wholly typhus; in Scotland, it was to some extent relapsing fever, but there also it was mainly typhus. It was more severe, while it lasted, than the epidemic of 1837 and following years; but it was of shorter duration, ceasing almost abruptly in 1848. The rise of the epidemic of 1847 in London is shown by the following quarterly returns of the deaths from fever:

1st Quarter	2nd Quarter	3rd Quarter	4th Quarter
442	568	895	1279

In the last quarter of 1846, the deaths from fever in London

[1] Dr Betty, of Lowtherstown, Fermanagh, *Dubl. Quart. Journ. Med. Sc.* VII. 125.

had been·619. In all England, the last quarter of 1846 was also
most unhealthy, its deaths from all causes being 53,055 (only
43,850 in the first quarter of the year). The summer of 1846 had
been remarkable for heat and drought, and the end of the year
was, according to precedent, an unwholesome time. It was just
the season for enteric fever, as in the still more memorable
circumstances of 1826. There is evidence from various parts
of England and Scotland that much of the fever of the end of
1846 was enteric ; and it was doubtless the unusual prevalence
of that disease, and of other maladies that are favoured, like it,
by extreme fluctuations of the ground-water, that explains the
very high mortality of the last quarter of 1846[1]. But it is
equally certain that it was typhus which raised the fever deaths
in London in the last quarter of 1847 to 1,279, and the deaths
from all causes in all England to the enormous total of 57,925.
In the whole of the year 1847, typhus alone claimed 30,320
deaths in England and Wales, the total in 1848 falling to 21,406.
Lancashire and Cheshire had the largest share of this epidemic,
and Liverpool the largest share in Lancashire. In that Registration Division (the North-western) the deaths from typhus in
1847 were 9,076, and in 1848 they were 3,380. Next in order
(excluding London and suburbs) came the West Midland Division, and next to that Yorkshire. At Liverpool, and in other
places of the north-west of England, the fever was very clearly
connected with the enormous Irish immigration, and was in
great part among the Irish. There were floating lazarettos on
the Mersey, filled with fever and dysentery, workhouses over-
flowing, and sheds hastily built to hold each 300 patients. The
following returns from the several sub-divisions of Liverpool
for the months of July, August and September, 1847, show the
proportions of dysentery and fever, as well as the mortality from

[1] Murchison says that the enteric fever of the end of 1846 was prevalent at many
places in England where the epidemic of typhus never made its appearance, and that
in Edinburgh (according to an unpublished essay by Waters) most of the enteric cases
not only occurred prior to the outbreak of the epidemic of Irish fever, but came from
localities in the neighbouring country and from the best houses of the New Town—
not from the crowded courts of the Old Town, to which the later epidemic of typhus
and relapsing fever was restricted. Murchison, u. s. p. 49. The following papers
relate to the autumnal typhoid of 1846 in England : Sibson, " Fever at Nottingham
and neighbourhood in Summer and Autumn of 1846," *Med. Gaz.* XXXIX.; Taylor,
" Fever at Old and New Lenton in 1846," *Med. Times,* XV. 159 and *Med. Gaz.*
XXXVIII. 127; Turner, " Fever at Minchinhampton in Autumn 1846," *Med. Gaz.*
XLII. 157; Brenchley, " Fever in Berkshire in 1846," *Med. Gaz.* XXXVIII. 1082; Bree,
" Epidemic Fever at Great Finborough in Autumn of 1846," *Prov. Med. and Surg.
Journ.* 1847, p. 676.

diarrhoea, which last was mostly an affair of the infants and young children[1]:

Liverpool deaths, July—Sept. 1847.

	Fever	Dysentery	Diarrhoea
St Martin's	291	82	174
Dale Street	250	20	111
St Thomas	(301 deaths on the floating lazarettos)		
Mount Pleasant	324	18	73
Islington	105	37	78
Great Howard Street	(the fever extending to the upper classes)		

In his report for the quarter before (April, May and June, 1847) the registrar of the Great Howard Street sub-district says: "Eight Roman Catholic priests, and one clergyman of the Church of England, have fallen victims to their indefatigable attentions to the poor of their church[2]."

In Manchester there were causes of fever independently of the Irish contagion. The registrar of the Deangate sub-district writes in the third quarter of 1847: "In the calamitous season just passed, manufactures have been almost at a stand-still; food has been unattainable by the poor, for employment they had none; Famine made her dwelling in their homes &c." The hardships of the children caused an immense mortality from summer diarrhoea. The same registrar gives an account of the epidemic fever in his report for the second quarter of 1847, from which it appears that, although nearly all the hospital cases were distinctly maculated, and the fever was undoubtedly typhus in all other respects and in its conditions, yet tympanitis, with abdominal tenderness and diarrhoea, were specially noted[3].

Besides Liverpool and Manchester, many other towns in Lancashire had the "Irish fever" in them; also Birmingham, Dudley, Wolverhampton, Shrewsbury, Leeds, Hull, York and Sunderland. Except in London, the fever mortality was not unusual in the southern half of England[4].

---

[1] In the *Report of the Registrar-General for the year* 1847.

[2] This was the occasion which furnished Father Newman with a famous argument for the *bona fides* of his co-religionists: "The Irish fever cut off between Liverpool and Leeds thirty priests and more, young men in the flower of their days, old men who seemed entitled to some quiet time after their long toil. There was a bishop cut off in the North; but what had a man of his ecclesiastical rank to do with the drudgery and danger of sick calls, except that Christian faith and charity constrained him?" John Henry Newman, D.D., *History of My Religious Opinions*, London, 1865, p. 272.

[3] Leigh, in *Report Reg.-Gen. for* 1847, X. p. xx.

[4] H. M. Hughes, "On the Continued Fever at present existing in the southern districts of the metropolis," *Lond. Med. Gaz.* Nov. 1847; Laycock, "Unusual

In Scotland the epidemic was a mixture of relapsing fever and typhus. The following were the proportions of each admitted to the Glasgow Royal Infirmary:

Year	Relapsing Fever	Typhus
1846	777	500
1847	2,333	2,399
1848	513	980
1849	168	342

In the Barony Fever Hospital, Glasgow, open from 5 August 1847 to July 1848, the relapsing cases were double the typhus cases at the opening of the hospital, at the end of 1847 they were nearly equal, and from February 1848 the typhus cases were double the relapsing. In Edinburgh, where the epidemic was less severe, the same relations were observed—relapsing fever most at the beginning, typhus fever (much more fatal) most at the end[1]. Some relapsing fever occurred also in London, among destitute Irish, which was often attended by a miliary eruption (Ormerod).

Subsequent Epidemics of Typhus and Relapsing Fevers.

By midsummer, 1848, there was a most marked improvement in the public health, corresponding with the great fall in the prices of food, under the influence of free trade, and with a good harvest and the commencement of an era of steady employment for workers. The improvement is strikingly shown in the following comparison of the deaths from all causes in

prevalence of Fever at York," *Lond. Med. Gaz.* Nov. 1847; Bottomley, "Notes on the Famine Fever at Croydon in 1847," *Prov. Med. and Surg. Journ.* 1847; Ormerod, *Clinical Observations on Continued Fever at Bartholomew's Hospital*, Lond. 1848; Art. in *Brit. and For. Med. Chir. Rev.* 1848, I. 285; Duncan, *Journ. Pub. Health*, I. 200 (Liverpool); Paxton, *Prov. Med. Journ.* 1847, pp. 533, 596 (Rugby).
[1] The following papers relate to the epidemic in Scotland in 1847: Orr, "Historical and Statistical Sketch of the progress of Epidemic Fever in Glasgow during 1847," *Edin. Med. and Surg. Journ.* LXIX.; Stark, "On the Mortality of Edinburgh and Leith for 1847," *Ibid.* and LXXI.; R. Paterson, "Account of the Epidemic Fever of 1847-8" in Edinburgh, *Ibid.* LXX.; W. Robertson, "Notes on the Epidemic Fever of 1847-8," *Month. Journ. of Med. Sc.* IX. 368; J. C. Steele, "View of the Sickness and Mortality in the Glasgow Royal Infirmary during 1847," *Edin. Med. and Surg. Journ.* LXX.; J. C. Steele, "Statistics of the Glasgow Infirmary for 1848," *Ibid.* LXXII. 241; J. Paterson, "Statistics of the Barony Parish Fever Hospital of Glasgow in 1847-8," *Ibid.* LXX. 357.

Lancashire and Cheshire in the third quarter of each of the years
1846, 1847 and 1848:

	1846	1847	1848
Deaths in the 3rd Quarter	15,221	17,080	11,720

Since the epidemic of 1847, which was not unfairly called
"the Irish fever," there has been no such extensive and fatal
outbreak of typhus or relapsing fever in England, Scotland or
Ireland.   The fever deaths rose somewhat in Ireland and in
Glasgow in 1851–53, the type of disease being relapsing and
typhus.   In London there was a considerable increase of typhus
in 1856, at the end of the Crimean War.   From 1861 to 1867
there was a considerable epidemic of the same fever in England
and Scotland (not much of it in Ireland until 1864), the chief
centres in England having been the Lancashire towns, Preston,
Manchester, Accrington, Chorley, Salford and Blackburn, and
the occasion of it the "cotton famine" of the American Civil
War[1].   Greenock was the chief seat of typhus in 1863–64 in
Scotland; indeed, in the whole kingdom, its death-rate from that
cause was approached by that of Liverpool only.   Fevers had
been very mortal there in the epidemic of 1847 (it is said 353
deaths); in the next fever-period they rose as follows[2]:

1860	1861	1862	1863	1864
19	57	63	98	274

This epidemic was more easily dealt with than those of the
same kind before it.   Very large sums were subscribed by the
wealthy, of which, indeed, a considerable balance remained
undistributed.   Rawlinson, as engineer, and Villiers, as Minister,
devised extensive relief works, in the form of main drainage for
the distressed Lancashire towns, the whole cost being defrayed
eventually by the municipalities themselves.   The following
table, from Murchison, shows the admissions for typhus to
the fever hospitals of various towns, subsequently to the great
epidemic of 1847–48.   The first rise in London was in 1856;
the next rise, which was somewhat prolonged, coincided with
the epidemic in Lancashire.

[1] Buchanan, *Report Med. Officer Privy Council, for* 1864, and *Trans. Epid. Soc.* 1865,
II. 17; Hamilton, *Lancet,* II. 1867, p. 608 (Liverpool); Martyn, *Brit. Med. Journ.*
July, 1863; Davies, *Med. Times and Gaz.* II. 1867, p. 427 (Bristol); Thompson,
St George's Hosp. Reports, I. (1866), p. 47 (London); Allbutt, *ibid.* p. 61 (Leeds).
[2] Buchanan, *Report Med. Off. Privy Council for* 1865, p. 210.

C. II.   14

Hospital Cases of Typhus, 1849—71.

Year	London Fever Hosp.	Edin. Royal Infirm.	Glasgow Royal Infirm.	Glasgow Fever Hosp.	Dundee Royal Infirm.	Aberdeen Royal Infirm.	Cork Fever Hosp.
1849	155	—	342	—	—	—	—
1850	130	—	382	—	—	—	—
1851	68	—	919	—	—	—	—
1852	204	—	1293	—	—	—	—
1853	408	—	1551	—	—	—	—
1854	337	—	760	—	—	—	—
1855	342	—	385	—	—	—	—
1856	1062	—	385	—	—	—	—
1857	274	—	314	—	—	—	—
1858	15	—	175	—	—	—	—
1859	48	—	175	—	17	—	—
1860	25	—	229	—	128	—	—
1861	86	—	509	—	67	—	—
1862	1827	14	780	—	129	—	116
1863	1309	74	1286	—	54	—	272
1864	2493	212	2150	—	236	379 (4 mos.)	692
1865	1950	447	2334	1154	264	811	1021
1866	1760	847	1055	384	891	422	791
1867	1396	303	761	795	706	167	247
1868	1964	280	620	1023	225	68	124
1869	1259	259	1430	2023	502	78	245
1870	631	287	947	702	402	170	136
1871	411	101	418	511	257	3	397

During the unusual prevalence of fever in Scotland, 1863–65, it was made clear by the diagnosis in hospitals, that the excess was caused by typhus, and not by enteric.

Of 440 cases of fever treated in the Royal Infirmary of Edinburgh, in 1864, 212 were cases of pure typhus, 140 were enteric fevers, while 88 were simple continued fever and febricula. In the Royal Infirmary of Glasgow in 1864, of 2,190 cases of fever, 2,150 were reported to be cases of typhus fever, while only 40 were cases of enteric fever. In the Aberdeen Royal Infirmary not a case of enteric fever was observed: of 396 cases in the year 1863, 387 were pure typhus, and 9 febricula; and in 1864, of 926 cases, 897 were pure typhus and 29 febricula. In the Royal Infirmary of Dundee, of 355 cases of fever treated in 1864, 318 were typhus, 16 enteric fever, and 21 febricula. It was only at Perth, and there not exclusively in hospital practice, that an excess of typhoid fever was observed; from 1st August, 1863, to 30th April, 1864 (months which included the special typhoid season), there were 101 cases of gastro-enteric or typhoid fever, 46 cases of typhus, 19 of relapsing fever, and 59 of simple continued fever[1].

The last considerable prevalence of contagious fever in England and Scotland was in 1869 and 1870. It was relapsing fever, mixed with some typhus, and it was restricted almost to

[1] James Stark, M.D., "Remarks on the Epidemic Fever of Scotland during 1863–64–65" etc., *Trans. Epidem. Soc.* N. S. II. 312. See also Russell, *Glasg. Med. Journ.* July, 1864, and R. Beveridge (for Aberdeen), *Lancet,* I. 1868, p. 630.

a few large towns, including London, Liverpool, Manchester, Leeds, Bradford, Glasgow, and Edinburgh[1]. It was first seen in London in 1868 among Polish Jews. It was heard of as late as 1872 at Newcastle. It was observed during this epidemic in Liverpool, Bradford and Edinburgh that the subjects of the relapsing fever were not suffering from want[2]. The same observation has been made in some foreign countries. Still, on the great scale and in a broad view, relapsing fever has been *typhus famelicus* or famine-fever, occurring in association with other maladies due to want, and especially in the circumstances which have been discussed fully in the chapter on fevers in Ireland.

Relative prevalence of Typhus and Enteric Fevers since 1869.

It was not until the year 1869, or about the time when typhus fever ceased to be epidemic or common, that the deaths from typhus fever, simple continued fever and enteric fever began to be tabulated separately in the Registrar-General's reports. The following tables show for England and Wales and for London a steady decline of the deaths from typhus and simple continued fever since the end of the epidemic period 1869–71, which was the last epidemic of typhus and relapsing fever in this country hitherto. The deaths from enteric fever, it will be seen, remained somewhat steady (in a growing population) for about ten years after the separation, and then began to decline.

---

[1] Weber, *Lancet*, I. 1869, pp. 221, 255; Murchison, *ibid.* II. 1869, pp. 503, 647; Gee (Liverpool), *Brit. Med. Journ.* II. 1870, p. 246; Robinson (Leeds), *Lancet*, I. 1871, p. 644; Muirhead (Edinburgh), *Edin. Med. Journ.* July, 1870, p. 1; Rabagliati (Bradford), *ibid.* Dec. 1873; Tennant (Glasgow), *Glasgow Med. Journ.* May, 1871, p. 354; Armstrong (Newcastle), *Lancet*, I. 1873, p. 48.

[2] Muirhead (l. c.) says: "In no single instance which came under my observation could starvation be said to be the immediate cause of the disease. Not one of those individuals could be said to be emaciated....On strict and repeated inquiry, not one of them would confess to having been in destitute circumstances." During the winter of 1870–71 I attended from the Edinburgh New Dispensary several relapsing-fever patients at their homes, and can clearly remember having been surprised at the condition of decency and comfort in which I found them. The appearance of comfort was certainly due in part to the district visitors, who were numerous and active during the epidemic.

Continued-fever Deaths in England and Wales, 1869-91.

Year	Typhus	Simple or Ill-defined	Enteric
1869	4281	5310	8659
1870	3297	5254	8731
1871	2754	4248	8461
1872	1864	3352	8741
1873	1638	3081	8793
1874	1762	3089	8861
1875	1499	2599	8913
1876	1192	1974	7550
1877	1104	1923	6879
1878	906	1776	7652
1879	533	1472	5860
1880	530	1490	6710
1881	552	1159	5529
1882	940	1016	6036
1883	877	963	6068
1884	328	768	6380
1885	318	662	4765
1886	245	505	5061
1887	211	502	5165
1888	168	436	4848
1889	140	413	4971
1890	160	361	6146
1891	148	325	5075

Continued-fever Deaths in London, 1869-91.

Year	Typhus	Simple or Ill-defined	Enteric
1869	716	615	1069
1870	472	570	976
1871	384	436	871
1872	174	322	867
1873	277	325	968
1874	312	337	879
1875	128	272	817
1876	159	202	769
1877	157	194	901
1878	151	197	1033
1879	71	160	849
1880	74	134	702
1881	92	134	971
1882	53	95	975
1883	55	102	963
1884	32	75	925
1885	28	78	597
1886	13	73	618
1887	19	44	612
1888	9	35	694
1889	16	42	538
1890	10	35	604
1891	11	44	557

Such being the proportions of typhus and enteric fever since 1869, when the separation was made, it remains to ask what share each of them may have had in the total of "typhus," or of continued fever generally, in the years before the two forms were distinguished in the annual registration reports. Of course, they were distinguished by many of the profession long before that; so that there are means of forming a judgment. At the London Fever Hospital, enteric fever and typhus were distinguished after 1849. If the admissions of each kind of fever to that hospital be assumed to have been proportionate to the prevalence of each in London from year to year, we should get in the following table a means of estimating which of the two forms of continued fever furnished most of the deaths in all London, as given in the first column :

Year	Deaths in London from both fevers	Admissions to London Fever Hospital	
		Typhus	Typhoid
1838	4078	—	—
1839	1819	—	—
1840	1262	—	—
1841	1151	—	—
1842	1184	—	—
1843	2094	—	—
1844	1721	—	—
1845	1324	—	—
1846	1838	—	—
1847	3297	—	—
1848	3685	—	—
1849	2564	155	138
1850	2032	130	137
1851	2374	68	234
1852	2183	204	140
1853	2617	408	212
1854	2816	337	228
1855	2410	342	217
1856	2717	1062	149
1857	2195	274	214
1858	1919	15	180
1859	1840	48	176
1860	1476	25	95
1861	1848	86	161
1862	3673	1827	220
1863	2871	1309	174
1864	3782	2493	253
1865	3217	1950	523
1866	2688	1760	582
1867	2184	1396	380
1868	2468	1964	459

From this it will appear that every great annual rise in the London deaths from "fever," since the last great typhus epidemic

of 1847–48, has corresponded to a greatly increased admission, not of enteric cases, but of typhus cases into the London Fever Hospital. On the other hand, enteric fever has been at a somewhat steady or endemic level for a good many years. Even at that level it would have had a small share of the whole fever-mortality in the old London; in modern London, especially in its residential quarters, its rate has probably been higher than in former times; while in recent years, owing to the absolute decline of typhus, it has been by far the most common continued fever. If the conditions were the same in London as in Edinburgh, it was the very creation of residential streets and new quarters of the town that called forth typhoid fever; while the more the town was remodelled, the more were the *fomites* of typhus destroyed. Thus it seems probable that the same progress in well-being among all classes, which has gradually brought typhus down almost to extinction (or apparently so for the present), has been attended with an increase of typhoid, an increase which has happily fallen within the last few years from its highest point.

The disappearance, during the last twenty years, of typhus and relapsing fevers from the observation of all but a few medical practitioners in England, Scotland and Ireland, is one of the most certain and most striking facts in our epidemiology. Most of the recent English cases have occurred in Lancashire, especially in Liverpool, and in Sunderland, Gateshead, Newcastle and other shipping places of the north. In the decennial period 1871–80 the death-rate from typhus, per 1000 living, was 0·58 in Liverpool and 0·33 in Sunderland, rates which were about the same as those from enteric fevers. The rates in 1881–83 were also high in the same group of towns. As to other industrial centres, including the coal-districts of Cumberland, Wales and Scotland, it is probable that a good deal of typhus passes under the name of "typhoid," the change in medical fashion having outrun somewhat the real change in the relative prevalence of each fever[1]. In Scotland the disease is still heard of from time to time in Glasgow, Edinburgh, Leith, Dundee, Aberdeen, Inverness and Thurso. In London the recent immunity from it is remarkable, but intelligible. First, the populace is better housed: we have got rid of the window-tax,

[1] Spear, "Typhus Fever in various parts of England, 1886–87." *Rep. Med. Off. Loc. Gov. Bd.* N. S. XVI. p. 169.

rebuilt the houses in regular streets opening upon wide thoroughfares, pulled down most of the back-to-back houses, dispersed the working population over square miles of suburbs easily accessible from the heart of the town by tramways and railways, perfected the sewerage and the water-supply. These great structural changes are so far an earnest that typhus cannot come back in the old way. Secondly, food has been for a long time cheap and wages good. During the remarkable lull in typhus from 1803 to 1816, Bateman pointed out that the unwholesome state of the dwellings of the working class remained the same as before, but that money was flowing freely among all classes (thanks to the special war-expenditure). Under free trade, the same abundance of the necessaries of life has been secured in another way. Typhus, it need hardly be said, is an indigenous or autochthonous infection ; the conditions of its engendering are never very far off. In a small and remote island off the coast of Skye, which I happened to know in its pleasing aspects from having landed upon it during a summer vacation, typhus fever was reported by the newspapers a few months after to have broken out in the hamlet of twenty or thirty families, the winter storms having prevented the fishers from leaving their cottages or any stranger from approaching the island. In a sparsely populated parish of the east coast of Scotland, two cases of genuine typhus (one of them fatal), and two only, have occurred, to medical knowledge, within the last ten years, each in a very poor cottage in a different part of the parish and in a different season. So long as our cheap supplies of food, fuel and clothing are uninterrupted, there is small chance of typhus or relapsing fever. But the population of England being now twice as great as the home-grown corn can feed, a return of those fevers on the great scale is not out of the question in the event of the foreign food-supply being interfered with, or the necessaries of life becoming permanently dearer from any other cause.

The following Table of the fever-deaths in Scotland since the beginning of Registration does not distinguish enteric from typhus, relapsing and simple continued during the first ten years of the period ; but it is probable, from all that is known non-statistically or by hospital figures only, as to the history of enteric fever in Scotland, that it made the smaller part of the generic total of fever-deaths so long as typhus and relapsing fevers were common.

Scotland—Deaths from the Continued Fevers since the beginning of Registration.

Year		
1855	2419	
1856	2363	
1857	3087	
1858	2790	
1859	2436	Inclusive of typhus, relapsing, enteric
1860	2344	and other continued fevers.
1861	2579	
1862	3021	
1863	3441	
1864	4804 [1]	

Year	Typhus	Enteric	Relapsing	Simple continued	Infantile Remittent	Cerebro-Spinal
1865	3272	1048	62	839	164	—
1866	2172	1404	34	249	159	—
1867	1745	1378	40	105	119	—
1868	1561	1404	45	100	132	—
1869	2059	1335	29	121	157	—
1870	1460	1207	205	151	141	—
1871	1129	1234	411	108	124	—
1872	795	1223	115	103	118	—
1873	628	1495	31	192	117	—
1874	726	1455	27	104	80	—
1875	615	1625	17	98	85	—
1876	471	1448	18	65	88	—
1877	265	1427	5	164	—	—
1878	263	1477	2	147	—	—
1879	210	1013	5	133	—	—
1880	170	1338	4	155	—	—
1881	229	1004	0	115	—	—
1882	180	1204	2	90	—	—
1883	152	998	1	71	—	—
1884	138	1050	2	63	—	7
1885	111	889	1	58	—	9
1886	80	755	2	62	—	8
1887	126	835	7	65	—	10
1888	102	665	6	58	—	4
1889	69	795	1	58	—	6
1890	77	777	—	45	—	2
1891	107	799	4	30	—	3
				23		6

Circumstances of Enteric Fever.

The circumstances of typhus and relapsing fevers need no general stating after what has been said of particular epidemics in England and Scotland, or remains to be said, for the most distinctive instances of all, in the chapter on fevers in Ireland. There has been so little typhus in the country at large since the

[1] 2303 of these fever deaths in 1864 occurred in the eight principal towns of Scotland, classified as follows: typhus, 1450, relapsing fever, 371, gastric, enteric, or typhoid, 382.

disease began to be registered apart in the mortality returns, in 1869, that hardly anything can be inferred except the fact of its disappearance. It is significant, however, that Sunderland, one of the two great towns which have kept typhus longest and in largest measure (Liverpool being the other) is distinguished for the overcrowding of its dwelling-houses (7·24 persons to a house in the Census of 1881, 7·00 in the Census of 1891).

But the circumstances of enteric fever are not only not so obvious as those of typhus in the historical way; they are also more complex and disputable. One fact in the natural history of enteric fever has been made clear in the chronology, namely, its greater frequency after a severe drought. It was in the autumn of 1826, after the driest and hottest summer of the century, that cases of fever with ulceration of the bowel were first described and figured in London. It was in the autumn of 1846, after the next very dry and hot summer, that cases of the same fever again became unusually common in many parts of England and Scotland. The same sequence has been remarked on more recent occasions and in various countries. It is explained by taking into account some other facts in the natural history of enteric fever. In nearly all countries in our latitudes, autumn is its principal season, and autumn is the season when the level of the water in the soil, or in the wells, is lowest. Virchow states the law of enteric fever in the following simple and concrete way: "We [in Berlin] have a certain number of cases of typhoid at all times. The number increases when the sub-soil water falls, and decreases when it rises. Every year, at the time of the lowest level of the sub-soil water, we have a small epidemic." A sharp rise above the mean level of the year, from the first week of September to the end of October, has been well shown for London from the admissions to the hospitals of the Metropolitan Asylums Board, 1875–1884. The curve has an equally sharp descent, passing below the mean line of the year in the second week of December[1]. There are indications that it is the partial filling of the pores of the sub-soil with water, after they have long been occupied with air only, that makes the virus of typhoid active, or, in other

---

[1] G. B. Longstaff, M.D., *Trans. Epid. Soc.* 1884-5, p. 72, reprinted in his *Studies in Statistics*, Lond. 1891, p. 402. The seasonal curve for the typhoid admissions to the London Fever Hospital over a longer period is nearly the same, as well as that of the registered deaths by typhoid in all London, 1869-84.

words, that the rains of late summer and autumn are the occasion of the seasonal increase of the infection.

Yet it is not the changes in the ground-water by themselves, just as it is not rainfall and temperature by themselves, that make enteric fever to prevail. The soil in which those vicissitudes of drought and saturation are potent for evil must be one that is befouled with animal organic matters, more especially with excremental matters. For that and other reasons (such as the geological formation), enteric fever shows, in its more steady or endemic prevalence from year to year or from decade to decade, certain marked preferences of locality. Since 1869, when the deaths from it began to be registered apart, it has been much more common, per head of the population, in the quick-growing manufacturing and mining towns than in any other parts of England and Wales, the districts with highest enteric death-rates being the mining region of the East Coast from the mouth of the Tees to somewhat north of the Tyne, the mining region of Glamorgan, certain manufacturing towns of Lancashire and the West Riding of Yorkshire, and some districts in the valley of the Trent in Staffordshire and Nottinghamshire. The following Table shows, by comparison with all England and Wales and with London, the excessive death-rates from enteric fever in the registration divisions which head the list:

Highest mortalities from Enteric Fever in Registration Divisions of England and Wales[1].

	Decennium 1871—80			Decennium 1881—90
	Annual death-rate, all causes per 1000 living	Annual death-rate, Enteric, per 1000 living	Enteric Deaths in 10 years	Deaths, Enteric, in 10 years
England and Wales London	21·27 22·37	0·32 0·24	78421 8536	53509 7497
Durham co.	23·77	0·56	4525	2590
South Wales	21·09	0·45	3715	2550
W. Riding, Yorks.	23·24	0·45	9166	5170
N. Riding, Yorks.	19·68	0·44	1259	896
Nottinghamshire	21·23	0·43	1707	1263
Lancashire	25·17	0·39	12388	9874

[1] The following large registration districts besides those in the Table, had enteric-fever death rates of ·5 and upwards per 1000 persons living, in the ten years 1871–80; in nearly all of them there has been a marked decline in the ten years 1881–90:—

Durham Mining Districts.

Stockton incl. part of Middlesborough (4¾ years)	26·64	1·09	561	—
Stockton (5¼ years)	22·49	0·62	208 (5¼ years)	258
Guisborough, incl. part of Middlesborough (4¾ years)	24·80	1·17	251	—
Guisborough (5¼ years)	20·45	0·38	71	106
Middlesborough[1] (5¼ years)	19·93	0·63	272 (5¼ years)	460
Auckland	24·52	0·71	541	318

South Wales Mining Districts.

Pontypridd[2]	23·16	0·71	515	541
Merthyr Tydvil	24·23	0·62	639	249
Swansea	22·38	0·63	505	387
Llanelly	20·93	0·83	330	165

In the second decennium of the Table, 1881–90, the total deaths from enteric fever (the death-rates are still unpublished) are much below those of 1871–80. All the counties of England and Wales have shared in that notable decline, including Durham and Glamorgan. But these two great districts of the coal and iron mining are, by the latest returns, still keeping the lead; and it is probable that we shall find in them, or in particular towns within them, the conditions that have been most favourable to enteric fever in the earlier decennia of this century and are still favourable to it. First it is to be observed that one of the most noted of the old typhoid centres in Glamorgan, namely Merthyr Tydvil, has ceased to be in that class; its enormous rate of growth has been checked (to 18·9 per cent. from 1881 to 1891) and it has at the same time become a more uniform and better-ordered municipality.

Durham, Hartlepool, Easington, Houghton-le-Spring, Darlington, Gateshead (county Durham); Morpeth (Northumberland); Aysgarth, Todmorden, Dewsbury, Pontefract, Barnsley, Rotherham (Yorkshire); Dudley, Leigh, Ormskirk (Lancashire); Crickhowell (Wales); Worksop, Radford (Nottingham); Shrewsbury; Peterborough; Portsea Island (Hants). Of the London districts, Hackney had the highest enteric fever, 0·46 per 1000 in a general death-rate of 20·78. The high rate of a decennium is not unfrequently brought up by one great explosion. In many of the Lancashire, Yorkshire and Midland towns, with rates about ·4 per 1000 persons, the rate has been somewhat steady from year to year. In the decennium 1871–80, many special outbreaks, some of them in villages, were reported on by the inspectors of the Medical Department, and traced for the most part to water-supplies tainted by the percolation of excrement.

[1] The Registration District of Middlesborough was carved out of Stockton and Guisborough in 1875.

[2] Registration District containing a population of 72,707 on a mean between the census of 1871 and that of 1881. In 1891 the population was 146,812.

On the other hand, on the same river Taff, and in the tributary valley of the Rhondda, there is an immense population of miners, among whom the enteric fever death-rate will probably be found to have been higher in 1881–90 than in any other registration district. The most populous part of the district is the town of Ystradyfodwg, which had 44,046 inhabitants in 1881 and 68,720 in 1891, an increase of over fifty per cent., the highest urban rate of increase in the country. On the mean of the last three years, 1891–93, its enteric fever death-rate has been ·62 per 1000. There are several populous towns or townships in the mining districts of the north-east which have in like manner kept their high rate of typhoid mortality—Auckland, Easington, Bellington (Morpeth) and Middlesborough. It is held by many that enteric fever has been most characteristically a product of the modern system of closet-pipes and sewers. It is, of course, the defects of the system that are, in this hypothesis, to blame, including its partial adoption, the transition-state from the older system, the tardy extension to new streets, as well as cheap and faulty construction. All those things, together with the inherent difficulty of connecting with a main sewerage the irregular squattings of a mining community, are probably to be found in highest degree in those districts of Durham and South Wales that are most subject to enteric fever. While enteric fever is in some places steady or endemic from year to year, in others its force is felt mostly in great and sudden explosions.

One such happened in the city and district of Bangor in the summer of 1882. The registration district had only 95 deaths from enteric fever in the ten years 1871–80, but in the single year 1882 it had 87 deaths registered under that name. Of 548 attacks (with 42 deaths) which were known from 22 May to 12 September, 407 fell in August and the first twelve days of September[1]. In the following year and throughout the rest of the decennium the district had its usual low average of enteric-fever deaths. One thing relevant to the explosion was probably the excessive rainfall of June and July (9·5 inches, as compared with 4·8 inches about London).

Another explosion, probably unique in the history of enteric fever, took place at Worthing, on the Sussex coast, in the summer of 1893. The enteric death-rate of the town had been much below the average of England and Wales from 1871 to 1880, the rate being 0·15 per 1000 and the whole deaths in ten years 36. During the next ten years, 1881–90, the whole enteric deaths were 43 in the entire registration district (population in 1891,

[1] F. W. Barry, M.D., in *Rep. Med. Off. Loc. Gov. Board for* 1882, p. 72. The contention of the inspector was that the water-supply had been tainted by enteric-fever evacuations from a case which began on 22 May in a cottage some half-mile distant from the reservoir but in communication with it through ditches and brooks. The area of the water-supply did not correspond with the area of the fever.

32,394). In 1891 the typhoid deaths were two, in 1892 they were six. In 1893 a severe outbreak of typhoid took place within the municipal borough (population 16,606): In the first quarter of the year Worthing was one of the places mentioned for typhoid, having had 5 deaths; in April there were no deaths, in May 25, in June 19, in July 61, in August 64, in September 11, and in the last quarter of the year 8, making 193 deaths in the year. The highest weekly number of cases notified was 253 in the second week of July. The enormously wide dispersion of the poison, in a town little subject to enteric fever, caused suspicion to fall on the water-supply, the more reasonably that the district of West Worthing, which had a separate water-supply, was said not to have suffered from the outbreak. A new water-supply was at once undertaken. A relief fund of £7000 was raised for the sufferers.

The towns of Middlesborough, Stockton and Darlington, in the lower valley o the Tees, were together the scene of two remarkable explosions of enteric fever, the first from 7 September to 18 October, 1890, the second from 28 December, 1890, to 7 February, 1891. The phenomenal nature of these outbreaks in the autumn and winter of 1890-91 will appear from the following table of deaths by enteric fever:

	Darlington	Stockton	Middlesborough
Ten years 1881-90	104	258	460
1890	21	66	130
1891	17	59	93

In the first of the two explosions the three towns were almost equally attacked per head of their populations; in the second explosion, in mid-winter, Darlington had relatively only half as many cases as each of the other two, which had about the same number of cases as in the former six-weeks' period. In both periods, of six weeks each, the three towns had together 1334 cases of typhoid, while the country districts near them had a mere sprinkling. A flooded state of the Tees appeared to be a relevant antecedent to each of the explosions. The Tees is a broad shallow river flowing rapidly, subject to frequent inundations, tortuous in its lower course, forming at its mouth, where Middlesborough stands, a wide estuary bordered by low flat grounds. The rainfall at Middlesborough was 6·3 inches in August, of which 2·2 inches fell on the 12th of the month, the river being high in flood thereafter. There were again high floods in November, chiefly caused by the melting of snow in the upper basin (5 inches fell at Barnard Castle in November, 3·1 inches at Middlesborough, while the December fall was 1·2 inches at the former and 1·4 inches at the latter). To apply correctly the ground-water doctrine of enteric fever to these explosions, other particulars would have to be known, more especially the extent of the previous dryness of the subsoil (the rainfall at Middlesborough was 9·3 inches in the first half of 1890, 15·6 in the second half, and below average for the whole year). But the flooded state of the Tees valley in August and November must have changed abruptly the state of the ground-ferments within the areas of the respective towns and so afforded, according to the general law, the conditions for an abrupt increase of enteric fever in these its endemic or perennial soils[1].

[1] The report for the Medical Department by F. W. Barry, M.D. (*Enteric Fever in the Tees Valley*, 1890-91, Parl. papers, Nov. 1893), is an elaborate argument to prove that the flooded state of the Tees was indeed the relevant antecedent, not as indexing the rise of the ground-water in the respective towns, but as dislodging and sweeping down the slops, sewage and dry refuse of the market town of Barnard Castle, in upper Teesdale, whereby the water taken in from the Tees two miles above Darlington to the tanks, filters and reservoirs of the Darlington Corporation, and of the Stockton and Middlesborough Water Board, was tainted in some unusual degree—a hypothesis the more remarkable that the refuse, such as it was, had been suspended or dissolved in an unusual volume of water, that little refuse could have collected between the

While the more or less steady or endemic prevalence of typhoid fever is due to the formation and reproduction in the soil of an infective principle (probably of faecal origin) which affects more or less sporadically the individuals living thereon, after the manner of a miasma rising from the ground, there have been some hardly disputable instances of the infection being conveyed to many at once from a single source in the drinking water and by the medium of milk[1]. But such instances, suggestive though they be and easy of apprehension by the laity, must not be understood as giving the rule for the bulk of enteric fever. In like manner, the escape or reflux of excremental gases from pipes or sewers, or the leakage into basements or foundations from faulty plumber-work, are causes, real no doubt, but of limited application, which do not conflict with, as they do not supersede, the more comprehensive and cognate explanation of enteric fever as an infection having its habitat in the soil and an incidence upon individuals after the manner of other miasmatic infections. Sex has little or nothing to do with the incidence of the infective virus. As to age, enteric fever rarely befalls infants, and, in the general belief of practitioners, is a less frequent cause of death among children than among adolescents and adults.

In the following Table from the Registrar-General's Decennial Review, 1871–80, enteric fever is not separated from other continued fevers. It is probable that a considerable ratio of the deaths from 0 to 5 years are due to febrile disorders other than enteric.

Annual Mortality per million living at all ages and at eleven groups of ages, males and females, from fever (including Typhus, Enteric Fever and Different Forms of Continued Fever) 1871–80.

	All ages	0—	5—	10—	15—	20—	25—	35—	45—	55—	65—	75+
Both sexes	484	651	518	439	543	509	411	379	402	458	553	498
Males	494	644	483	390	513	579	436	395	437	503	629	593
Females	477	658	550	487	573	445	387	362	369	418	488	425

first floods and the second, and that no cases of enteric fever were known in the upper valley of the Tees. This judicial deliverance has not been accepted by the authorities of Darlington, Stockton and Middlesborough, nor by the Royal Commission on Water Supply, before whom it was laid.

[1] Besides the epidemic at Worthing in 1893, which is still *sub judice*, the best known instance of typhoid following a certain water-supply is the explosion at Redhill and Caterham in Jan.—Feb. 1879, *Rep. Med. Off. Loc. Gov. Board, for* 1879, Parl. papers, 1880, p. 78. The first instance alleged of the distribution by milk was the Islington explosion in July—August 1870 (Ballard, *Med. Times and Gaz.* 1870, II. 611). It was soon followed by the Marylebone explosion in the summer of 1873 (*Rep. Med. Off. L. G. B.*, N.S. II. 193); but such instances have become less common, while instances of scarlatina and diphtheria following a milk-supply have become more common.

The cases notified under the Act in 1891 and 1892 have been found to average five or six for every death registered in the corresponding districts, the rate of fatality ranging widely. It is matter of familiar knowledge that many of the attacks and fatalities occur among the richer classes. New comers to an endemic seat of the disease are most apt to take it (this has been elaborately shown for Munich, and holds good for the British troops in India). There are undoubtedly constitutional proclivities to it among individuals, which may run strongly in families. As in other miasmatic infective diseases, such as yellow fever, Asiatic cholera, and (formerly) plague, there seem to be occasions in the varying states of body and mind, as well as in the external circumstances, when the infection of enteric fever is specially apt to find a lodgement and to become effective. The old plague-books gave lists of the things that were apt to invite venom or to stir venom (see former volume pp. 212, 674); and it is probable that some of these hold good also for the incidence of enteric fever.

CHAPTER II.

FEVER AND DYSENTERY IN IRELAND.

THE history of the public health in Ireland has been so remarkable that it may be useful to take a continuous view of it in a chapter apart, so far as concerns flux, or dysentery, and typhus with relapsing fever.

Ireland is a country which would have given Hume, had he thought of it, the best of all his illustrations of the difficult problem handled in the essay "Of National Characters"—how far the habits, customs, temperaments and, he might have added, morbid infections have been determined by climate, and how far by laws and government, by revolutions in public affairs, or by the situation of the nation with regard to its neighbours. Not only is there something special and peculiar in the actual epidemiology of Ireland, but its political and social history has been apt to borrow the phrases of medicine in a figure. "First the physicians are to take care," says Burke, "that they do nothing to irritate this epidemical distemper. It is a foolish thing to have the better of the patient in a dispute. The complaint, or its cause, ought to be removed, and wise and lenient arts ought to precede the measures of vigour[1]." And this singular use of the imagery of disease in Irish history might be illustrated from many other passages of the same orator and essayist, just as it may be seen any day in the columns of newspapers in our own time. Giraldus Cambrensis began it, within a few years of the first English conquest of Irish territory by Henry II. Writing of that singular effect upon the English settlers by contact with the native Irish, whereby they

[1] *Second Letter to Sir Hercules Langrishe*, May, 1795.

became, in the words of another medieval author, *ipsis Hibernis hiberniores*, he resorts to the medical figure of "contagion" as the best way to account for it. So again, to overleap six centuries, Bishop Berkeley in his query "whether idleness be the mother or daughter of spleen[1]," is .trying upon the Irish both Hume's problem of national character and the use of the medical figure. And, to take a modern instance, Lord Beaconsfield used the same figure of the old humoral pathology, and gave his adhesion to a theory of national characters adverse to the sense of Hume, when he ascribed the habits and manners of the Iris.1, and the course of their national history, to their propinquity to a "melancholy" ocean.

As far back as we can go in the history, two diseases are conspicuous—the flux or "the country disease," and the sharp fever or "Irish ague." When Henry II. invaded Ireland in 1172, his army suffered from flux, which the contemporary chronicler, Radulphus de Diceto, dean of St Paul's, set down to the unwonted eating of fresh meat (*recentium esus carnium*), the drinking of water, and the want of bread[2]. Less than a generation after, Giraldus of Wales wrote his "Topography of Ireland," wherein he remarks that hardly any stranger, on his first coming to the country, escapes the flux by reason of the juicy food (*ob humida nutrimenta*)[3]. At that time Ireland was almost wholly a pastoral country, and a pastoral country it has remained to a far greater extent than England or Scotland. It is to this comparative want of tillage, an almost absolute want when Giraldus was there, that we shall probably have to look in the last resort for an explanation of the two national maladies that here concern us—the "country disease" and the "Irish ague." The same dietetic reason that the dean of St Paul's gave in 1172 for the prevalence of flux in the army of Henry II., the want of bread and the eating of fresh meat, can be assigned for the country disease long after, and, in some periods, on the explicit testimony of observers. As to the Irish ague, or typhus fever, Giraldus mentions it in the medieval period; and Higden, copying him exactly, says: "The inhabitants of Ireland are vexed by no kind of fever except the

---

[1] Berkeley's *Querist*, Q. 362.

[2] Radulphus de Diceto, *Imag. Histor.* Eng. Hist. Soc. ed. I. 350.

[3] "Topogr. Hiberniae" in *Opera*, Rolls ed. v. 67. This and the preceding reference had escaped the notice of Dr John O'Brien, in the historical introduction to his *Observations on the Acute and Chronic Dysentery of Ireland.* Dublin, 1822.

C. II.   15

acute, and that seldom "—the word *acuta* being the original of "the ague," or, as in another translation of the passage, "the sharp axes[1]." In this pastoral country, according to Giraldus, there was little sickness and little need of physicians; but there is hardly an instance of military operations by the English unattended with sickness among the troops, and famine with sickness among the native Irish.

The generalities of Fynes Moryson, a traveller of the time of James I., who included Ireland among the many countries that he visited and described, throw light upon the dietetic peculiarities of the Irish. Having little agriculture, and at that time no general cultivation of the potato (although they adopted it much sooner than the English and Scots), they lived, says Moryson, mostly on milk (as Giraldus Cambrensis also records in the twelfth century), and upon the flesh of unfed calves, which they cooked and ate in a barbarous fashion. "The country disease" is also noted. The experience in Ireland from time immemorial, that a bellyful was a windfall, must have been the origin of a habit observed by Moryson:

"I have known some of these Irish footemen serving in England to lay meate aside for many meales to devoure it all at one time." And again: "The wilde Irish in time of greatest peace impute covetousnesse and base birth to him that hath any corne after Christmas, as if it were a point of nobility to consume all within these festivall dayes." The Irish slovenliness or filthiness in their food, raiment and lodging was apt, he says, "to infect" the English who came to reside in their country[2].

About a generation after we come to the earliest medical account of the sicknesses of Ireland, by Gerard Boate, compiled during the Cromwellian occupation[3]. The following occurs under the head of The Looseness:

[1] *Polychronicon*, Rolls ed. I. 332–3.

[2] "Many of the English-Irish have by little and little been infected with the Irish filthinesse, and that in the very cities, excepting Dublin and some of the better sort in Waterford, where the English continually lodging in their houses, they more retain the English diet." And again: "In like sort the degenerated citizens are somewhat infected with the Irish filthinesse, as well in lowsie beds, foule sheetes, and all linnen, as in many other particulars...Touching the meere or wild Irish, it may truely be said of them, which was of old spoken of the Germans, namely, that they wander slovenly and naked, and lodge in the same house (if it may be called a house) with their beasts." Fynes Moryson, *Itinerary*, Pt. IV. p. 180.

[3] *Ireland's Natural History, &c.* Written by Gerard Boate, late Doctor of Physick to the State in Ireland. And now published by Samuel Hartlib, Esquire. Lond. 1652. The author died at Dublin, shortly after his arrival there, on $\frac{9}{19}$ January $16\frac{50}{49}$. His information would seem to have come in part from his brother Arnold Boate, resident in Ireland.

The English have given it the name of the Country Disease. The subjects of it are often troubled a great while, but take no great harm. It is easily cured by good medicines: "But they that let the looseness take its course do commonly after some days get the bleeding with it ;......and last it useth to turn to the bloody flux, the which in some persons having lasted a great while, leaveth them of itself; but in far the greatest number is very dangerous, and killeth the most part of the sick; except they be carefully assisted with good remedies."

The other reigning disease is the "Irish Ague," a continued fever of the nature of typhus:

"As Ireland is subject to most diseases in common with other countries, so there are some whereunto it is peculiarly obnoxious, being at all times so rife there that they may justly be reputed for Ireland *endemii morbi*, or reigning diseases, a: indeed they are generally reputed for such. Of this number is a certain sort of malignant feavers, vulgarly in Ireland called Irish agues, because that at all times they are so common in Ireland, as well among the inhabitants and the natives, as among those who are newly come thither from other countries. This feaver, commonly accompanied with a great pain in the head and in all the bones, great weakness, drought, loss of all manner of appetite, and want of sleep, and for the most part idleness or raving, and restlessness or tossings, but no very great nor constant heat, is hard to be cured." If blood-letting be avoided and cordial remedies given, "very few persons do lose their lives, except when some extraordinary and pestilent malignity cometh to it, as it befalleth in some years." Those who recover "are forced to keep their beds a long time in extreme weakness, being a great while before they can recover their perfect health and strength."

The occasion of Boate's writing was the subjugation of Ireland by Cromwell, in the course of which we hear from time to time of sickness. The greatest of the calamities was the utter destruction of the prosperity of Galway by the frightful plague of 1649–50, and by the suppression of the Catholics, who had brought the port of Connaught to be a place of foreign commerce[1].

Cromwell's troops in 1649 incurred dysentery through the hardships of campaigning. On 17 September, 1649, the Lord General writes from Dublin to Mr Speaker Lenthall after the storming of Tredah or Drogheda: "We keep the field much; our tents sheltering us from the wet and cold. But yet the country-sickness overtakes many: and therefore we desire recruits, and some fresh regiments of foot, may be sent us." And on 25 October, "Colonel Horton is dead of the country-disease[2]."

---

[1] Hardiman, *History of Galway*, p. 126 *seq.* The plague from July 1649 to Lady Day 1650 is said to have swept away 3700 of the inhabitants, including 210 of the most respectable burgesses and freemen, with their families. The capitulation on 5 April, 1652, was followed by famine throughout the country, and by a revival of plague for two years, "during which upwards of one-third of the population of the province was swept away."

[2] *Cromwell's Letters and Speeches*, II. 55, 77.

Another general reference to the "country disease" of Ireland, by Borlase, is very nearly the same as Boate's. It is introduced early in the history, on the occasion of the death in 1591 of Walter, Earl of Essex, earl marshal of Ireland:

"The dysentery, or flux, so fatal to this worthy person, is commonly termed the country disease; and well it may, for it reigns nowhere so epidemically as in Ireland; tainting strangers as well as natives. But whether it proceeds from the peculiar disposition of the air, errour in diet, the laxity and waterishness of the meat, or some occult cause, no venomous creature living there to suck that which may be thought (in other countries) well distributed amongst reptilious animals, I shall not determine, though each of these circumstances may well conduce to its strength and vigour. Certain it is that regular diet preserves most from the violence, and many from the infection of this disease; yet as that which is thought very soveraign—I might say that the stronger cordial liquors (viz. brandy, usquebeh, treacle and Mithridate waters) are very proper, or the electuaries themselves, and the like[1]."

From the Restoration to the Revolution little is known of epidemics in Ireland. It is probable that Dublin and the other considerable towns fared much the same as English towns. A Dublin physician writing to Robert Boyle on 27 February, 1682, speaks of a petechial fever, marked by leaping of the tendons, which had been fatal to very many in that city for these twelve or fourteen months[2]. With the Revolution the troubles of the country begin again, and enter on their peculiarly modern phase. For our history, two characteristic incidents come at the very beginning of the new period of disorder among the Irish— the sicknesses of the siege of Londonderry and the unparalleled havoc of disease among the troops of Schomberg in the camp of Dundalk. In both, the old "country disease," which had affected Cromwell's troops, was the primary malady, occurring, of course, in circumstances special enough to have bred it anywhere; in both, the dysentery was attended or followed by typhus fever, the old "Irish ague;" and although the epidemics of Londonderry and Dundalk in 1689 are properly examples of war sickness, yet the circumstances of each may help to realize the connexion between dysentery and typhus in the ordinary history of the Irish.

---

[1] Edmund Borlase, *History of the Reduction of Ireland to the Crown of England.* 1675, p. 172.
[2] Boyle's *Works*, fol. Lond. 1744, V. 92.

Dysentery and Fever at Londonderry and Dundalk, 1689.

The siege of Londonderry[1] by the Catholic Irish army of James II. began in April and ended on 28 July, having lasted 105 days. On 19 April the garrison numbered 7020 men, and the total of men, women and children in the town was estimated at 30,000, a number which included refugees from the neighbouring country and would have been more but for many Protestants at the beginning of the siege leaving the city and taking "protection" at the hands of the besiegers. On 21 May, a collection was made for the poor, who began to be in want. Sickness is heard of on 5 June, when several that were sick were killed in their beds by the enemy's bombs. The dread of the bombs in the houses caused the people to lie about the walls or in places remote from the houses all night, so that many of them, especially the women and children, caught cold, which along with the want of rest and failing food, threw them into fluxes and fevers. The pinch of hunger began to be felt before the middle of June, about which time and for six weeks after the fluxes and fevers were rife. A great mortality spread through the garrison as well as the inhabitants ; fifteen captains and lieutenants died in one day, and it was estimated that ten thousand died during the siege, " besides those who died soon after." The want, the dysentery, the fever and the vast numbers of dead every day must have produced a horrible state of things ; when, on 2 July, five hundred useless persons were put outside the walls, to disperse as they best could, the besiegers are said to have recognized them when they met them " by the smell."

---

[1] The war-pestilence at Londonderry in 1689 is the third recorded epidemic of the kind there, not including what may have happened in the capture of the town by the Catholics in O'Neill's rebellion, when Derry was destroyed, to be rebuilt in 1613 by the London Companies with a new charter under the name of Londonderry. The first historical occasion of sickness was in 1566. The troops of Elizabeth were landed on Loch Foyle in October and built their huts on the site of the old monastery. In the course of the winter the greater part of a force of 1100 men perished by dysentery and the infection which it breeds (see former volume, p. 372). On 12 Dec. 1642, a year after the outbreak of the Rebellion of Confederate Catholics, a petition of the agents of the distressed city of Londonderry to the Commons represented that there were 6059 persons in the city, whereof 5123 were women and children, or sick, aged or impotent ; only 2000 were inhabitants of the city, the rest having fled there for safety. Spotted fever had broken out. (*Hist. MSS. Comis.* v. "MSS. of the House of Lords.")

About the middle of June large quantities of provisions were found in cellars and places of concealment under ground; after that the garrison had always bread, although the allowance was small. An ingenious man discovered how to make pancakes of starch and tallow, of which articles there was no lack; the pancakes not only proved nutritious, but are said to have been an infallible cure of the flux, or preservative from it. At length, on 28 July some of the victuallers and ships of war which had been in Lough Foyle since the 15th of June, sailed up to the head of the Lough on the evening flood tide, finding little resistance from the enemy's batteries and none from "what was left of" the tide-tossed boom of logs across the mouth of the river. Provisions poured in, and the siege was raised; but it is clear that the infection continued for some time after, having been found among such of the released garrison as repaired to Schomberg's camp at Dundalk.

The Catholic army is said (by the Protestants) to have lost 8000 or 9000 before the walls of Londonderry, "most by the sword, the rest of fever and flux, and the French pox, which was very remarkable on the bodies of several of the dead officers and soldiers[1]."

Not far off, at Dundalk, there began, a few weeks after, an extraordinary outbreak of war-sickness, which, unlike the pestilence in Londonderry, was altogether inglorious in its circumstances. In many respects it resembled the disaster to Cromwell's troops at the first occupying of Jamaica in 1655–56[2]; but it was worse than that, and it is probably unexampled in the military annals of Britain[3].

Supplies had been voted in Parliament for quelling the Catholic rebellion in Ireland, and an expedition was got together under the illustrious Marshal, Duke of Schomberg. The force consisted of some ten thousand foot, most of them raw levies from the English peasantry, with one regiment of seasoned

[1] With the exception of the last quoted piece of information, the most minute particulars of the siege of Londonderry are in an essay by an army chaplain, John Mackenzie, *A Narrative of the Siege of Londonderry*, London, 1690, which was written to correct and augment *A True Account of the Siege of Londonderry* by the Rev. Mr George Walker, rector of Donoghmoore in the county of Tyrone, and late Governor of Derry. London, 1689.

[2] See former volume, pp. 634–43.

[3] Minute particulars of it are given in *An Impartial History of the Wars in Ireland* [1689–1692]. By George Story, Chaplain to Sir Thomas Gower's Regiment. London, 1693. Part I.

Dutch troops ("the blue Dutch"), and cavalry. While the bulk of the force was undisciplined, their clothes, food, tents and other munitions of war were bad or insufficient through the fraud of contractors. The expedition embarked at Hoylake on the Dee and landed on the 15th of August, 1689, nearly three weeks after the relief of Londonderry, at Bangor, on the south side of Belfast Lough. Schomberg took Carrickfergus, and began to advance on Dublin; but finding the towns burned and the country turned into a desert, he threw himself into an entrenched camp around the head of Dundalk Bay, nearly a mile from the town of Dundalk. His camp was on a low moist bottom at the foot of the hills. The Irish Catholic army took up a position among the hills "on high sound ground," not more than two miles distant from the English lines, and, being in superior force, in due time they offered battle, which was declined. Schomberg, who had been joined by the Enniskillen regiments of dragoons and by men from Londonderry, had under him some 2000 horse and not less than 12,000 foot at the time when James II. offered battle. The undisciplined state of his English troops and the suspected treachery of a body of French Protestants were among the causes that held Schomberg back; but he had to reckon also with sickness almost from the moment of sitting down at Dundalk. At a muster on 25 September, several of the regiments were grown thin "by reason of the distemper then beginning to seize our men." The distemper was dysentery and fever. The two maladies were mixed up, as they usually are in war and famines, the flux commonly preceding the fever, and perhaps affording the virulent matters in the soil and in the air upon which the epidemic prevalence of the fever depends. It was easy to account for the dysentery among the troops at Dundalk; but as to the fever, there was an ambiguity at the outset which Story is careful to note: "And yet I cannot but think that the feaver was partly brought to our camp by some of those people that came from Derry; for it was observable that after some of them were come amongst us, it was presently spread over the whole army, yet I did not find many of themselves died of it." Where the cause of death is specially named, it is fever, as in the cases of Sir Thomas Gower, Colonel Wharton and other officers on the 28th and 29th October. The fever was a most malignant form of typhus, marked by the worst of all symptoms, gangrene of the extremities, so that the toes or a

whole foot would fall off when the surgeon was applying a dressing[1].

It seems probable that most of the enormous mortality was caused by infection, and not by dysentery due to primary exciting causes.

The primary exciting causes were obvious, but seemingly irremovable. Schomberg had a great military reputation, but he was now over eighty, and it does not appear that he made himself personally felt in the camp, although he issued incessantly orders to inspect and report. As the mortality proceeded apace during the six or eight weeks of inactivity, murmurings arose against the commander. He was unfortunate in his choice of a camping ground, and in an unusually cold and wet season. The newly raised English troops seem to have been lacking equally in intelligence and in moral qualities. Their foul language and debauchery were the occasion of a special proclamation; their laziness and inability to make themselves comfortable called forth numerous orders, but all to no purpose. The regiment of Dutch troops were so well hutted that not above eleven of them died in the whole campaign; but the English would not be troubled to gather fern or anything else to keep themselves dry and clean withal: "many of them, when they were dead, were incredibly lousy."

The camping ground not only received the drainage of the hills, but, strange to say, the rain would be falling there all day while the camp of the enemy, only a few miles farther inland, would not be getting a drop. On 1 October the tents on the low ground were moved a little higher up. On the same date there were distributed among the regiments casks of brandy—Macaulay says it was of bad quality—which appears to have been the trusted remedy against camp sickness, as in the Jamaica expedition of 1655. There were twenty-seven victuallers or other ships riding in Dundalk Bay; but the stores were bad, and the regimental surgeons had come unprovided with drugs that might have been useful in flux or fever. While the weather continued cold and wet, there was also a scarcity of firing and forage. On 14 October all the regimental surgeons were ordered to meet at ten in the morning to consult with

[1] Gangrene of the extremities was one of the symptoms of the "plague of Athens" as described by Thucydides. There is no need to invoke ergotism for an explanation of it, as some have done.

Dr Lawrence how to check the sickness[1]. Several officers having died on the 16th and 17th, the camp was shifted on the 20th to new ground, the huts being left full of the sick. Gower's regiment had sixty-seven men unable to march, besides a good many dead before or sent away sick. Story, the chaplain, went every day from the new camp to visit the sick of his regiment in the huts, and always at his going found some dead. He found the survivors in a state of brutal callousness, utterly indifferent to each other, but objecting to part with their dead comrades as they wanted the bodies to sit or lie on, or to keep off the cold wind. The ships at anchor had now received as many sick as they could hold, and the deaths on board soon became as many as on shore. On 25–27 October, the camp was again shifted, but the sickness continued apace. At length on 3 November, the Catholic army having dispersed to winter quarters, the sick were ordered to be removed to Carlingford and Newry. "The poor men were brought down from all places towards the Bridge End, and several of them died by the way. The rest were put upon waggons, which was the most lamentable sight in the world, for all the rodes from Dundalk to Newry and Carlingford were next day full of nothing but dead men, who, even as the waggons joulted, some of them died and were thrown off as fast." Some sixteen or seventeen hundred had been left dead at Dundalk. The ships were ordered to sail for Belfast with the first wind, and the camp was broken up. There was snow on the hills and rain in the valleys; on the march to Newry, men fell out of the ranks and died at the road side. When the ships weighed anchor from Dundalk and Carlingford, they had 1970 sick men on board, but not more than 1100 of these came ashore in Belfast Lough, the rest having died at sea in coming round the coast of County Down. Such was the violence of the infection on board that several ships had all the men in them dead and nobody to look after them whilst they lay in the bay at Carrickfergus. An infective principle, once engendered in circumstances

---

[1] At that time there was little systematic knowledge of military hygiene. Nearly two generations after, the experiences of Pringle, Donald Monro and Brocklesby in the campaigns of 1743–48 and 1758–63 in Germany and the Netherlands, yielded many valuable hints, some of which Virchow made use of in compiling his "Rules of Health for the Army in the Field," in the Franco-Prussian War of 1870–71. See his *Gesammelte Abhandlungen aus dem Gebiete der öffentlichen Medicin und Seuchenlehre.* 2 Bde. Berlin, 1879, II. 193.

of aggravation such as these, is not soon extinguished. Belfast was the winter quarters, and in the great hospital there from 1 November, 1689, to 1 May, 1690, there died 3762, "as appears by the tallies given in by the men that buried them." These numbers together make fully six thousand deaths, which agrees with the general statement that Schomberg lost one half of the men whom he had embarked at Hoylake in August. The Irish Catholic army began to sicken in their camp in the hills above Dundalk Bay just before they broke up, and they are said to have lost heavily by sickness in their winter quarters.

The war ended with the Treaty of Limerick, in 1691. The Seven Ill Years followed,—ill years to Scotland, in a measure to England, and almost certainly to Ireland also; but it does not appear that the end of the 17th century was a time of special sickness and famine to the Irish, and it may be inferred from the fact of Scots migrating to Ireland during the ill years that the distress was not so sharp there. The epidemiology of Ireland is, indeed, a blank until we come to the writings of Dr Rogers, of Cork, in some respects the best epidemiologist of his time, which cover the period from 1708 to 1734. His account of the dysentery and typhus of the chief city of Munster in the beginning of the 18th century will show that the old dietetic errors of the Irish, noted in medieval times, had hardly changed in the course of centuries.

A generation of Fevers in Cork.

Rogers is clear that typhus fever was never extinct, while the three several times when it "made its appearance amongst us in a very signal manner," are the same as its seasons in England, namely 1708–10, 1718–21 and 1728–30[1]. His experience relates only to the city of Cork, and, so far as his clinical histories go, only to the well-to-do classes therein; and although those seasons were years of scarcity and distress all over Ireland, yet Rogers does not seem to associate insufficient food with the fever, and never mentions scarcity. The fevers were in the winter, for the most part, and were usually accompanied by epidemic smallpox of a bad type, which in 1708 "swept away multitudes." Nothing is said of dysentery for the earliest of the

[1] Joseph Rogers, M.D. *Essay on Epidemic Diseases.* Dublin, 1734.

three fever-periods; but for 1718 and following years we read that "dysentery of a very malignant sort, frequently producing mortification in the bowels," prevailed during the same space; and that the winters of the third fever-period, namely, those of 1728, 1729 and 1730 were "infamous for bloody fluxes of the worst kind." It is clear that the fever spread to the richer classes in Cork, for his five clinical histories are all from those classes. The following is his general account of the symptoms:

The patient is suddenly seized with slight horrors or rather chilliness, to which succeed a glowing warmth, a weight and fixed pain in the head, just over the eyebrows; soreness all over his flesh, as if bruised, the limbs heavy, the heart oppressed, the breathing laboured, the pulse not much alte ed, but in some slower; the urine mostly crude, pale and limpid, at first, or even throughout, the tongue moist and not very white at first, afterwards drier, but rarely black. An universal petechial effloresence not unlike the measles paints the whole surface of the bo y, limbs, and sometimes the very face; in some few appear interspersed eruptions exactly like the *pustulae miliares*, filled with a limpid serum. The earlier these petechiae appear, the fresher in colour, and the longer they continue out, the better (p. 5). The fixed pain in the head increasing, ends commonly in a coma or stupor, or in a delirium with some. Some few have had haemorrhage at the nose, a severe cough, and sore throat. In some he had observed a great tendency to sweats, even from the beginning: these are colliquative and symptomatic, not to be encouraged. In but few there have appeared purple and livid spots, as in haemorrhagic smallpox: some as large as a vetch, others not bigger than a middling pin's head, thick set all over the breast, back and sometimes the limbs, the pulse in these cases being much below normal. The extremities cold from the 6th or 7th day, delirium constant, tongue dry and black, urine limpid and crude, oppression greater, and difficulty of breathing more. It is a slow nervous fever (p. 18).

Rogers believed that mere atmospheric changes could not be the cause of these epidemics: "they may favour, encourage and propagate such diseases when once begun; but for the productive cause of them we must have recourse to such morbid effluvia as above described [particles of all kinds detached from the animal, vegetable and mineral kingdoms]; or resolve all into the θεῖον τί so often appealed to by Hippocrates[1]."

But, as regards Cork itself, special interest attaches to the following "four concurring causes:"

"1st, the great quantities of filth, ordure and animal offals that crowd our streets, and particularly the close confined alleys and lanes, at the very season that our endemial epidemics rage amongst us.

[1] In further illustration of the power of morbid effluvia, he says: "We see how small a portion of a putrid animal juice, taken into the blood by inoculation, like a most active *leaven* sets all in a ferment; and in a very short time brings the whole juices of a sound body into an equal state of corruption with itself,"—instancing war-typhus, plague from cadaveric corruption (according to Paré), the Oxford gaol fever, and "a later instance at Taunton not more than five or six years ago."

2nd, the great number of slaughter-houses, both in the north and south suburbs, especially on the north ridge of hills, where are vast pits for containing the putrefying blood and ordure, which discharge by the declivities of those hills, upon great rains, their fetid contents into the river.

3rd, the unwholesome, foul, I had almost said corrupted water that great numbers of the inhabitants are necessitated to use during the dry months of the summer.

4th, the vast quantities of animal offals used by the meaner sort, during the slaughtering seasons: which occasion still more mischief by the quick and sudden transition from a diet of another kind."

In farther explanation of the fourth concurring cause, he says that in no part of the earth is a greater quantity of flesh meat consumed than in Cork by all sorts of people during the slaughtering season—one of the chief industries of the place being the export of barrelled beef for the navy and mercantile marine. The meat, he says, is plentiful and cheap, and tempts the poorer sort "to riot in this luxurious diet," the sudden change from a meagre diet, with the want of bread and of fermented liquors, being injurious to them[1].

Famine and Fevers in Ireland in 1718 and 1728.

Thus far Rogers, for the city of Cork in the three epidemic periods, 1708–10, 1718–21, and 1728–30, two of which, if not all three, were periods of dysentery as well as of typhus. But it was usual in Ireland for the country districts and small towns to suffer equally with the cities. The circumstances of the Irish peasantry in the very severe winter of 1708–9 are not particularly known; if there was famine with famine-fever, it was not such as to have become historical. But for the next fever-period, 1718–20, we have some particulars. Bishop Nicholson, of Derry, writes: "Never did I behold even in Picardy, Westphalia or Scotland, such dismal marks of hunger and want as appeared

[1] Dr Rogan of Strabane, in his *Condition of the Middle and Lower Classes in the North of Ireland*, 1819, was of a different opinion (p. 90): "No police regulations exist in Strabane to prevent the slaughtering of cattle in any part of the town. The butchers, therefore, most of whom live in the narrow streets near the shambles, have their slaughter-houses immediately behind their dwellings. The garbage is thrown into a large pit, which is generally cleaned but once in the year, at the season when the manure is required for planting potatoes, and at this time an offensive smell pervades the whole town, and is perceptible for a considerable distance around. The families exposed constantly to the effluvia arising from these heaps of putrid offal might have been expected to suffer severely from fever; but on the contrary, they were found to be much less liable to it than others in the same rank of life. This was no doubt owing to their living chiefly on animal food, and thus escaping the debility induced by deficient nourishment, which certainly had the chief share in creating a predisposition to the disease."

in the countenances of most of the poor creatures I met with on the road." One of the bishop's carriage horses having been accidentally killed, it was at once surrounded by fifty or sixty famished cottagers struggling desperately to obtain a morsel of flesh for themselves and their children[1].

This was a time when the population was increasing, but agriculture, so far from increasing in proportion to the number of mouths to feed, was positively declining, unless it were the culture of the potato. In a pamphlet of about 1724, on promoting agriculture and employing the poor, the complaint is of beef and mutton everywhere, and an insufficiency of corn. "Such a want of policy," says one, "is there, in Dublin especially, on the most important affair of bread, without a plenty of which the poor must starve." Another, a Protestant, has the following threat for the clergymen of the Established Church: "I'll immediately stock one part of my land with bullocks, and the other with potatoes—so farewell tithes[2]!" From this it is to be inferred that potatoes were not made tithable until a later period, pasture being exempted to the last. For whatever reason, grazing, and not corn-growing, was then more general in Ireland than in the generations immediately preceding, much land having gone out of tillage. The culture of the potato was driven out of the fertile lowlands to the hill-sides, so as to leave the ground clear for ranges of pasture. Rack-renting was the rule, doubtless owing to the same reason as afterwards, the competition for farms. While the Protestants emigrated in thousands, the Catholics multiplied at home in beggary. A pamphleteer of 1727 says: "Where the plough has no work, one family can do the business of fifty, and you may send away the other forty-nine." Thus we find the pasturing of cattle preferred to agriculture long after the barbaric or uncivilized period had passed, preferred indeed by English landlords or farmers[3].

There were three bad harvests in succession, 1726, 1727 and 1728, culminating in a famine in the latter year. Boulter, archbishop of Armagh, who then ruled Ireland, was able to buy oats or oatmeal in the south and west so as to sell it below

[1] Bp. Nicholson to Archbp. of Canterbury, cited by Lecky (II. 216) from *Brit. Mus. Add. MS.* 6116.
[2] Cited by O'Rourke, *History of the Great Irish Famine of 1847.* Dublin, 1875, from pamphlet in the Halliday Collection of the Royal Irish Academy.
[3] See Boulter's *Letters to the English Ministers.*

the market price to the starving Protestants of Ulster, an interference with the distribution of food which led to serious rioting in Cork, Limerick, Clonmel and Waterford in the first months of 1728[1]. No full accounts of the epidemic fever of that famine remain. Rutty, of Dublin, says it was "mild and deceitful in its first attack, attended with a depressed pulse, and frequently with petechiae[2];" while, according to Rogers and O'Connell[3], the epidemic fever of Munster was the same. Of the famine itself we have a glimpse or two. Primate Boulter writes to the Duke of Newcastle on 7 March, 1727:

"Last year the dearness of corn was such that thousands of families quitted their habitations to seek bread elsewhere, and many hundreds perished; this year the poor had consumed their potatoes, which is their winter subsistence, near two months sooner than ordinary, and are already, through the dearness of corn, in that want that in some places they begin already to quit their habitations."

Quitting their habitations to beg was a regular thing at a later time of the year. It was in the course of these bad years, in 1729, that Swift wrote his 'Modest Proposal for preventing the Children of Poor People in Ireland from being a Burden to their Parents or Country.' The scheme to use the tender babes as delicate morsels of food for the rich, was a somewhat extreme flight of irony, not so finished as in Swift's other satires, but the circumstances out of which the proposal grew were more real than usual.

"It is a melancholy object," says the Dean of St Patrick's, "to those who walk through this great town, or travel in the country, when they see the streets, the roads and cabin doors crowded with beggars of the female sex followed by three, four, or six children, all in rags, and importuning every passenger for an alms." Having ventilated his project for the children, he proceeds to show that "their elders are every day dying and rotting by cold and famine, filth and vermin, as fast as can be reasonably expected."

All the while there was a considerable export of corn from Ireland. In the beginning of 1730, two ships laden with barley were stopped at Drogheda by a fierce mob and were compelled to unload[5].

The interval between those years of epidemic typhus in

---

[1] Wakefield's *Ireland*, II. 6, cited by Barker and Cheyne.
[2] John Rutty, M.D. *Chronological History of the Weather and Seasons and prevailing Diseases in Dublin during Forty Years.* London, 1770.
[3] Maurice O'Connell, M.D. *Morborum acutorum et chronicorum Observationes.* Dublin, 1746.
[4] Boulter's *Letters.* Oxford, 1769, I. 226.
[5] Lecky, II. 217.

Ireland and the next, 1740–41, was filled, we may be sure, with at least an average amount of the endemial fever. Rutty specially mentions it in Dublin in the autumn and winter of 1734–35 : "We had the low fever, called nervous (and sometimes petechial from the spots that frequently attended, although probably not essential)." He then adds : "It is no new thing with us for this low kind of fever to prevail in the winter season ;" and gives figures from the Dublin Bills of Mortality for forty years. He mentions the petechial fever as being frequent next in January and February, 1736, corresponding to a bad time of it in Huxham's Plymouth annals. In 1738 and 1739 the type of the Dublin fever was relapsing, in part at least, the same type having been seen at Edinburgh shortly before.

The economics of Ireland, at this time, gave occasion to Berkeley's *Querist*, a series of weekly essays written in 1737 and 1738, and collected in 1740, on the eve of the next great famine and mortality[1]. A few of the bishop's sarcasms, in the form of queries, will serve to show how anomalous was the economic condition of the country, and how easily a crisis of famine and pestilence could arise.

"169. Whether it is possible the country should be well improved while our beef is exported, and our labourers live upon potatoes?

"173. Whether the quantities of beef, butter, wool and leather, exported from this island, can be reckoned the superfluities of a country, where there are so many natives naked and famished?

"174. Whether it would not be wise so to order our trade as to export manufactures rather than provisions, and of those such as employ most hands?

"466. Whether our exports do not consist of such necessaries as other countries cannot well be without?

"353. Whether hearty food and warm clothing would not enable and encourage the lower sort to labour?

"354. Whether in such a soil as ours, if there was industry, there would be want?

"418. Whether it be not a new spectacle under the sun, to behold in such a climate and such a soil, and under such a gentle government, so many roads untrodden, fields untilled, houses desolate, and hands unemployed?

"514. Whether the wisdom of the State should not wrestle with this hereditary disposition of our Tartars, and with a high hand introduce agriculture?

"534. Why we do not make tiles of our own, for flooring and roofing, rather than bring them from Holland?

"539. Whether it be not wonderful that with such pastures, and so many black cattle, we do not find ourselves in cheese?"

[1] Berkeley's *Works*. Ed. Fraser, Oxford, 1871, III. 369.

In several of his queries (381, 383) Bishop Berkeley is driving at the expediency of domestic slavery. It was two hundred years since the same expedient had been tried by Protector Somerset in England, during the intolerable state of vaga-bondage which followed the rage for pasture farming under the first Tudors. In Scotland, it was hardly more than a generation since the institution of domestic slavery had commended itself to Fletcher of Saltoun, as the only expedient that could free that country from the vagabondage of a tenth, or more, of the population. England had surmounted the difficulty long ago, Scotland got over it easily and speedily when she was admitted to the English and colonial markets for her linen manufacture by the Treaty of Union[1]. But in Ireland in the year 1740, and until long after, disabilities of all kinds, not only economic, but political and religious, were fastened upon the weaker nation by the stronger, the unfortunate cause of their long continuance having been the costly inheritance of loyalty to James II. and the Mass.

The Famine and Fever of 1740–41.

At the time when the bishop of Cloyne was issuing his economic queries from week to week (not much to the satis-faction of Primate Boulter), things were making up for the greatest crisis of famine and pestilence that Ireland experienced in the 18th century. There had been relapsing fever among the poor in Dublin in the autumn of 1738, and it appeared among them again in the summer and autumn of 1739. Rutty's account of it is as follows:

"It was attended with an intense pain in the head. It terminated some-times in four, for the most part in five or six days, sometimes in nine, and commonly in a critical sweat. It was far from being mortal. I was assured of seventy of the poorer sort at the same time in this fever, abandoned to the use of whey and God's good providence, who all recovered. The crisis, however, was very imperfect, for they were subject to relapses, even some-times to the third time, nor did their urine come to a complete separation."

In October 1739, there appeared some dysenteries in Dublin. The winter of 1739 set in severely with cold and wet in November, and about Christmas there began a frost of many

[1] Lord John Russell used these historical parallels from England and Scotland in his great speech in the House of Commons, during the debate on Ireland, 25th January, 1847.

weeks' duration which was more intense than anyone remembered. It is said to have made the ground like iron to the depth of nine inches; the ice on all the rivers stopped the corn mills, trees and shrubs were destroyed, and even the wool fell out of the sheep's backs. In January 1740 the destitution was such that subscription-lists were opened in Dublin, Cork, Limerick, Waterford, Clonmel, Wexford and other places. Bishop Berkeley distributed every Monday morning twenty pounds sterling among the poor of Cloyne (near Cork) besides what they got from his kitchen. One morning he came down without powder on his wig, and all the domestics of the episcopal palace followed suit[1]. The distress became more acute as the spring advanced. The potato crop of 1739 had been ruined, not by disease as in 1845–46, but by the long and intense frost. It was usual at that time to leave the tubers in the ridges through most of the winter, with the earth heaped up around them. The frost of December found them with only that slight covering, and rotted them: "a dirissimo hoc et diuturno gelu penitus putrescebant," says Dr O'Connell. Besides putrid potatoes, the people ate the flesh of cattle which had died from the rigours of the season. Owing to the want of sound seed-potatoes, the crop of 1740 was almost a blank. The summer was excessively dry and hot. In Dublin, the price of provisions had doubled or trebled, and some of the poor had died of actual starvation. In July dysenteries became common, and extended to the richer classes in the capital. Smallpox was rife at the same time, and peculiarly fatal in Cork. Dysentery continued in Dublin throughout the autumn and winter of 1740 (the latter being again frosty), and became the prevailing malady elsewhere.

On 8 February, 1741, Berkeley writes that the bloody flux had appeared lately in the town of Cloyne, having made great progress before that date in other parts of the country. A week after he writes (15 Feb.), "Our weather is grown fine and warm: but the bloody flux has increased in this neighbourhood, and raged most violently in other parts of this and the adjacent counties[2]." This prevalence of dysentery, and not of fever, as the reigning malady of the winter of 1740–41 in Munster is

---

[1] Fraser, "Life and Letters of Berkeley," in *Works*, IV. 262.
[2] Berkeley to Prior, Feb. 8 and 15, 174$\frac{0}{1}$.

confirmed by Dr Maurice O'Connell, who says that the typhus of the previous summer gave place to it. Dysentery in the winter and spring, preceding the fever of summer, was also the experience in the famine of 1817. Berkeley treated the subjects of dysentery, not with tar water, but with a spoonful of powdered resin dissolved in oil by heat and mixed in a clyster of broth[1].

As the year 1741 proceeded, with great drought in April and May, typhus fever (which had appeared the autumn before) and dysentery were both widely epidemic, so that it is impossible to say which form of disease caused most deaths. In Dublin during the month of March, 1741, the deaths from dysentery reached a maximum of twenty-one in a week, "though it was less mortal than in the country, to which the better care taken of the poor and of their food undoubtedly contributed." Bishop Berkeley writes on the 19th of May:

"The distresses of the sick and poor are endless. The havoc of mankind in the counties of Cork, Limerick and some adjacent places, hath been incredible. The nation probably will not recover this loss in a century. The other day I heard one from county Limerick say that whole villages were entirely depeopled. About two months since I heard Sir Richard Cox say that five hundred were dead in the parish where he lives, though in a country I believe not very populous. It were to be wished that people of condition were at their seats in the country during these calamitous times, which might provide relief and employment for the poor[2]."

It was said that there were twenty-five cases of fever in the bishop's own household, which were cured by the panacea, tar-water, drunk copiously—a large glass, milk-warm, every hour in bed, the same method being practised by several of his poor neighbours with equal success[3]. In a "Letter from a country gentleman in the Province of Munster to his Grace the Lord Primate[4]" it is said:

"By a moderate computation, very near one-third of the poor cottiers of Munster have perished by fevers, fluxes and downright want...The charity of the landlords and farmers is almost quite exhausted. Multitudes have perished, and are daily perishing, under hedges and ditches, some by fevers, some by fluxes, and some through downright cruel want in the utmost agonies of despair. I have seen the labourer endeavouring to work at his spade, but fainting for want of food," etc.

[1] He published the receipt in a Dublin journal.
[2] Berkeley to Thomas Prior, in "Life and Letters," u. s., p. 265. Some attempts at relief-works had been made the year before, two of which are still to be seen in the obelisks on Killiney Hill near Dublin and on a hill near Maynooth ("Lady Conolly's Folly." O'Rourke, u. s.).
[3] Rutty, p. 93.
[4] (Dublin, 1741).

The loss of life must have been great also in Connaught. A letter of 8 July, 1741, from Galway, says: "The fever so rages here that the physicians say it is more like a plague than a fever, and refuse to visit patients for any fee whatever[1]." The Galway Assizes were held at Tuam[2], the races also being transferred to the same neighbourhood, not without their usual evening accompaniments of balls and plays.

Of this famine and sickness it might have been said, in the stock medieval phrase, that the living were hardly able to bury the dead[3].

As in later Irish famines, there appear to have been, in 1740–41, three main types of sickness—dysentery, relapsing fever and typhus fever. In Dublin, as we know from the direct testimony of Rutty, there was relapsing fever in 1739, before the distress had well begun, and again in the summer of 1741, when the worst was over. So much is said of dysentery that we may well set down to it, and to its attendant dropsy, a great part of the deaths, as in the famine of 1846–47. But it is probable that true typhus fever, sometimes of a malignant type, as at Galway, was the chief infection in 1741, which was the year of its great prevalence in England. It was characterized by a mild and deceitful onset, like a cold. Spots were not invariable or essential; they were mostly of a dusky red, sometimes purple, and sometimes intermixed with miliary pustules. O'Connell mentions, for Munster, bleeding from the nose, a mottled rash as in measles, and pains like those of lumbago. One of the worst features of the Irish epidemic of 1740–41 was the prevalence of fever in the gaols. At Tralee above a hundred were tried, most of them for stealing the means of subsistence; the gaol was so full that there was no room to lie down, and fifty prisoners died

[1] Cited by O'Rourke. Short, a contemporary, also says that the fever in Galway was like a plague.

[2] Dutton, *Statistical Survey of the County of Galway.* Dublin, 1824, p. 313: "1741. A fever raged this year that occasioned the judges to hold the assizes in Tuam. Numbers of the merchants of Galway died this year, and multitudes of poor people, caused partly by fever and by the scarcity, as wheat was 28*s.* per cwt."

[3] The author of *The Groans of Ireland* (Dublin, 1741) says: "On my return to this country I found it the most miserable scene of distress that I ever read of in history: want and misery in every face; the rich unable to relieve the poor; the road spread with dead and dying bodies; mankind of the colour of the docks and nettles which they fed on; two or three, sometimes more, on a car going to the grave for want of bearers to carry them, and many buried only in the fields and ditches where they perished." Skelton, a Protestant clergyman, says: "Whole parishes in some places were almost desolate; the dead have been eaten in the fields by dogs, for want of people to bury them." Skelton's *Works*, Vol. v. Cited by Lecky.

16—2

in six weeks. Limerick gaol had dysentery and fever among its inmates, and the judge who held the Munster Circuit died of fever on his return to Dublin[1].

Rutty says that the fever fell most upon strong middle-aged men, less upon women, and least of all upon children. The number of orphans was so great after the famine that Boulter, the Anglican primate, seized the opportunity to start the afterwards notorious Charter Schools for the education of the rising generation according to the Protestant creed. In all the subsequent Irish famines it was the enormous swarms of people begging at a distance from their own parishes that spread the infection of fever; and there seems to have been as much of beggary in 1741, when Ireland was underpeopled with two millions, as in 1817–18, when it was overpeopled with six millions. A few years after the famine, Berkeley wrote in 1749:

"In every road the ragged ensigns of poverty are displayed; you often meet caravans of poor, whole families in a drove, without clothes to cover, or bread to feed them, both which might be easily procured by moderate labour. They are encouraged in their vagabond life by the miserable hospitality they meet with in every cottage, whose inhabitants expect the same kind reception in their turn when they become beggars themselves."

The estimates of the Irish mortality in 1741 varied greatly, as they have done in the Irish famines of more recent times. One guessed a third of the cottiers of Munster, another said one-fifth; and it is known that, whereas in Kerry the hearth-money was paid in 1733 by 14,346, it was paid in 1744 by only 9372[2]. The largest estimates are 200,000 deaths or even 400,000 deaths in all Ireland in a population of less than two millions. But Dr Maurice O'Connell, who practised in Cork, and saw in Munster the mortality at its worst, estimated the deaths in all Ireland, in the two years 1740 and 1741, from fevers, fluxes and absolute want, at 80,000. Those who saw the famine, fever and dysentery of 1817–18 in a population increased by three times were inclined to doubt whether even the smallest estimate of 80,000 for 1740–41 was not too large; but it is clear that the famished and fever-stricken in the 18th century were in many places allowed to perish owing to the

[1] Report by Dr Phipps to Baron Wainwright, 10 March, 1741. Cited by F. C. Webb, *Trans. Epidem. Soc.* 1857, p. 67.
[2] Smith's *Kerry*, p. 77. He adds that many were excused the hearth-tax on account of their poverty, by certificate of the magistrates; so that the decrease in 1744 may mean a greater proportion excused the tax, as well as a depopulation.

indifference of the ruling class or the exhaustion of their means, so that a much higher rate of fatality may be assumed for that epidemic than for the first of the 19th century Irish famines.

The distress came to an end before the winter of 1741, when food was so cheap in Dublin that a shilling bought twenty-one pounds of bread. The subsequent prevalence of typhus fever and dysentery in Ireland, whether epidemic or endemic, is very imperfectly known to the end of the century. It may be inferred that there was in that period no epidemic so great as that of 1740–41; but it is clear from the records kept by Rutty in Dublin down to 1764, and by Sims in Tyrone to 1772, that the indigenous fevers and fluxes of the country were never long absent, being more common in some years than in others[1].

The year 1744 was remarkable for a destructive throat distemper among children, described elsewhere, and the year 1745 for smallpox dispersed by swarms of beggars. In 1746 and 1748, the Dublin fever was relapsing in part, "terminating," says Rutty, "the fifth, sixth, seventh or eighth day with a critical sweat. A relapse commonly attended, which however was commonly carried off by a second critical sweat." In 1748, though the season was sickly, the diseases were not mortal, several of the fevers being "happily terminated by a sweat the fifth or sixth day." But there were also fevers of the low kind, sometimes with petechiae, sometimes with miliary pustules, though not essentially with either. In the autumn of 1754 Rutty begins to adopt the language of the time concerning a "putrid" constitution, identifying the fever with the dangerous remittents which Fothergill was then writing about in London; "it is probable that ours was akin to them and owing to the same general causes." In February, 1755, the fevers were fatal to many, raising the deaths to double the usual number; they attacked all ages, were of the low, depressed kind, and commonly attended with miliary pustules. He again identifies them with the low, putrid fever in London. From that time on to 1758, Rutty has frequent references to the same fever, under

[1] How near the verge of want the people were is brought out by an experience in Galway county in 1745: a great fall of snow smothered vast numbers of cattle and sheep, which caused a great many farmers to surrender their lands. Wheat rose from six to eighteen shillings the hundredweight, while, after the distress, the best land in Connaught could be rented for five shillings an acre. Dutton's *Galway*, p. 313.

the names of low, putrid, petechial and miliary. It was at its worst in 1757, and was marked by the remarkable tremors described by Johnstone at Kidderminster, as well as by miliary eruptions and by a gangrenous tendency at the spots where blisters had been applied. In November, 1757, it was fatal to not a few of the young and strong in Dublin, "and we received accounts of a like malignity attending this fever in the country[1]." It was still prevalent in the North and West of Ireland in the spring of 1758. He describes also an unusual amount of fever in the end of 1762. Sims, of Tyrone, an epidemiologist in the same manner as Rutty, does not begin his full annals until 1765; but he sums up the years from 1751 to 1760 as unhealthy by agues in spring, dysenteries and cholera morbus in autumn, and "low, putrid or nervous fevers throughout the year[2]." He adds:

"To the unhealthiness of these years the bad state and dearth of provisions might not a little contribute; the poor, being incapable to procure sufficient sustenance, were often obliged to be contented with things at which nature almost revolted; and even the wealthy could not by all their art and power render wholesome those fruits of the earth which had been damaged by an untoward season."

Much of the distress, however, was owing to the continual spread of pasture-farming, which made the labour of villagers unnecessary[3].

The nearest approach to a great Irish epidemic in the second half of the 18th century was in 1771, as described by Sims, the type of fever being clearly the same low, putrid or nervous fever, with offensive sweats and muscular tremors, that was commonly observed in England also in the middle third of the 18th century. Early in the summer of 1771 a fever began to appear which, as autumn advanced, raged with the greatest violence; nor was it overcome by a severe winter. It claimed the prerogative of the plague, almost all others vanishing from before its presence. It began twelve months sooner in the

[1] For Kinsale, Cork and Bandon, see Marjoribanks, *Med. Press and Circ.* 1867, II. 8.
[2] James Sims, M.D. *Observations on Epidemic Disorders, with Remarks on Nervous and Malignant Fevers.* London, 1773, p. 10. The preface is dated from London, whither Sims had removed from Tyrone. He rose to eminence in the London profession.
[3] *A Letter to a Member of the Irish Parliament relative to the present State of Ireland.* By Philo-Irene. London, 20 May, 1755. The turning of hundreds of acres into one dairy-farm had caused the depopulation which Goldsmith described in the *Deserted Village*: "By this unhappy policy several villages have been deserted at different times by the inhabitants, and numbers of them set a-begging," p. 6.

eastern parts of the kingdom, pursuing a regular course from
East to West.   Some symptoms suggest cerebro-spinal fever.

The symptoms were languor, precordial oppression, want of appetite,
slight nausea, pains in the head, back and loins, a thin bluish film on the
tongue, turbid urine, eyes lifeless and dejected.   After the fourth day,
constant watchfulness, the eyes wild, melancholy, sometimes with bloody
water in them, constant involuntary sighing, the tendons of the wrists
tremulous, the pulse quick and weak, most profuse sweats, small dun petechiae
principally at the bend of the arm and about the neck.   At the height of the
fever, on the ninth or tenth day, the tremulousness of the wrists spread to all
the members, "insomuch that I have seen the bed-curtains dancing for three
or four days to the no small terror of the superstitious attendants, who on
first perceiving it, thought some evil spirits shook the bed.   This agitation was
so constant a concomitant of the fever as to be almost a distinguishing
symptom."   The patients lay grinding their teeth; when awake, they would
often convulsively bite off the edges of the vessel in which drink was given
them.   They knew no one, their delirium being incessant, low, muttering,
their fingers picking the bed covering.   The face was pale and sunk, the
eyes hollow, the tongue and lips black and parched.   Profuse clammy sweats
flowed from them; the urine was as if mixed with blood: the stools were
involuntary.   Petechiae almost black came out, having an outer circle with
an inner dark speck; sometimes there were the larger vibice..   Bleedings at
the nose were frequent.   Those who were put to bed and sweated almost
all died.   Death took place about the 13th day.

Curiously enough this disease showed itself even among the
middle ranks of the people, especially those who lived an
irregular life, used flesh diet and drank much.   Among the
poorer sort, who used vegetable food, the fever was more
protracted and less malignant, but in the winter and spring it
made much greater havoc among them.   "Bleeding, that first
and grand auxiliary of the physician in treating inflammatory
disorders, seemed here to lose much of its influence."   It was,
indeed, the long prevalence of this low or nervous type of fever
in Britain and Ireland in the middle of the 18th century that
drove blood-letting in fevers out of fashion until the return of a
more inflammatory type (often relapsing fever) in the epidemic
of 1817.   In 1770, while such fevers more or less nervous,
putrid, miliary, were beginning to be prevalent among the
adults, there was a good deal of "worm fever" among children.
They suffered from heat, thirst, quick, full pulse, vomiting, coma,
and sometimes slight convulsions, universal soreness to the touch,
and a troublesome phlegmy cough.   When not comatose they
were peevish.   The fever was remitting, the cheeks being highly
flushed at its acme, pale in its remission.   It lasted several days,
but seldom over a week, nor was it often fatal.   In children
under five or six years, it could hardly be distinguished from

hydrocephalus internus[1]. The same association of the worm fever or remittent fever of children with the putrid or nervous fever of adults had been noticed at Edinburgh in 1735. Neither the fever of the adults nor that of the children will be found, on close scrutiny, to have had much in common with our modern enteric fever.

The Epidemic Fevers of 1799-1801.

Sims left Tyrone to practise as a physician in London, and with his departure what seems to have been the only contemporary record of epidemics in Ireland ceased. The last quarter of the 18th century in Ireland had probably as much epidemic fever as in England; but it is not until the years 1797–1801 that we again hear of fever and dysentery, on the testimony of the records of the Army Medical Board, of the Dublin House of Industry, and of the Waterford Fever Hospital. At the end of the year 1796 the health of the regiments in Ireland was everywhere good; but in December of that year, and in January 1797, the poor in the towns began to suffer more than usual from fever, and in the course of the year 1797 fever appeared in several cantonments of troops—at Armagh as early as February or March, at Limerick, at Waterford and in Dublin[2]. The summer and autumn were unusually wet, so that the peasantry of the southern and western counties were unable to lay in their usual supply of turf for fuel. In the course of the winter 1797–98 a considerable increase of fever and dysentery was remarked among them, and these two maladies appeared in various regiments in the early months of 1798. This was the year of the rebellion in the south-east of Ireland, pending the efforts for the union with England. The British troops were much engaged with the insurgents throughout the summer, and got rid in great part of the maladies of their quarters while they were campaigning. But in the end of the year fever began to spread, both among the inhabitants and among the troops. It was nothing new for English and Scots regiments to suffer from fever or dysentery during the greater part of their first year in Ireland; but the

---

[1] Sims, u. s. pp. 164–5.

[2] F. Barker and J. Cheyne, *Account of the Fever lately epidemical in Ireland.* 2 vols. London, 1821. This work relates mainly to the epidemic of 1817–19, but there is a short retrospect, the valuable part of which is for the years 1797–1802.

epidemics in the end of 1798 were more than ordinary. The Buckinghamshire Militia quartered in the Palatine Square of the Royal barracks, Dublin, lost by "malignant contagious fever" 13 men in October, 13 in November, and 15 in December. From November to January, the Warwick regiment suffered greatly in the same barrack. The Herefordshire regiment, 833 strong, lost 47 men at Fermoy, mostly from fever contracted in bad barracks; the Coldstream Guards at Limerick, the 92nd regiment at Athlone, and the Northamptonshire Fencibles at Carrick-on-Shannon, also lost men by fever. In July, 1799, not a single regiment in Ireland was sickly; but a wet and very cold autumn made a bad harvest, aggravating the distresses of the poor and causing much sickness, which the troops shared. The county of Wexford, the principal scene of the rebellion, suffered most, and next to it the adjacent county of Waterford. The fever-hospital of the latter town, the earliest in Ireland[1], was projected in 1799; the statement made in the report of a plan for the new charity, that fifteen hundred dependent persons suffered from contagious fever every year there, showed that the need for it was nothing new, although hardly a tenth part of the number sought admission to the hospital when it was at work. Next year, 1800, the managers of the newly-opened hospital gave some particulars of the causes of fever in Waterford—want of food, causing weakness of body and depression of mind, but above all the excessive pawning of clothes and bedding, whereby they suffered from cold and slept for warmth several in a bed. In the winter and spring of 1799–1800 the poor of Waterford had epidemic among them fever and dysentery, as well as smallpox. In Donagh-a-gow's Lane nine persons died of dysentery between October 1799 and March 1800. The harvest of 1800 was again a failure, from cold and wet, bread and potatoes being dear and of bad quality. In the autumn and winter the distress, with the attendant fever and dysentery, became worse. At that time in Dublin all fever cases among the poor were received into the House of Industry (the Cork Street and Hardwick Hospitals were soon after built for fever-cases), at which the deaths for four years were as follows:

[1] The history of the Limerick and Belfast fever-hospitals is carried back to a few years before the founding of the Waterford hospital; but the latter was the first that was formally organised as a fever-hospital.

Year	Died in the Dublin House of Industry
1799	627
1800	1315
1801	1352
1802	384

The enormous rise of the deaths in 1800 and 1801 shows how severe the epidemic of fever must have been. Compared with the epidemic of 1817–18, it has few records, perhaps because the political changes of the union engrossed all attention. But the significant fact remains that the deaths in the Dublin House of Industry in 1800 and 1801 were nearly as many as in all the special fever-hospitals of Dublin during the two years, 1 Sept. 1817 to 1 Sept. 1819. At Cork, in 1800, there were 4000 cases of fever treated from the Dispensary; at Limerick the state of matters is said to have been as bad as in the great famine of 1817–18; and there is some reason to think that the same might have been said of other places. All the relief in 1800–1801 came from private sources, the example of Dublin in opening soup-kitchens having been followed by other towns. The troops shared in the reigning diseases, especially at Belfast and Dublin; in the latter city, the spotted fever was severe both among the military and all ranks of the civil population in August, 1801. The harvest of 1801 was abundant, and the fever quickly declined. It had been often of the relapsing type[1]. Dysentery appeared in the end of September, and became severe in many places in October and November, being attributed to the rains after a long tract of dry, hot weather. Ophthalmias and scarlatinal malignant sore-throats were common at the same time.

The Growth of Population in Ireland.

When the history of the great famine and epidemic sicknesses of 1817-18 was written, it was found that this calamity had fallen upon a population that had grown imperceptibly until it had reached the enormous figure of over six millions, the census of 1821 showing the inhabitants of Ireland to be 6,801,827. The increase from an estimated one

---

[1] "The fever in 1800 and 1801 very generally terminated on the fifth or seventh day by perspiration; the disease was then very liable to recur. The poor were the chief sufferers by it; and it was much more fatal amongst the middling and upper classes in proportion to the number attacked." Barker and Cheyne, *op. cit.* p. 20.

million and thirty-four thousand in 1695 was, according to Malthus, probably without parallel in Europe. According to Petty, the inhabitants in 1672 numbered about one million one hundred thousand, living in two hundred thousand houses, of which 160,000 were "wretched, nasty cabins without chimney, window or door-shut, and wholly unfit for making merchantable butter, cheese, or the manufacture of woollen, linen or leather." In 1695, the war on behalf of James II. having intervened, the population as estimated by South was 1,034,000. When the people were next counted in 1731, by a not incorrect method in the hands of the magistracy and Protestant clergy, they were found to have almost doubled, the total being 2,010,221. This increase, the exactness of which depends naturally upon the accuracy of Petty's and South's 17th century estimates, had been made notwithstanding the famines and epidemics of 1718 and 1728, and an excessive emigration, mostly of Protestants, to the West Indian and American colonies, which was itself attended by a great loss of life through disease. For the rest of the 18th century, the estimates of population are based upon the number of houses that paid the hearth-tax. In the following figures six persons are reckoned to each taxed hearth:

Year	Persons
1754	2,372,634
1767	2,544,276
1777	2,690,556
1785	2,845,932

The hearth-money was not altogether a safe basis of reckoning, for the reason that many were excused it on account of their poverty by certificate from the magistrates, and that hamlets in the hills, perhaps those which held their lands in rungale or joint-lease, often compounded with the collectors for a fixed sum; so that cabins might multiply and no more hearth-tax be paid[1]. It is probable that a considerable increase had taken place which was not represented in the books of the tax-collectors; for in 1788, only three years from the last date given, the number of hearths suddenly leapt up to the round figure of 650,000 (from 474,322), giving a population of 3,900,000, at the rate of six persons to a cabin or house. But it is undoubted that a new impulse was given to population in the last twenty years of the 18th century, firstly by the bounties on

[1] Smith's *Kerry.* Dublin, 1756, p. 77.

Irish corn exported, dating from 1780, which caused much grazing land to be brought under the plough, and secondly by the gradual removal, after 1791, of various penalties and disabilities which had rested on the Roman Catholics since the reign of Anne, affecting their tenure of land, and serving in various ways to repress the multiplication of families. Accordingly we find the hearths rated in 1791 at the number of 701,102, equal to a population of 4,206,612. The estimates or enumerations from 1788, to the census of 1831, show an increase as follows:

Year	Persons	Year	Persons
1788	3,900,000	1812	5,937,856
1791	4,206,612	1821	6,801,827
1805	5,395,456	1831	7,784,539

The secret of this enormous increase was the habit that the Irish peasantry had begun to learn early in the 17th century of living upon potatoes. From that dietetic peculiarity, it is well known, much of the economic and political history of Ireland depends. At the time when it was losing its tribal organization (rather late in the day, although not so late as in the Highlands of Scotland), the country was in a fair way to pass from the pastoral state to the agricultural and industrial. It is conceivable that, if Ireland had peacefully become an agricultural country, wheaten bread would have become the staple food of the people, as in England in early times and again in later times; or that the standard might have been oatmeal in the northern province, as in Scotland: in which case one may be sure that the population would not have increased as it did. "Since the culture of the potatoes was known," says a topographer of Kerry in 1756, "which was not before the beginning of the last century, the herdsmen find out small dry spots to plant a sufficient quantity of those roots in for their sustenance, whereby considerable tracts of these mountains are grazed and inhabited, which could not be done if the herdsmen had only corn to subsist on[1]." Twenty years later Arthur Young found an enormous extension of potato culture, the pigs being fed on the surplus crop[2]. The motive, on the part of the landlord or the farmer, was to have the peat bogs on the hill-sides reclaimed by the spade; the surface of peat having

[1] Smith's *Kerry*, p. 88.
[2] *A Tour in Ireland...in* 1776–78. London, 1780.

been removed, a poor subsoil was exposed, which might be made something of after it had grown several crops of potatoes, but hardly in any other way. Another motive was political; namely, the multiplication by landlords of forty-shilling freeholder dependent votes among the Catholics as soon as they became free to exercise the franchise[1].

Malthus relied so much upon statistics, that he found the case of Ireland, notable though it was, little suited to his method, and dismissed it in a few sentences. But he indicated correctly the grand cause of over-population:

"I shall only observe, therefore, that the extended use of potatoes has allowed of a very rapid increase of population during the last century (18th). But the cheapness of this nourishing root, and the small piece of ground which, under this kind of cultivation, will in average years produce the food for a family, joined to the ignorance and depressed state of the people, which have prompted them to follow their inclinations with no other prospect than an immediate bare subsistence, have encouraged marriage to such a degree that the population is pushed much beyond the industry and present resources of the country; and the consequence naturally is, that the lower classes of people are in the most impoverished and miserable state."

In another section he showed that the cheapness of the staple food of Ireland tended to keep down the rate of wages:

"The Irish labourer paid in potatoes has earned perhaps the means of subsistence for double the number of persons that could be supported by an English labourer paid in wheat...The great quantity of food which land will bear when planted with potatoes, and the consequent cheapness of the labour supported by them, tends rather to raise than to lower the rents of land, and as far as rent goes, to keep up the price of the materials of manufacture and all other sorts of raw produce except potatoes. The indolence and want of skill which usually accompany such a state of things tend further to render all wrought commodities comparatively dear...The value of the food which the Irish labourer earns above what he and his family consume will go but a very little way in the purchase of clothing, lodging and other conveniences...In Ireland the money price of labour is not much more than the half of what it is in England."

Lastly, in a passage quoted in the sequel, he showed how disastrous a failure of the crop must needs be when the staple was potatoes; the people then had nothing between them and starvation but the garbage of the fields[2].

What the growth of population could come to on these terms was carefully shown for the district of Strabane, on the borders of Tyrone and Donegal, by Dr Francis Rogan, a writer

[1] The forty-shillings freeholder of Ireland was a life-renter whose farm was worth forty shillings annual rent more than the rent reserved in his lease.

[2] Malthus, *Essay on the Principle of Population.* Bk. II. chap. 10, Bk. III. chap. 8, and Bk. IV. chap. 11.

on the famine and epidemic fever of 1817–18[1]. Strabane stood at the meeting of the rivers Mourne and Fin to form the Foyle; and in the three valleys the land was fertile. All round was an amphitheatre of hills, in the glens of which and among the peat bogs on their sides was an immense population. The farms were small, from ten to thirty acres, a farm of fifty acres being reckoned a large holding. The tendency had been to minute subdivisions of the land, the sons dividing a farm among them on the death of the father:

"The Munterloney mountains," says Rogan, "lie to the south and east of the Strabane Dispensary district. They extend nearly twenty miles, and contain in the numerous glens by which they are intersected so great a population that, except in the most favourable years, the produce of their farms is unequal to their support. In seasons of dearth they procure a considerable part of their food from the more cultivated districts around them; and this, as well as the payment of their rents, is accomplished by the sale of butter, black cattle, and sheep, and by the manufacture of linen cloth and yarn, which they carry on to a considerable extent."

These small farmers dwelt in thatched cottages of three or four rooms, in which they brought up large families[2]. Besides the farmers, there were the cottiers, who lived in cabins of the poorest construction, sometimes built against the sides of a peat-cutting in the bog. The following table shows the proportion of cottiers to small farmers on certain manors of the Marquis of Abercorn, near Strabane, at the date of the famine in 1817–18 (Rogan, p. 96):

[1] Francis Rogan, M.D., *Observations on the Condition of the Middle and Lower Classes in the North of Ireland, as it tends to promote the diffusion of Contagious Fever; with the History and Treatment of the late Epidemic Disorders.* London, 1819.

[2] William Carleton, the *vates sacer* of the Irish peasantry, was born, in 1798, in one of those Tyrone thatched cottages, in the parish of Clogher. His father had changed his holding three times before William, the youngest child, was fourteen years old; the last of the four was a farm of sixteen or eighteen acres in the north of Clogher parish, and "nearer the mountains." Carleton says that he "lived among the people as one of themselves" until he was twenty-two, which would have been until the year 1820; so that he probably saw the famine and fever of 1817–18 among that very Tyrone peasantry whom Dr Rogan brings before us from the medical side. The scenes of famine and fever in the 'Black Prophet' are those "which he himself witnessed in 1817, 1822, and other subsequent years," having been recalled by him in the form of a tale which was published in 1846, at the beginning of the Great Famine of that and the following year. His early recollections of famine and fever come into other tales, such as the 'Clarionet,' the 'Poor Scholar' and 'Tubber Derg,' in which last is related the almost inevitable reduction to poverty and at length to beggary of a most upright and industrious farmer owing to the fall of prices, without fall of rents, after the Peace of 1815. Carleton's work has always the quality of fidelity, and he may be credited when he says that the scenes of famine and fever are not exaggerated.

Manors	Number of Families	
	Farmers	Cottiers
Derrygoon	368	335
Donelong	243	322
Magevelin and		
Lismulmughray	319	668
Strabane	302	415
Cloughognal	328	279

The cottiers rented their cabins and potato gardens from the farmers, paying their rent, on terms not advantageous to themselves, by labour on the farm. For a time about the beginning of the century the practice by farmers of taking land on speculation to sublet to cottiers was so common that a class of "middlemen" arose. One pamphleteer during the distress of 1822 speaks of the class of middlemen as an advantage to the cottiers, and regrets that they should have been personally so disreputable as to have become extinct. It is not easy to understand how they served the interests of the cottiers: for the latter were answerable to the landlord for the middleman's rent, and were themselves over-rented and underpaid for their labour. The system of middlemen did not in matter of fact answer; they hoped to make a profit from the tenants under them, and neglected to work on their own farms; it appears that they were a drunken class, and that they were at length swallowed up in bankruptcy. After the first quarter of the century the cottiers and the landlords (with the agents and the tithe proctors) stood face to face; but at the date of the famine of 1817 there was subletting going on, of which Rogan gives an instructive instance in his district of Ulster[1].

Under this system of subdividing farms and subletting potato gardens with cabins to cottiers, the following enormous populations had sprung up in four parishes within the

[1] Rogan, u. s. p. 95: "A farmer within my knowledge, who holds fifteen acres of arable land, with nearly an equal quantity of cut-out bog, for which he pays £28 per annum, has erected six cabins for labourers. They are built with mud, instead of lime, and are thatched, so that they cannot each have cost more than three or four pounds. For some time he received from three of his tenants six guineas per annum, and from the others two guineas each, the latter only holding a cottage and a small garden [the former three having also grazing for a milch cow, half a rood of land for flax, and half an acre for oats, with privileges of cutting turf and planting as many potatoes as they could each provide manure for]; but they have been all so reduced in circumstances by the late scarcity as to be now unable to keep a cow, and for the two last years have rented their cabins and potato gardens alone. All the straw raised on the farm would scarcely suffice to keep the houses water-fast if applied solely to this purpose." One of the first things that the Marquis of Abercorn did in the epidemic of 1817 was to call upon the subletting farmers on his manors to repair the roofs of their cottiers' cabins.

Dispensary district of Strabane and in four manors of the Marquis of Abercorn adjoining them, but not included in the Dispensary District :

Town of Strabane	3896
Parish of Camus	2384
,, ,, Leck	5092
,, ,, Urney	4886
Manor of Magevelin and Lismulmughray	5548
Manor of Donelong	3126
,, ,, Derrygoon	2568
,, ,, Part of Strabane	2796

In the language of the end of the 19th century, this would have been called a "congested district" of Ireland; but all Ireland was then congested to within a million and a half of the utmost limit, so that the famine, which we shall now proceed to follow in this part of Ulster, has to be imagined as equally severe in Connaught, in Munster, and even in parts of Leinster.

The Famine and Fevers of 1817–18.

The winter of 1815–16 had been unusually prolonged, so that the sowing and planting of 1816 were late. They were hardly over when a rainy summer began, which led to a ruined harvest. The oats never filled, and were given as green fodder to the cattle; in wheat-growing districts, the grain sprouted in the sheaf; the potatoes were a poor yield and watery; such of them as came to the starch-manufacturers were found to contain much less starch than usual. The peat bogs were so wet that the usual quantity of turf for fuel was not secured[1]. This failure of the harvest came at a critical time. The Peace of Paris in 1815 had depressed prices and wages and thrown commerce into confusion. During the booming period of war-prices, from 1803 to 1815, farms and small holdings had doubled or even trebled in rent, and had withal yielded a handsome profit to the farmers and steady work to the labourers. When the extraordinary war expenditure stopped, this factitious prosperity came to a sudden end. The sons of Irish cottiers were not wanted for the war, and the daughters were no longer

---

[1] Carleton, in one of his tales, has given a vivid picture of the lurid or gloomy appearance of the country in the late autumn of 1816, as if it foreboded the distress of the following spring.

profitable as flax-spinners to the small farmers. Weavers could hardly earn more than threepence a day, and labourers who could find employment at all had to be content with fourpence or sixpence, without their food. A stone of small watery potatoes cost tenpence; but the value of cattle fell to one-third, and butter brought little. By Christmas the produce of the peasants' harvest of 1816 was mostly consumed. "Many hundred families holding small farms in the mountains of Tyrone," says Rogan, "had been obliged to abandon their dwellings in the spring of 1817 and betake themselves to begging, as the only resource left to preserve their lives[1]." At Galway, in January, a mob gathered to stop the sailing of a vessel laden with oatmeal. At Ballyshannon the peasants took to the shore to gather cockles, mussels, limpets and the remains of fish. In some parts the seed potatoes were taken up and consumed. The people wandered about in search of nettles, wild mustard, cabbage-stalks and the like garbage, to stay their stomachs. It was painful, says Carleton, to see a number of people collected at one of the larger dairy farms waiting for the cattle to be blooded (according to custom), so that they might take home some of the blood to eat mixed with a little oat meal. The want of fuel caused the pot to be set aside, windows and crevices to be stopped, washing of clothes and persons to cease, and the inmates of a cabin to huddle together for warmth. This was far from being the normal state of the cottages or even of the cabins, but cold and hunger made their inmates apathetic. Admitted later to the hospitals for fever, they were found bronzed with dirt, their hair full of vermin, their ragged clothes so foul and rotten that it was more economical to destroy them and replace them than to clean them.

Some months passed before this state of things produced fever. The first effect of the bad food through the winter, such as watery potatoes eaten half-cooked for want of fuel, had been dysentery, which became common in February, and was aggravated by the cold in and out of doors. It was confined

[1] Probably their cattle had been impounded for rent and tithe. The author of the pamphlet *Lachrymae Hiberniae* (Dublin, 1822), a resident on the western coast, says (p. 8), with reference to the seizures for rent and tithe: "Oh what scenes of misery were exhibited in Ireland in this way during the years 1817, '18 and '19; by that time the people were left without cattle; after this their potatoes and corn were seized and sold, and in some cases their household furniture, even to their blankets." The hardness of landlords in general is alleged by Dr Rogan, with an exception in favour of the Marquis of Abercorn in his own district.

to the very poorest, and was not contagious, attacking perhaps one or two only in a large family. Comparatively few of those who were attacked by it in the country places came to the Strabane Dispensary; but the dropsy which often attended or followed it brought in a larger number. The following table of cases at the Dispensary shows clearly enough that dysentery and dropsy preceded the fever, which became at length the chief epidemic malady[1]:

Cases at Strabane Dispensary.

1817	Dropsy	Dysentery	Typhus
June	23	2	10
July	107	31	60
August	40	22	206
September	9	23	287

At a few of the larger towns in each of the provinces typhus had risen in the autumn of 1816 somewhat above the ordinary low level which characterized the years from 1803 to 1816 in Ireland as well as in Britain. At that time there was steadily from year to year a certain amount of typhus in the poorest parts of the towns and here or there among the cabins of the cottiers. Statistically this may be shown by the table of regular admissions to the fever hospitals of some of the chief towns from the date of their opening.

Admissions to Irish Fever Hospitals, 1799–1818.

Year	Dublin, Cork St. Hospital	Dublin House of Industry	Cork Fever Hospitals	Waterford Fever Hospital	Limerick Fever Hospital	Kilkenny Fever Hospital
1799	—	—	—	146	—	—
1800	—	—	—	409	—	—
1801	—	—	—	875	—	—
1802	—	—	—	419	—	—
1803	—	—	254	188	446	—
1804	415	82	190	223	86	73
1805	1024	709	200	297	95	80
1806	1264	1276	441	165	90	69
1807	1100	1289	191	166	86	56
1808	1071	1473	232	157	84	81
1809	1051	1176	278	222	100	96
1810	1774	1474	432	410	109	116
1811	1471	1316	646	331	120	135
1812	2265	2006	617	323	196	153
1813	2627	1870	550	252	146	156
1814	2392	2398	845	175	227	183
1815	3780	2451	717	403	221	236
1816	2763	1669	1026	307	394	249
1817	3682	2860	4866	390	659	162
1818	7608	17894	10408	2729	2586	1100
					4829	1924

[1] There was dysentery also in the autumn of 1818. Cheyne, *Dubl. Hosp. Rep.* III. I.

In 1812 the first step was taken towards the adoption of the Poor Law, namely the division of the country into Dispensary Districts, which remained the units of charitable relief until 1839, when the old English system of a poor-rate and parochial Unions was applied to Ireland. During that intermediate period much was left to the medical profession, which contained many well-educated and humane men, to the priests and clergy, and to charitable persons among the laity. There was fever in many places where there were no fever hospitals. A physician at Tralee reported that the back lanes of the town, crowded with cabins, were seldom free from typhus. Rogan gives two instances from the Strabane district in the summer and winter of 1815, at a time when the district was remarkably healthy. A beggar boy was given a night's lodging by a cottier at Artigarvan, three miles from Strabane. Next morning he was too ill to leave; he lay three weeks in typhus, and gave the disease to twenty-seven persons in the eight cabins which formed the hamlet. A few months after, about a mile from Strabane, a mother fell into typhus and was visited many times by her two married daughters and by others of her children at service in the neighbourhood. Nineteen cases were traced to this focus; "but the actual number attacked was probably more than three times this, as the disease, when once introduced into the town, spread so widely among the lower orders as to create general alarm, and led to the establishment of the small fever ward attached to the Dispensary." It was in April, 1816, that this was done, two rooms, each with four beds, having been provided at Strabane for fever cases; but at no time until the summer of 1817 were they all occupied at once.

The epidemic really began there in May, 1817, in a large house which had been occupied during the winter by a number of families from the mountains; they had brought no furniture with them, nor bedding except their blankets, and lay so close together as to cover the floors. Each room was rented at a shilling a week, the tenant of a room making up his rent by taking in beggars at a penny a night. The floors and stairs were covered with the gathered filth of a whole winter; the straw bedding, never renewed, was thrown into a corner during the day to be spread again at night. Every crevice was stopped to keep out the cold; the rain came in through the roof, the floors were damp, and the cellars of the house full of stagnant

water turned putrid.   Meanwhile more than a fourth part of the families resident in Strabane, to the number of 1026 persons, were being fed from a soup-house opened early in the spring of 1817, while there were others equally destitute but too proud to ask relief.   The rumour of this charity soon brought crowds of people from the surrounding country, with gaunt cheeks, says Carleton, hollow eyes, tottering gait and a look of "painful abstraction" from the unsatisfied craving for food.   In the crowd round the soup-shop, the timid girl, the modest mother, the decent farmer scrambled "with as much turbulent solicitation and outcry as if they had been trained, since their very infancy, to all the forms of impudent cant and imposture."   These soup-shops were opened in all the Irish towns.   At Strabane some of the richer class lent money to procure supplies, for sale at cost price, of oatmeal, rice and rye-flour, the last being in much request in the form of loaves of black bread.

The fever, having begun among the houseful of vagrants above mentioned, made slow progress until June, when it spread through the town, and in the autumn became a serious epidemic.   Meantime the soup-kitchen was closed, the supplies having ceased, and the country people returned to their cabins carrying the infection of typhus everywhere with them.   By the middle of October, 1817, the epidemic was general in the country round Strabane.

The following table shows the rise and decline of the epidemic of typhus in the town itself.

Cases of Fever attended from Strabane Dispensary[1].

	1817	1818		1817	1818
Jan.	9	83	July	60	106
Feb.	13	46	Aug.	206	90
March	6	60	Sept.	287	57
April	13	48	Oct.	233	49
May	3	39	Nov.	193	40
June	10	71	Dec.	140	38

The exact particulars from the Dispensary district of Strabane show clearly how famine in Ireland is related to fever. The epidemic of typhus was an indirect result of the famine, and was due most of all to the vagrancy which a famine was bound to produce in Ireland, in the absence of a Poor Law.   In the

[1] Rogan, p. 31.

spring of 1817, said a gentleman near Tralee, "the whole country appeared to be in motion." "It was lamentable," said Peel, in the Commons debate, on 22 April, 1818, "at least it was affecting, that this contagion should have arisen from the open character and feelings of hospitality for which the Irish character was so peculiarly remarkable." They gathered also at funerals, and, as Graves said of a later epidemic, they were "scrupulous in the performance of wakes." The concourse of people at the daily distributions of soup was another cause of spreading infection, many of them having come out of infected houses[1]. Of such houses, the lodging-houses of the towns, we have several particular instances. At Strabane, there were four such, which sent ninety-six patients to the fever hospital in eighteen months. At Dublin, a house in Cathedral-lane sent fifty cases to the fever hospitals in a twelvemonth; the house No. 4, Patrick's close sent thirty cases in eight months; No. 52½ Kevin-street sent from five rooms nineteen persons in six weeks.

The spread of the disease was much aided by the ordinary annual migration of harvest labourers. It was the custom every year for cottiers in Connaught to shut up their cabins after the potatoes were planted, and to travel to the country round Dublin in search of work at the hay and corn harvests, leaving their families to beg; in the same way there was an annual migration from Clare to Kilkenny, from Cavan, Longford and Leitrim into Meath, and from Derry into Antrim, Down and Armagh[2]. In the summer of 1817 some parishes of Derry were left with only four or five families. The keeper of the bridge at Toome, over the Bann, counted more than a hundred vagrants every day passing into Antrim, from the middle of May to the

---

[1] The following is an instance, from Boyle, in Roscommon: "In the middle of June, 1817, or a little earlier, a soup-shop was established here by subscription, where soup was daily given out to one thousand persons, who, naturally anxious to procure it in time, crowded together during its distribution, though every pains was taken to keep order amongst them. From the 16th to the 23rd of that month the weather became suddenly and unusually hot, and the disease about that period spread rapidly among those persons, the greater number of whom attributed the origin of their complaint to attendance at the soup-shop; among that crowd, many of whom I have seen faint from absolute want during exposure to the sun, there were persons from houses where the disease existed." Report by Dr Verdon of Boyle, 26 June, 1818, in Barker and Cheyne, I. 325.

[2] Dr King of Tralee (Barker and Cheyne, I. p. 177) wrote as follows: "It is a custom in this country for very poor persons, living in the country parts, and possessing a miserable hovel with a small garden, after they have sowed their potatoes, to shut up their hut and carrying their families with them, to roam about the country, trusting to the known hospitality of the towns and villages for shelter and subsistence till the time for digging the potatoes shall have arrived."

beginning of July; and the same might have been seen at the other bridge over the Bann at Portglenone.

As the spread of contagion came to be realized, the ordinary hospitality to vagrants ceased. Rogan was struck with the apathy which at length arose towards sick or dead relatives; even parents became callous at the death of their children (of whom many died from smallpox). "For some time," he says, "it has been as difficult for a pauper bearing the symptoms of ill-health to procure shelter for the night, as it was formerly rare to be refused it." In Strabane they extemporised a poor's fund by voluntary contributions of £30 a month, by means of which eighty poor families were kept from begging in the streets. In Dublin there was so much alarm of infection from the number of beggars entering the shops that trade was checked. The following, relating to a town in the centre of Ireland, is an extreme instance of the panic which the idea of contagion at length caused:

"In Tullamore, when measures were proposed for arresting the progress of fever, by the establishment of a fever hospital, so little was the alarm that the design was regarded by most of the inhabitants as a well-intentioned project, uncalled for by the circumstances of the community. But when the death of some persons of note excited a sense of danger, alarm commenced, which ended in general dismay: military guards were posted in every avenue leading to this place, for the purpose of intercepting sickly itinerants. The town, from the shops of which the neighbouring country is supplied with articles of all kinds, was thus in a state of blockade. It was apprehended that woollen and cotton goods might be the vehicles of infection, and all intercourse between the shops and purchasers was suspended. Passengers who inadvertently entered the town considered themselves already victims of fever. No person would stop at the public inns, nor hire a carriage for travelling; in a word all communication between the town and the adjacent country was completely interrupted. Apprehension did not proceed in most other places to the same extent as in Tullamore[1]."

Several isolated places escaped the epidemic of typhus, either for a time or altogether. The island of Rathlin, seven miles to the west of Antrim, which was as famished as the mainland, had no typhus at the time when it was epidemic along the nearest shore; the island of Cape Clear, at the southernmost point of Ireland, had a similar experience. The whole county of Wexford, where the soil was dry and the harvest of 1816 had been fair, kept free from typhus until 1818, partly because it was out of the way of vagrants. The town of Dingle, at the head of a bay in Kerry, with old Spanish

---

[1] Barker and Cheyne, I. 60.

traditions, was totally free from typhus at a time when its near neighbour, Tralee, was full of it, the immunity being set down to the well-being of the population from their industry at the linen manufacture (and fisheries) and their thrifty habits.   But the counties of Wexford and Waterford, and other places more or less exempted in 1817, had a full share of the epidemic in 1818, which was the season of its greatest prevalence in most parts of Ireland except Ulster.   The harvest of 1817 had been little better than that of the year before, although the potato crop was hardly a failure.   The fine summer of 1818 brought out crowds of vagrants who slept in the open, and, when they took the infection, were placed in "fever-huts" erected near the roads[1]. The harvest of that year was abundant, and by the end of 1718 the epidemic had declined everywhere except in Waterford.

The most carefully kept statistics of the sickness and mortality were those by Rogan for the Strabane Dispensary district, and the adjoining manors of the Marquis of Abercorn, for each of which a private dispensary was established under the care of a physician.

Abstract of Returns of the Dispensary district of Strabane, shewing the numbers ill of fever from the commencement of the epidemic in the summer of 1817, till the end of September, 1818, the numbers labouring under the fever at that date, and the mortality caused by the disease (Rogan, p. 72).

	Population	Ill of Fever	Dead	Remaining ill
Town of Strabane	3896	639	59	13
Parish of Camus	2384	685	61	37
„ „ Leck	5092	1462	96	57
„ „ Urney	4886	1381	86	42
	16,258	4167	302	149

Similar return for those parts of the Marquis of Abercorn's estates not within the Dispensary district:

Manors	Population	Ill of fever (to Oct. 1818)	Dead
Magevelin and Lismulmughray	5548	1666	101
Donelong	3126	1217	71
Derrygoon	2568	1215	90
Part of Strabane	2796	990	75
Totals	14,038	5088	337

[1] In Carleton's tale of 'The Poor Scholar,' it is related how the hay-mowers stopped in their work to erect a hut for the fever-stricken youth, and a much larger hut not far from the first for the numerous persons who ministered to his wants under a kind of quarantine arrangement.   The stealing of milk from rich men's cows for the sick youth is the subject of a dialogue between the Roman Catholic bishop and the leader of the kindly party of mowers, in which the latter shows a skill in casuistry creditable to his religious instructors.

The proportion of attacks in these tables for a part of Tyrone, one-third to one-fourth of the whole population, is believed to have been a fair average for the whole of Ireland. Each attack, with the weakness that it left behind, lasted about six weeks; cases would occur in a family one after another for several months; in some cottages, says Rogan, only the grandmother escaped.

One hundred thousand cases were known to have passed through the hospitals. Harty thought that seven times as many were sick in their cabins or houses, making 800,000 cases in all Ireland in two years; Barker and Cheyne estimated the whole number of cases at a million and a half (1,500,000). The mortality was comparatively small. It comes out greater in the tables for the Strabane district than anywhere else in Ireland except the hospital at Mallow. The following table, compiled by Harty, shows how widely the fatality ranged (if the figures can be trusted), from place to place and from season to season:

Proportions of fatal cases of typhus in the chief hospitals of Ireland 1817, 1818 and 1819 (Harty)[1].

	1817	1818	1819	Average
	One in	One in	One in	One in
Dublin	$14\frac{1}{2}$	24	$18\frac{1}{4}$	20
Kilkenny	$16\frac{1}{2}$	14 [illegible]	$12\frac{2}{3}$	$14\frac{1}{4}$
Dundalk	$20\frac{6}{7}$	54	25	30
Belfast	$19\frac{1}{5}$	$15\frac{4}{5}$	19	$17\frac{1}{3}$
Newry	$21\frac{1}{9}$	$34\frac{1}{2}$	$13\frac{1}{2}$	26
Cork	29	35	35	$33\frac{1}{5}$
Limerick	$13\frac{1}{2}$	$15\frac{2}{3}$	$30\frac{2}{3}$	$16\frac{1}{2}$
Waterford	$27\frac{1}{3}$	25	$23\frac{1}{3}$	$24\frac{3}{5}$
Clonmel	27	18	$18\frac{1}{4}$	$19\frac{1}{3}$
Mallow	$22\frac{1}{2}$	$9\frac{3}{5}$		12
Killarney	74	67	33	62
Tralee	$20\frac{3}{4}$	69	43	39

What this meant to particular places will appear from some instances. In the parish of Ardstraw, Tyrone, with a population of about twenty thousand, 504 coffins are stated by the parish minister to have been given to paupers in eighteen months. The burials were about twice as many as in ordinary years,

[1] William Harty, M.D. *Historic Sketch of the Contagious Fever Epidemic in Ireland during* 1817–19. Dublin, 1820. This work contains information collected by a circular of queries addressed to practitioners in the several provinces. It was undertaken by Dr Harty at the instance of Sir John Newport, M.P. for Waterford. The work by Barker and Cheyne on the same epidemic took longer to prepare, having been published in 1821. See also Cheyne, *Dubl. Hosp. Rep.* II. 1—147.

according to the register of the Cathedral churchyard of Armagh:

1815	247 burials	
1816	312	,,
1817	571	,,
1 May—25 Dec. } 1818 }	463	,,

Of the 463 burials in eight months of 1818, there were 165 from fever, 180 from smallpox, and 118 from other causes.

Barker and Cheyne make the whole mortality of the two years from fever and dysentery to have been 65,000; Harty makes it 44,300. But not more than a sixth part of the latter total were registered deaths, and the estimate of the whole may be wide of the mark. In the county of Kerry, ten Catholic priests died of it. Many medical men took it, as well as apothecaries and nurses, and several physicians died, of whom Dr Gillichan, of Dundalk, a young man of good fortune, made a notable sacrifice of his life. Everyone bore willing testimony to the devotion of the Roman Catholic clergy. Some harrowing incidents were reported, such as those from Kanturk, in county Cork:

Dr O'Leary visited a low hut in which lay a father and three children: "There were also two grown-up daughters who were obliged to remain for several nights in the open air, not having room in the hut till the father died, when the stronger of the two girls forced herself into his place. On the road leading to Cork, within a mile of this town, I visited a woman of the name of Vaughan, labouring under typhus; on her left lay a child very ill, at the foot of the bed another child just able to crawl about, and on her right the corpse of a third child, who had died two days previously, and which the unhappy mother could not get removed. When the grant arrived from Government, I visited a man of the name of Brahill near the chapel gate, who with his wife and six children occupied a very small house, all of them ill of fever with the exception of one boy, who was so far convalescent as to creep to the door to receive charity from the passengers."

Infants rarely took the fever. Dr Osborne, of Cork, stated that in one instance a physician in attendance on the poor had to separate two children from the bed of their dead brother, the father and mother being already in a fever hospital; in another instance, he had to remove an infant from the corpse of its mother who had just expired in a hovel[1].

Nosologically the epidemic of 1817–18 presented several features of interest. It began with dysentery, and ended with the same in autumn, 1818. It was in great part typhus, but

---

[1] Barker and Cheyne, p. 65. A similar incident comes into Carleton's tale of 'The Clarionet': "At length, out of compassion, the few neighbours who feared not to attend a feverish death-bed, acting on the popular belief that children under a certain age are not liable to catch a fever, placed the boy in her arms." This popular belief was well founded.

towards the end of the epidemic, in Dublin, at Strabane, and doubtless elsewhere, it changed to relapsing fever, that is to say, the sick person "got the cool" about the fifth or seventh day instead of the tenth or twelfth, but was apt to have one or more relapses or recurrences of the fever. The relapsing type was milder in its symptoms and was more rarely fatal. The average fatality of typhus was much less than in ordinary years, while a good many of the fatal cases came from the richer classes, to whom the contagion reached, the proportion of fatalities among them being noted everywhere as very high, up to one death in three or four cases[1]. The fatalities were most common, as usual, at ages from forty to sixty. A full share of the women and children took the fever, perhaps an excess of women, allowing for their excess in the population. The following were the numbers at each period of life among 18,891 cases treated in the hospitals of Dublin and Waterford:

Years of age	1—10	10—20	20—30	30—40	40—50	50 and over
Cases	2426	6116	5230	2476	1415	1228

The action of the English Government was thought by some to have been apathetic. Nothing was done to check the export of corn from Irish ports. Peel, who held the office of Irish Secretary in 1817, was probably actuated in this by the same constitutional and economic considerations which led him, as Prime Minister in 1845, to refuse O'Connell's demand for a proclamation against the export of corn.

Carleton says that there were scattered over the country "vast numbers of strong farmers with bursting granaries and immense haggards," and that long lines of provision carts on their way to the ports met or intermingled with the funerals on the roads, the sight of which exasperated the famishing people. Several carts were attacked and pillaged, some "strong farmers" were visited, and here or there a "miser" or meal-monger was obliged to be charitable with a bad grace; but on the whole there was little lawlessness, less indeed than in England in 1756 and 1766, or in Edinburgh in 1741. In September, 1817, Peel commissioned four Dublin physicians to visit the respective provinces and report on the causes and extent of the epidemic

[1] Accounts from various places in Barker and Cheyne, and in Harty. Rogan (u. s. p. 45) says: "The cases of typhus gravior were infinitely more numerous among the rich and well-fed than among the poor; and with them also the head was most frequently the seat of diseased action."

fever. On 22 April, 1818, Sir John Newport, member for Waterford, for whom Dr Harty had been collecting information, raised a debate on the epidemic in the House of Commons, and moved for a Select Committee. The debate, after the opening speech and a sensible brief reply by Peel, degenerated at once into irrelevant talk on the inadequacy of the fever hospital of London. The Select Committee was named, and quickly reported on the 8th of May.

A Bill embodying the recommendations of the Committee received the royal assent on 30th May. The Act provided for the extension of fever hospitals, the exemption of lodging-houses, under certain regulations, from the hearth-tax and the window-tax, and the formation of Boards of Health with powers to abate and remove nuisances. The Boards of Health were found unworkable, partly by reason of expense, partly of excessive powers. The epidemic having visited Waterford somewhat late in its progress, Sir John Newport again called attention to it on 6th April, 1819, and moved for the revival of last year's Committee. Mr Charles Grant, afterwards Lord Glenelg, who was now Irish Secretary, gave much satisfaction to the patriotic members both by his sympathetic speech on the occasion and by his previous action at the Irish Office in the way of pecuniary help to the fever hospitals or Dispensary district officers. The Second Report of the Committee remarked that the rich absentee landlords had given nothing. Another Act, of June, 1819 (59 Geo. III. cap 41), defined the duties of officers of health, and contained an important clause (ix.) relating to the spread of contagion by vagrants. By that time the epidemic was over; nor can it be said that the action of the Government from first to last had made much difference to its progress.

Vagrancy was the principal direct cause; and behind the vagrancy were usages and traditions, with interests centuries old, which made the landlords resolute not to pay poor-rates on their rentals. It was not until twenty years after that the English Poor Law was applied to Ireland (in 1839), whereby the pauper class were dealt with as far as possible in their respective parishes. How far that measure was effective in checking the spread of contagion will appear when we come to the great famine and epidemic of dysentery and fever in 1846–49.

It will not be necessary to follow with equal minuteness the successive famines and epidemics of typhus, relapsing fever and dysentery in Ireland, to the great famine of 1846–49. After 1817 distress became chronic among the cottiers and small farmers. Leases had been entered into at high rents during the years of war prices, and in the struggle for holdings tenants at will offered the highest rate. When peace came and prices fell, rents were found to be excessive, not to say impossible. But in Ireland with a rapidly increasing population it was easier to put the rents up than to bring them down. Other things helped to embarrass the poor cottager: he paid twice over for his religion, tithes to the parson, dues to the priest; and he paid all the more of the tithe in that the graziers, who were mostly of the established Church and the occupiers of the fertile plains, had taken care to make potato land titheable (at what date this innovation arose is not stated) but had used their power in the Irish Parliament to resist the tithe on arable pastures. Again the cottiers or cottagers paid, in effect, the whole of the poor rate in the form of alms; for the dogs of the gentry kept all beggars from their gates.

Famine and Fever in the West of Ireland, 1821–22.

The next famine in 1821–22 is remarkable for two things besides its purely medical interest. Owing to the number of desperate evicted tenants, it gave occasion to an increased activity of the secret associations, especially the Whiteboys of Tipperary and Cork[1]; and it called forth the first great dole of English charity in the form of princely subscriptions to a Famine Fund. The English charity in 1822 was prompt and large-hearted, contrasting with the tardy help from the exchequer in the much more serious famine of 1817–18. The true explanation of it is, doubtless, that England on the second occasion had more money to spare. The trouble in 1821–22 came from the total loss of the potato crop in Mayo, Galway, Clare and Kerry, and from a partial loss of it in some other counties of the south and west. There was no corn famine, and no general dearth. Accordingly it affected the poorest class only, and the most remote districts chiefly. The planting season of 1821 had

---

[1] *Report on the Present State of the Distressed District in the South of Ireland: with an Enquiry into the Causes of the Distresses of the Peasantry and Farmers.* Dublin, 1822.

not been favourable, and the yield of potatoes had been poor. But the autumn was so wet in the west that the floods in some places washed away the soil with the potatoes in it, and in other places drowned the potatoes after they had been pitted. The flooded state of the basin of the Shannon was a natural calamity on the great scale that touched the imagination and loosened the purse-strings. A Committee was formed at the London Tavern, which sat through the spring of 1822, and quickly raised an immense sum. The great mercantile firms of the City and of Liverpool gave each a thousand pounds; a ball at the Opera House under the patronage of the king (George IV.) brought six thousand, and from all sources the Committee found themselves with three hundred thousand pounds at their disposal (forty-four thousand of it from Ireland), while a fund at the Dublin Mansion House amounted to thirty thousand more. Much of this was sent to Galway, Mayo, Clare and Kerry, in time to save many thousands of families from starvation[1]; it was, no doubt, wastefully given away, and there was a balance of sixty thousand pounds sterling unused. More tardily in June, 1822, Parliament voted one hundred thousand "for the employment of the poor in Ireland," and in July two hundred thousand to meet contingencies of the famine. It was generally admitted that the Government grants were jobbed and mis-appropriated to a scandalous extent. The towns had to be made the centres of relief and the depôts of provisions; and yet the towns were not suffering from famine or fever but only from penury. The fever hospital at Ennis, the county town of Clare, was constantly filled by strangers, the townspeople remaining healthy. Kerry was one of the most afflicted counties, but Tralee and Killarney had no unusual sickness. Limerick town had hardly more fever than in an ordinary year. In Dublin the admissions for fever in 1822 were a good deal below the usual number. On the other hand, Sligo town had much fever, and Galway town had an altogether unique experience, the history of which, as related by Dr Graves, will be the best possible view of the peculiar circumstances of 1821–22[2].

[1] *Lachrymae Hiberniae, or the Grievances of the Peasantry of Ireland, especially in the Western Counties.* By a Resident Native. Dublin, 1822 (September). The author, a resident of the west coast, was concerned in the distribution of relief, and positively asserts the saving of thousands "from his own personal knowledge."

[2] Robert James Graves, M.D., "Report on the Fever lately prevalent in Galway and the West of Ireland." *Trans. K. and Q. Col. Phys.* IV. (1824), p. 408.

In Connemara, where the distress was acute, there were no roads over which the provisions from England could be carted to the famished districts. Accordingly a great store was made in Galway, to which crowds flocked from the country in boats and on foot. Many died a few days after they arrived, from exhaustion or from the surfeit of food after long hunger. Galway, a crowded place at best, with narrow streets and lanes, contained thousands of strangers, who slept about the quays and the fish-market, or in the lanes and entries, or in crowded lodging-houses four or five in a bed. The fever began in May, and quickly spread so much that the priests were kept fully employed by calls to the dying. In June and July the sixty beds of the fever hospital were filled, principally with the fugitives from Connemara. Sixty more beds were added, and these by the middle of September were insufficient. The infection had now spread to many good houses. When Dr Graves and three other Dublin physicians arrived, on 26 September, they found ropes stretched across the streets to stop the wheel traffic. The shops of tradesmen were avoided. The town was like a place in the plague; people passing along the streets put their handkerchiefs to their noses when they came to a house with fever in it. Yet the number of cases was not remarkable; on 3 October, there were 404 sick in a population of 30,000, of whom 130 were in the fever hospital and 274 at their homes, the new cases occurring at the rate of 29 per diem. At length it was found practicable to set up depôts of provisions in country places, and the crowd of strangers left Galway. The fever was mild but tedious among the poor, more violent and fatal among the well-to-do. In many country places dysentery and choleraic diarrhœa were prevalent, as well as fever. In Erris, county Mayo, dysentery and dropsy were more common than fever, many of the cottiers having subsisted on weeds, shell-fish, or new potatoes dug six weeks after the seed was planted. In this famine the people ate the flesh of black cattle dead of disease. Excepting in Connemara the county of Galway was not so soon affected as some other parts of Ireland; but, as in 1818, the contagion of fever was spread abroad by vagrants. After Mayo, Galway, Clare and Kerry, the counties most affected were Roscommon and Sligo, and next to these Leitrim, Tipperary and Cork.

Dysentery and Relapsing Fever, 1826–27.

Fever and dysentery decreased to an ordinary level in 1823, but rose somewhat again in 1824, the summer of which was hot and moist. But it was in the hot and dry summers of 1825 and 1826 that dysentery became notably common in Ireland generally and in Dublin in particular. It began in the capital in June—among the richer class of people. About the middle of August admissions for dysentery were perceptibly raising the number of patients in the Cork Street Fever Hospital, and continued to do so throughout the autumn. At one dispensary three out of four applicants had dysentery. All those admitted to hospital were over twenty years of age; of thirty-five cases under Dr O'Brien, nine died, all of which had ulceration of the great intestine, in one case gangrenous. The mortality was not nearly so great among the richer classes, in which respect dysentery reversed the rule of typhus fever. O'Brien had one obvious case illustrating the curious connexion between dysentery and rheumatic fever, originally remarked by English observers in the 18th century. A hospital porter was admitted with "fever of a mixed catarrhal and rheumatic type." Having been blooded and subjected to free evacuations, his fever left him on the fourth day, but he was at once seized with dysentery, which ran its course[1].

It is to be noted that this epidemic of dysentery began in Dublin in the hot June weather of 1825 among the richer classes, and that there was no notable increase of fever while it lasted. It appears to have declined in Dublin in the early part of 1826. After a cold and dry spring there began one of the hottest and driest summers on record. The first rain for four months fell on the 15th of July, 1826, the thermometer rose as high as 86°, and was on a mean several degrees above summer temperature in Dublin. In the spring labour had become slack, and before long it was estimated that 20,000 artizans in the Liberties (weavers and others) were out of work. Early in May there began a most extraordinary epidemic of relapsing fever, with which some typhus was mixed. By the 9th of May, the 220 beds of the Cork Street Hospital were full,

[1] John O'Brien, M.D., "On the Epidemic Dysentery which prevailed in Dublin in the year 1825." *Trans. K. and Q. Col. Phys.* V. (1828) p. 221; Burke, *Ed. Med. Surg. Journ.* July, 1826, p. 56; Speer, *Med. Phys. Journ.* N. S. VI. 199.

and applicants were sent away daily. On 4 August, a temporary hospital of 240 beds was opened in the garden of the Meath Hospital; on the 18th, the Wellesley Hospital, in North King Street, was opened with 113 beds; on the 15th, tents to hold 180 patients were erected on the lawn of the Cork Street Hospital, raising its accommodation to 400; a warehouse in Kevin Street was furnished with beds for 230 patients, and some increase was made to the beds in Sir Patrick Dun's and Stevens's Hospitals. The whole number of fever-beds in Dublin hospitals at length reached 1400; but not half the number of cases was provided for. At a meeting in the Mansion House on 26 October, it was stated that there were at that date 3200 persons sick of the fever at their homes, besides the 1400 in the hospitals. Funds were subscribed, soup-kitchens and dispensaries opened in various districts of Dublin, and kept open most of the winter, "but they made little impression on the epidemic, which continued with unabated violence." In March, 1827, it began suddenly to decline, and fell rapidly until it was nearly extinct in May; and that, too, although "the complaints of distress and want are to the full as loud as at the commencement of the epidemic, and provisions are dearer[1]." The corresponding sicknesses in Edinburgh and Glasgow were later—the fever chiefly in 1828, the dysentery in 1827 and 1828.

This great epidemic was mainly one of relapsing fever. The patient "got the cool," or passed the crisis of the fever, usually on the evening of the fifth or seventh day, sometimes on the ninth, the evening exacerbation, which was to prove critical, being ushered in generally with a rigor, and passing off in profuse perspiration throughout the night. The five-day fever was more certain to relapse than that of seven days, the seven-day fever was more likely to relapse than that of nine days. The relapses might be one or two or three or more, prolonging the illness for weeks. The clear interval varied from twenty-four hours to fourteen days. There were some cases with jaundice which led Stokes and Graves to speak loosely of "yellow fever[2]." O'Brien saw only four cases with exquisite icterus in fifteen hundred cases of relapsing fever. There was a small proportion of cases of ordinary typhus of a severe kind,

---

[1] John O'Brien, "Med. Rep. of the H. of Recovery, Cork Street, Dublin, for the year ending 4 Jan. 1827." *Trans. K. and Q. Col. Phys.* v. 512.
[2] Graves, *Clinical Medicine*, 1843. Lect. XVIII.

marked by unusual delirium or phrensy and the absence of sordes on the teeth or petechiae on the skin; the typhus cases became more numerous in the winter season, or, in other words, the original attack lasted to nine, eleven, or thirteen days, with little or no tendency to relapse. Gangrene was not uncommon in one part of the body or another, and in four cases the feet became gangrenous[1].

Even with the admixture of pure typhus cases, and with dysenteric complications in the autumn and winter, the mortality of the whole epidemic was small—not more than it would have been among a third part the number of fever cases in an ordinary year. At the Cork Street Hospital alone (including the tents) there were 8453 admissions from 4th August, 1826, to 4th April, 1827, with 332 deaths, or four deaths in a hundred cases. The proportion of recoveries was quite as remarkable in known instances in the squalid homes of the poor, where two or three would be found ill of fever on one pallet, or a father and six children in one room, shunned by the neighbours.

The strangest thing in this epidemic was the sequel of it. In the spring of 1827, intermittent fever, which had not made its appearance for several years in Dublin, began to prevail pretty generally; whilst the ordinary continued fever showed a strong tendency to assume the intermittent and remittent forms. It is not surprising, therefore, that Dr O'Brien, who had these varied experiences of epidemic dysentery in 1825, of epidemic relapsing fever and typhus in 1826, and of intermittent fever in 1827, should adopt Sydenham's language of epidemic constitutions, and revert to the old Sydenhamian doctrine of causes. While the sequence of epidemic diseases in Dublin was some dysentery in the autumn and winter of 1825 and relapsing fever on a vast scale during the excessively dry spring and summer of 1826, in country districts of Ireland, such as Skibbereen, dysentery became epidemic after the great drought and heat of 1826, while "fever disappeared altogether," and indeed all other prevalent forms of sickness gave way before it, so general was it. Such is the report from Skibbereen, county Cork, a district that became early notorious, in the great famine of 1846–47, and was perhaps a kind of barometer of Irish distress twenty years earlier. The epidemic dysentery of 1826 attacked all classes

---

[1] O'Brien, u. s.

there, but chiefly the poorest; it was apt to begin insidiously, and, as it was often neglected, so it often became obstinate and hard to cure. Dr McCarthy attributed it to the drought of 1826, the commercial distress of 1825, the lack of employment for labourers, the overgrowth of population, and the alarming rise in the prices of food[1]. He uses the same economic illustrations as O'Connell and Smith O'Brien in the Great Famine twenty years after, which were, indeed, as old as the time of Bishop Berkeley[2].

Although little is heard of the fever of 1826–27 except in Dublin, it is probable that the same causes which produced it there were operative in other large towns. The admissions to the Limerick Fever Hospital rose rapidly in the end of 1826. Geary, who was appointed one of its physicians that year, estimates that about one in twelve of the population of Limerick (63,310) were treated for fever in 1827 at public institutions, besides those treated in private practice. It was relapsing fever, as in Dublin[3].

Perennial Distress and Fever.

According to all the figures of Irish fever-hospitals, and the generalities of their physicians, fever was now constantly present in the towns. After the relapsing epidemic of 1826–27 had subsided, there was no rise above the steady level until the years 1831 and 1832, when a considerable increase appears in the admissions to the hospitals of Dublin, Limerick and Belfast. But the fever of 1831–32 was totally eclipsed by the cholera, and little is heard of typhus in Irish writings until 1835–36, when an epidemic arose, purely of typhus fever, which is said to have been as severe upon some districts as that of 1817–18 had

1 "Remarks on the Epidemic Dysentery of the Autumn of 1826 in the South of Ireland." By Alexander McCarthy, M.D. *Edin. Med. and Surg. Journ.* April, 1827, p. 289.
2 "It is a melancholy picture of society to witness the increase of wealth and luxury on one side, and the greatest want and wretchedness on the other; to meet famine and exhaustion in the great body of the people, in a country that produces as much food as would afford a full supply for once and a half its present population; to see the granaries full of corn and flour, and the great body of the people scarcely existing on a half supply of bad potatoes. Such is the miserable situation of the Irish, a race of people distinguished for their intellect, and above all for their resignation and patience under afflictions the most trying."
3 *Dub. Quart. Journ. Med. Sc.* XI. 385.

been. This outbreak fell at the time of the Commission presided over by the Earl of Devon, the report of which is authoritative for the state of the Irish lower class and the causes of the same. The country cottiers and the poor of the towns were always on the verge of starvation. Dr Geary, of Limerick, in 1836 estimated as follows the proportion of poor to the whole population, "the poor" being taken to mean "those who would require aid if a Poor Law existed[1]:"

Proportion of "Poor" in the several Parishes of Limerick, 1836.

	St Nicholas and St Mary	St John and St Laurence	St Munchin	St Michael
Population	14,629	15,667	4,071	16,226
Number of Poor	7,000	6,400	930	2,500

Most of the poor lived in the old town of Limerick in lofty and closely-built houses which the better classes had abandoned. These dilapidated barracks were the abodes of misery and filth, two and often three families occupying a single room: "It is here, as in the decayed Liberties of Dublin[2], that the indigent room-keeper, the ruined artisan, the unemployed labourer, and the ejected country cottier, with their famishing families retreat." Their degradation, Dr Geary thought, was owing to the delay of Parliament in giving Ireland the Poor Law. The sanitary state of the old town was disgraceful. Heaps of manure were carefully kept in back yards, to be sold to farmers in the spring —"a very principal source of livelihood" for those who collected it. Certain houses near these depôts had always fever in them, dysentery was frequent, and Exchange-lane never free from it[3]. An extensive glue-mill in the Abbey poisoned the air with the effluvia of putrid animal matters. The following table shows the number of fever-cases admitted to the Hospital or attended from the Dispensary in 1827 and in four ordinary years thereafter :

[1] W. J. Geary, M.D., "Report of the St John's Fever and Lock Hospitals." *Dub. Quart. Journ. Med. Sc.* XI. 378: XII. 94.

[2] Various descriptions of these exist, of which that by Carleton in the tale 'Barney Branagan,' is probably not overdone.

[3] The Report of the Roscrea Fever Hospital for 1827 says: "In March, when the dung is being removed from the back yards for the purpose of planting the potatoes, the number of patients becomes double in the Fever Hospital." *Dublin Medical Press*, Jan. 1846, p. 235.

Limerick:—Table of Hospital Cases of Fever and Cases at their Homes attended from the Dispensary.

	Hospital Cases			Dispensary Cases			
Year	Admitted	Died	Average mortality. One in	Attended	Died	Average mortality. One in	Total
1827	2781	137	20	2800	80	35	5581
1828	854	37	23	960	22	39	1714
1829	506	23	22	640	18	35	1146
1830	806	34	23½	910	25	36	1716
1831	1015	65	15½	920	31	29	1935
Totals	5962	296	20	6130	176	. 34	12092

From 1831 to 1836 the admissions to hospitals were as follows:

Year	Admitted	Died
1832	1028	57
1833	824	42
1834	906	55
1835	1484	121
1836	3227	235

The last lines show the epidemic increase, which began in the autumn of 1835. It will appear from the following (by Geary) that it was largely an epidemic of young people, and that the fatality was by far the greatest among the comparatively small number of persons attacked at the higher ages—a well-known law of typhus of which this Limerick demonstration was perhaps the first numerically precise:

Table of the Numbers admitted to Limerick Fever Hospital at stated ages of five years, with the deaths, from 6 Jan. 1836 to 6 Jan. 1837.

Ages in Years	Admitted	Died	Average mortality per cent.	Ages in Years	Admitted	Died	Average mortality per cent.
1—5	81	2	2¼	40—45	70	13	18½
5—10	489	13	2½	45—50	82	22	27
10—15	762	18	2¼	50—55	23	5	21½
15—20	701	37	5¼	55—60	36	12	33¼
20—25	362	22	6	60—65	2	1	50
25—30	304	27	8¾	65—70	10	5	50
30—35	100	12	12	Over 70	2	1	50
35—40	203	45	23¼	Total	3227	235	7¼

One-sixth of these Limerick hospital cases, to the number of 567, came from the county, chiefly from the damp, boggy districts five to sixteen miles from the city. The whole admissions were rather more than the same hospital received in the famine year, 1817. But, although 1836 was not a year of

special scarcity, there must have been some cause at work to raise the perennial typhus to the height of an epidemic, not only in Limerick, but in Dublin, Cork, Waterford, Ennis, Belfast, and other towns.   In the country, an epidemic outburst during the months of March, April and May, 1836, in the parish of Donoughmore, Donegal, is perhaps only a sample of others unrecorded: it was remarkable in that nine-tenths of the cases of fever had as a sequel large boils on various parts of the body, but principally on the limbs[1].

In Dublin, the influenza of the first months of 1837 seemed to check the prevalence of typhus for a time ; but the latter increased greatly when the influenza was over, so that the admissions to the Cork Street Hospital until the end of 1838 nearly equalled those of the worst epidemics since the hospital was opened in 1804[2].   Females in typhus were admitted greatly in excess of males ; a large proportion (1847 in two years) were under fifteen years of age ; the fever rarely relapsed, so that it was mostly typhus, as in England and Scotland at the same time.   In twelve months of the same period (Oct. 1837 to Sept. 1838) there were 1786 admissions for fever at Cork, 1840 at Limerick, and 1706 at Belfast[3].

In Dublin, as in London, Edinburgh and Glasgow, the continued fevers of the "thirties" were distinctively spotted typhus, which was a new constitution.   Graves, lecturing at Dublin in November, 1836, said: "We are now at a point of time possessing no common interest for the reflection of medical observers.   It is now nearly two years since my attention was first arrested by the appearance of maculated fever, of which the first examples were observed in some hospital cases from the neighbourhood of Kingstown.   This form of fever has lasted ever since, prevailing universally, as if it had banished all other forms of fever, and being almost the only type noticed in our wards[4]."

[1] Babington, "Epidemic Typhous Fever in Donoughmore." *Dub. Quart. Journ.* x. 404.
[2] G. A. Kennedy, "Report of Cork St. Fever Hosp. 1837–38." *Ibid.* xiii. 311. Graves, *Ibid.* xiv. 363.
[3] Lynch, *Ibid.* N. s. vii. 388, gives some particulars of it also at Loughrea, Galway, in 1840.
[4] *System of Clinical Medicine.* Dublin, 1843, p. 57. The "change of type," with special reference to treatment, is discussed more fully in Lecture xxxiv. pp. 492–500. See also *Dub. Quart. Journ. Med. Sc.* xiv. 502, where a letter on the changed character of fever at Sligo is cited.

This increase of fever in Ireland, as well as the change in its type, corresponded closely to the great epidemic outburst in Scotland and England. The census of Ireland, taken in June, 1841, for the ten years preceding, gave a somewhat loose return of the causes of death in each year of the decennial period[1].

The worst years for fever were 1837 and 1840, the best year 1841. The deaths from fever in ten years were 112,072, being 1 in 10·59 of the deaths from all causes. The counties with highest fever mortality were Cavan, Mayo, Galway and Clare; the worst towns were Belfast, Kilkenny, Dublin, Limerick and Carrickfergus. Of these deaths from typhus-like fevers, 14,501 occurred in 86 fever-hospitals, which were open, or which kept records, for more or less of the decennial period. The following table shows the proportions of rural, urban and hospital fever-deaths in each of the four provinces:

Deaths from fever in ten years, 1831–41.

	Leinster	Munster	Ulster	Connaught
Rural fever-deaths	16,159	23,718	21,616	19,319
Urban	4,626	4,878	3,183	1,262
Hospital	9,030	5,465	2,439	386
	29,815	34,061	27,238	20,958
Rural population in 1841	1,531,106	2,009,220	2,160,698	1,338,635
Ratio of do. per sq. mile	247	332	406	386

The following detailed table for the province of Leinster shows the enormous preponderance of fever-deaths in the cottages or cabins[2]. Only Dublin and Kilkenny have most of the deaths in their fever hospitals or public institutions; it was not until near the end of this decennial period, the year 1839, that workhouses, with their infirmaries, began to be provided for all the poor-law unions:

---

[1] *The Census of Ireland,* 1841, Parl. Papers, 1843. "Report on the Table of Deaths," by W. R. Wilde. The deaths in the family, with their causes, &c., in each of the previous ten years were entered on the census paper by the head of the family, or by the parish priest for him. These returns were, of course, far from exhaustive or correct.

[2] Graves, *Clinical Medicine,* 1843, p. 46. Remarking on the much greater frequency of fever in Ireland than in England, he says (p. 47): "Nothing can be more remarkable than the facility with which a simple cold (which in England would be perfectly devoid of danger), runs into maculated fever in Ireland, and that, too, under circumstances quite free from even the suspicion of contagion—in truth, except when fever is epidemic, catching cold is its most usual cause."

Fever Mortality in Leinster, 1831–41.

Localities	Deaths from Fever in Hospitals and Public Institutions	Deaths from Fever at home	Total
Carlow County	202	891	1093
Drogheda Town	1	238	239
Dublin County	111	1248	1359
Dublin City	6393	2369	8762
Kildare County	276	1068	1284
Kilkenny County	114	2378	2492
Kilkenny City	487	204	691
King's County	126	1754	1880
Longford County	3	1265	1268
Louth County	1	1201	1202
Meath County	294	2151	2445
Queen's County	84	1763	1847
Westmeath County	54	1550	1604
Wexford County	637	1736	2373
Wicklow County	280	1002	1282
	9063	20,758	29,821

The Great Famine and Epidemic Sicknesses of 1846–49.

The great epidemic of relapsing fever, typhus, dysentery, anasarca and purpura, which arose in Ireland in the end of 1846 or spring of 1847 and lasted until the beginning of 1849, had for its direct antecedents the more or less complete loss of the potato-crop through blight in two successive autumns, 1845 and 1846, while the state of distress and sickness was prolonged by the potato disease in 1847 and 1848[1]. The potato-blight, which caused so much alarm in Ireland for the first time in September, 1845, had been seen in Germany several years before, in Belgium in 1842, in Canada in 1844, and in England about the 19th of August, 1845. Shortly after the last date, it attacked the Irish potato-fields, first in Wexford, and before the end of the year it was estimated that one-third to one-half of the yield, which was a fifth larger than usual from the greater breadth planted and the abundant crop, was lost by absolute rottenness or unfitness for food, the process of decay being of a kind to make great progress after the tubers were pitted. The loss to Ireland was estimated at about one pound sterling per head of the population. Sir Robert Peel was keenly alive to the magnitude of the calamity which threatened the Irish

[1] The principal work on the general circumstances of the Irish famine of 1846–47 is *The History of the Great Irish Famine of* 1847, *with notices of Earlier Irish Famines.* By Rev. John O'Rourke, P.P., M.R.I.A. Dublin, 1875.

peasantry. His first step was to summon to his aid a botanist,
Dr Lindley, and a chemist, Dr Playfair; the latter went down
to Drayton Manor, and joined the prime minister in examining
samples of the diseased potatoes. The question was whether
some chemical process could not be found to arrest the decay of
the tubers. Sir Robert Peel, in a much talked-of address at the
opening of the Tamworth Reading-Room in the winter of 1840,
had hailed the rising sun of science and useful knowledge. It
was only in reference to morals and religion that Peel's
deliverance called forth criticism, more particularly the memorable series of letters to the *Times* by John Henry Newman.
But one of Newman's gibes was in a manner prophetic of Peel's
attitude in approaching the material distress of Ireland: " Let
us, in consistency, take chemists for our cooks, and mineralogists
for our masons." The two professors proceeded to Ireland, but
could only confirm the fact, already known, that one-third, or
one-half, of the potato-crop would be lost.

Botany and chemistry being powerless to stay the effects of
the potato-blight, the appeal was next to economics. Ireland
produced not only potatoes but also corn. But for the most
part the cottiers and cottagers tasted little of the oats or wheat
which they grew; as soon as the harvest was gathered, the corn
was sold to pay the November rents, and was exported. Ireland
was still in the paradoxical condition which Bishop Berkeley
puzzled over a hundred years before: "whether our exports do
not consist of such necessaries as other countries cannot well be
without?" The industry and trade of Irish ports was largely
that of corn-milling and shipping of oatmeal, flour and other
produce; thus Skibbereen in the extreme south-west, where the
horrors of famine were felt first, had several flour-mills and a
considerable export trade in corn, meal, flour and provisions.
The Irish corn harvest of 1845 had been abundant: O'Connell
cited the *Mark Lane Express* for the fact that 16,000 quarters of
oats from Ireland had arrived in the Thames in a single week of
October; on the 23rd of the same month the parish priest of
Kells saw fifty dray-loads of oatmeal on the road to Drogheda
for shipment. Ireland paid its rent to absentee landlords in
corn and butter, just as a century before it had paid it largely
in barrelled beef, keeping little for its own use besides potatoes
and milk. In the face of the potato famine, the measure
approved by the Irish leaders of all parties, O'Connell and

Smith O'Brien as well as ducal proprietors, was to keep some of the oatmeal at home. A committee which sat at the Dublin Mansion House were of opinion, on 19 November, 1845, that the quantity of oats already exported of that harvest would have sufficed to feed the entire population of Ireland. O'Connell's plan was to raise a million and a half on the annual revenue of the Irish woods and forests (£74,000), and to impose a tax on landlords, both absentee and resident, and with the moneys so obtained to buy up what remained of the Irish corn harvest for use at home. In the ensuing session of Parliament, both he and Smith O'Brien protested that Ireland had no need of English doles, having resources of her own if the landlords were compelled to do their duty.

About the same time Lord John Russell, leader of the Opposition, was led by the danger of famine in Ireland to pronounce for the repeal of the Corn Laws of 1815; and at the meetings of the Cabinet in December, Peel urged the same policy upon his colleagues for the same reason. The political history does not concern us beyond the fact that the threatened Irish distress caused by the first partial potato-blight of 1845 was the occasion of the Corn and Customs Act of June, 1846, by which the Corn Laws were repealed, and that an Irish Coercion Bill, brought in on account of outrages following an unusual number of evictions, was made the occasion of turning out Peel's ministry at the moment of its Free Trade victory, by a combination of Tory protectionists, Whigs and Irish patriots.

The direct effects of the potato-blight of 1845 were not so serious as had been expected. The Government quietly bought Indian meal (maize flour) in America without disturbing the market, and had it distributed from twenty principal food-depots in Ireland, to the amount of 11,503 tons, along with 528 tons of oatmeal. This governmental action ceased on the 15th of August, 1846, by which time £733,372 had been spent, £368,000 being loans and the rest grants. The people were set to road-making, so as to pay by labour for their food, the number employed reaching a maximum of 97,000 in August. The Government, having been led by physicians in Dublin to expect an epidemic of fever, passed a Fever Act in March, 1846, by which a Board of Health was constituted. But no notable increase of sickness took place, and the Board was dissolved. There was a small outbreak of dysentery and

diarrhoea at Kilkenny (and possibly elsewhere) in the spring of 1846, which the physician to the workhouse set down to the use of the Indian meal "and other substitutes for potatoes[1]."

It was the total loss of the potato crop in the summer and autumn following, 1846, together with a failure of the harvest in England and in other countries of Northern Europe, that brought the real Irish distress. A large breadth of potatoes had been planted as usual, but doubtless with a good deal of the seed tainted. An ordinary crop would have been worth, according to one estimate, sixteen millions sterling, according to another, twice as much. The crop was a total loss. The fields looked well in the summer, but those who dug the early potatoes found them unusually small. About the beginning of August the blight began suddenly and spread swiftly. A letter of the celebrated Father Mathew, the temperance reformer, brings this out:

"On the 29th of last month (July) I passed from Cork to Dublin, and this doomed plant bloomed in all the luxuriance of an abundant harvest. Returning on the 3rd instant (August) I beheld with sorrow one wide waste of putrefying vegetation. In many places the wretched people were seated on the fences of the decaying gardens wringing their hands and wailing bitterly the destruction that had left them foodless[2]."

The relief-works and distribution of Indian meal, which had been estimated by the Government to last only to August, 1846, at a cost of £476,000 (one-half of it being a free grant), were resumed under the pressure of public opinion, in the winter of 1846 and spring of 1847, at a cost of £4,850,000, one-half of the sum being again a free grant. Before the distress was over, other free grants and advances were made; so that, on 15 February, 1850, Lord John Russell summed up the famine-indebtedness of Ireland to the Consolidated Fund at £3,350,000, (which was to be repaid out of the rates in forty years from that date). Allowing an equal sum freely gifted from the national exchequer, the whole public cost of the famine would have been about seven millions sterling.

The short crops in Britain in 1846 were an excuse for not interfering with the export of oats from Ireland. The imports of Indian meal were left to the ordinary course of the market, and the distribution to retail traders. The corn merchants of Cork, Limerick and other ports made fortunes out of the

---

[1] Joseph Lalor, M.D., *Dub. Quart. Journ. Med. Sc.* N. S. III. 38.
[2] Cited by O'Rourke, p. 152.

American cargoes, and the dealers throughout the country made large profits.

To encourage the influx of foreign food-supplies, and to lower freights, the Navigation Laws were suspended for a few months, so that corn could be carried in other than British bottoms. When Parliament met in January, 1847, the distress in Ireland occupied the greater part of the Queen's Speech.

Lord George Bentinck proposed that sixteen millions should be advanced for the construction of railroads, so as to give employment and wages to the starving multitudes. The Government, however, objected that such relief would operate at too great a distance, in most cases, from the homes of the people; and it was urged by independent critics that a State loan for railways would really be for the relief of the landlords more than of the peasantry. The large sums actually voted were spent in road-making and in procuring food and medical relief. A Board of Works directed the relief-works. A Commissariat, with two thousand Relief Committees under it, directed the distribution of food. A Board of Health provided temporary fever-hospitals and additional physicians. It was not to be expected that this machinery would work well, and, in fact, the public relief was costly in its administration and often misdirected in its objects. Private charities, especially that of the Society of Friends, gave invaluable help, money being subscribed by all classes at home and sent from distant countries, including a thousand pounds from the Sultan of Turkey. On one day, the third of July, 1847, nearly three millions in Ireland received food gratuitously from the hands of the relieving officers. In March, 1847, the public works were employing 734,000. The number relieved out of the poor rates at one time reached 800,000. Workhouses were enlarged, and temporary fever-hospitals were built to the number of 207, which in the two years 1847 and 1848, received 279,723 patients.

Emigration to the United States and Canada, which had averaged 61,242 persons per annum from the last half of 1841 to the end of 1845, rose steadily all through the famine until it reached a total of 214,425 in the year 1849, the passage money to the amount of millions sterling having come largely from the savings of the Irish already settled in the New World.

The grand effect of the famine upon the population of Ireland was revealed by the census of 1851. The people in 1841

had numbered 8,175,124; in 1851 they numbered 6,515,794. The decrease was 28·6 per cent. in Connaught, 23·5 per cent. in Munster, 16 per cent. in Ulster, and 15·5 per cent. in Leinster. In many remote parishes the number of inhabitants, and of cabins, fell to nearly a half. The depopulation was wholly rural, so much so that there was a positive increase of inhabitants not only in the large county towns, but even in small towns such as Skull and Kanturk, situated in Poor Law unions where the famine and epidemics had made the greatest clearances all over[1]. Our business here is with the epidemical maladies, which contributed to this depopulation; but a few words remain to be said on the subject at large.

Malthus had been prophetic about this crisis in the history of Ireland. Criticizing Arthur Young's project to encourage the use of potatoes and milk as the staple food of the English labourer instead of wheat, so as to escape the troubles of scarcity and high prices of corn, Malthus says:

"When, from the increasing population, and diminishing sources of subsistence, the average growth of potatoes was not more than the average consumption, a scarcity of potatoes would be, in every respect, as probable as a scarcity of wheat at present; and when it did arrive it would be beyond

---

[1] *The Census of Ireland*, 1851. Part V. Table of deaths, vol. I. Dublin, 1856, p. 235.

The following are a few instances of depopulation between 1841 and 1851.

Union of Loughrea, Co. Galway.
1841   65,636
1851   38,698

Union of Clonakilty, Co. Cork.
1841   52,185
1851   31,473

Union of Kanturk, Co. Cork.
1841   61,238
1851   41,801

Parish of Kanturk.
1841   4,096
1851   6,754

Union of Portumna, Co. Galway.
1841   30,714
1851   19,747

Union of Skibbereen, Co. Cork.
1841   57,439
1851   37,283

Parish of Skibbereen.
1841   9,557
1851   8,931

Union of Skull, Co. Cork.
1841   26,620
1851   16,866

Parish of Skull.
1841   2,895
1851   3,226

all comparison more dreadful. When the common people of a country live principally upon the dearest grain, as they do in England on wheat, they have great resources in scarcity; and barley, oats, rice, cheap soups and potatoes, all present themselves as less expensive, yet at the same time wholesome means of nourishment; but when their habitual food is the lowest in this scale, they appear to be absolutely without resource, except in the bark of trees, like the poor Swedes; and a great portion of them must necessarily be starved[1]."

The forecast of Malthus was repeated in his own way by Cobbett, although neither of them foresaw the potato-blight as the means.

"The dirty weed," said Cobbett in a conversation in 1834, "will be the curse of Ireland. The potato will not last twenty years more. It will work itself out; and then you will see to what a state Ireland will be reduced... You must return to the grain crops; and then Ireland, instead of being the most degraded, will become one of the finest countries in the world. You may live to see my words prove true; but I never shall[2]."

This is what has come to pass in a measure, and will come to pass more and more. Only in some remote parts do the Irish cottiers now live upon potatoes and milk. It has come to be quite common for them to grow an Irish half acre of wheat, and, what is more to the purpose, to consume what they thus produce instead of selling it to pay the rent. Doubtless the enormous imports of American, Australian and Black Sea wheat have made it easier for the Irish to have wheaten bread. But, whatever the reason, they have at length adopted the ancient English staff of life, a staple or standard which they were in a fair way to have achieved long ago, had not their addiction to "lost causes and impossible loyalties" given an unfavourable turn to the natural progress of the nation[3].

We come at length to the purely medical side of the great famine of 1846–47[4]. The distress in the latter part of the year

---

[1] *Essay on the Principle of Population.* Bk. IV. chap. XI. Thorold Rogers has in many passages emphasized the advantages of the English practice from medieval times of living on the dearest kind of corn; but he seems to have overlooked the priority of Malthus throughout the whole of the eleventh chapter of his fourth book. In *Six Centuries of Work and Wages* (p. 62), Rogers says: "Hence a high standard of subsistence is a more important factor in the theory of population than any of those checks which Malthus has enumerated."

[2] Cited in Thomas Doubleday's *Political Life of Sir Robert Peel.* London, 1856, II. 398 *note.*

[3] It is a doctrine of economics that the higher standard of living checks population. Thus Marshall says of England: "The growth of population was checked by that rise in the standard of comfort which took effect in the general adoption of wheat as the staple food of Englishmen during the first half of the 18th century." *Economics,* p. 230.

[4] Vol. VII. (1849) pp. 64–126, 340–404, and Vol. VIII. pp. 1–86, 270–339 of the *Dublin Quart. Journ. of Medical Science,* N.S. contain numerous reports collected

1846 was felt first in the west and south-west—in the districts to which the famine of 1822 had been almost confined. It happened that the state of matters around Skibbereen, the extreme south-western point of Ireland, was brought most under public notice; but it is believed that there were parts of the western sea-board counties of Mayo, Galway, Clare and Kerry from which equally terrible scenes might have been reported at an equally early period. It was in Clare that relief at the national charges was longest needed.

Dr Popham, one of the visiting physicians to the Cork Workhouse, wrote as follows:

"The pressure from without upon the city began to be felt in October [1846], and in November and December the influx of paupers from all parts of this vast county was so overwhelming that, to prevent them from dying in the streets, the doors of the workhouse were thrown open, and in one week 500 persons were admitted, without any provision, either of space or clothing, to meet so fearful an emergency. All these were suffering from famine, and most of them from malignant dysentery or fever. The fever was in the first instance undoubtedly confined to persons badly fed or crowded into unwholesome habitations; and as it originated with the vast migratory hordes of labourers and their families congregated upon the public roads, it was commonly termed 'the road fever'[1]."

It was the same in the smaller towns of the county, such as Skibbereen; in the month of December, 1846, there were one hundred and forty deaths in the workhouse; on one day there were fifteen funerals waiting their turn for the religious offices. Still farther afield, in the country parishes, the state of matters was the same. The sea-board parish of Skull was a typical poor district, populous with cabins along the numerous bays of the Atlantic, but with few residential seats of the gentry. On the 2nd of February, 1847, the parish clergyman, the Rev. Traill Hall (himself at length a victim to the contagion), wrote as follows:

"Frightful and fearful is the havock around me. Our medical friend, Dr Sweetman, a gentleman of unimpeachable veracity, informed me yesterday that if he stated the mortality of my parish at an average of thirty-five daily, he would be within the truth. The children in particular, he remarked, were disappearing with awful rapidity. And to this I may add the aged, who, with the young—neglected, perhaps, amidst the wide-spread destitution—are almost without exception swollen and ripening for the grave[2]."

by the editors from all parts of Ireland, and published either in abstract or in full. These are the chief medical sources. Some particulars are given also in the *Dublin Med. Press*, 1846 to 1849 in several papers on dysentery.

[1] John Popham, M.D., *Dub. Quart. Journ. Med. Sc.* N.S. VIII. 279.
[2] Cited by Dr Jones Lamprey, *Dub. Quart. Journ.* VII. 101.

They were "swollen" by the anasarca or general dropsy, which was reported from nearly all parts of Ireland as being, along with dysentery and diarrhoea, the prevalent kind of sickness before the epidemic fever became general in the spring of 1847. The same had been remarked as the precursor of the fever of 1817–18. In the end of March, Dr Jones Lamprey, sent by the Board of Health, found the parish of Skull "in a frightful state of famine, dysentery and fever." Dysentery had been by far more prevalent than fever in this district, as in many others. "It was easily known," says Dr Lamprey, "if any of the inmates in the cabins of the poor were suffering from this disease, as the ground in such places was usually found marked with clots of blood." The malady was most inveterate and often fatal. It must have had a contagious property, for the physician himself went through an attack of it[1].

In the Skibbereen district the dead were sometimes buried near their cabins; at the town itself many were carried out in a shell and laid without coffins in a large pit[2]. Along the coast of Connemara for thirty miles there was no town, but only small villages and hundreds of detached cabins; this district is said to have been almost depopulated[3].

Besides the dysentery and dropsy, which caused most of the mortality in the winter of 1846–47, another early effect of the famine was scurvy, a disease rarely seen in Ireland and unknown to most of the medical men. It was by no means general, but undoubtedly true scurvy did occur in some parts: thus in the Ballinrobe district, county Mayo[4], it was very prevalent in 1846 for some months before the epidemic fever appeared, being "evidenced by the purple hue of the gums, with ulceration along their upper thin margin, bleeding on the slightest touch, and deep sloughing ulcers of the inside of the fauces, with intolerable foetor"—affecting men, women, and children. In some places, as at Kilkenny early in 1846, there was much purpura[5]. These earlier effects of the famine (dysentery and diarrhoea, dropsy, scurvy and purpura), were seen in varying degrees before the end of 1846 in most parts of Ireland. The counties least touched by them were in Leinster and Ulster,

---

[1] Lamprey, *Dub. Quart. Journ.* VII. 101.
[2] O'Rourke.   [3] Ormsbey, *Dub. Quart. Journ.* VII. 382.
[4] Pemberton, *ibid.* VII. 369.
[5] Lalor, u. s.

such as Down, Derry, Tyrone, Fermanagh and some others, where the peasantry lived upon oatmeal as well as on potatoes. But even these were invaded by the ensuing epidemic of fever, the only place in all Ireland which is reported to have escaped both the primary and the secondary effects of the famine having been Rostrevor, on the coast of Down, a watering-place with a rich population, which was also one of the very small number of localities that escaped in 1817–18.

According to the following samples of admissions to the Fever Hospital of Ennis in the several months, the summers were the season of greatest sickness, a fact which was noted also in the epidemic of 1817–18 :

Year	Month	Patients		Year	Month	Patients
1846	November	93		1848	February	210
,,	December	224		,,	May	705
1847	June	757		,,	November	400

The almost uniform report of medical men was that the epidemic of fever began in 1847, in the spring months in most places, in the summer in others. Relapsing fever was the common type. It was usually called the famine fever for the reason that it was constantly seen to arise in persons " recovering from famine," on receiving food from the Relief Committees[1]. It was a mild or "short" fever, apt to leave weakness, but rarely fatal. Dr Dillon, of Castlebar, reports that he would be told by the head of a family: " We have been *three times down* in the fever, and have all, thank God, got through it." Dr Starkey, of Newry, "knew many families, living in wretched poverty on the mountains near the town, who were attacked with fever, and who without any medical attendance, and but little attendance of any kind, passed through the fever without a single death." The doctor of Bryansford and Castlewellan, county Down, (where there was no famine), declared that the recoveries of the poor in their own cottages destitute of almost every comfort, were astonishing. In the Skibbereen district, Dr Lamprey was "often struck with the rarity of the ordinary types of fever among the thousands suffering from starvation." In some of the most famine-stricken places, such as the islands off the coast

---

[1] This epidemic called forth two pamphlets on the relation of famine to fever, one by Dominic Corrigan, M.D., *On Famine and Fever as Cause and Effect in Ireland* ("no famine, no fever"), and a reply to it by H. Kennedy, M.D., *On the Connexion of Famine and Fever.*

of Mayo and Galway, and in Gweedore, Donegal, not more than one in a hundred cases of relapsing fever proved fatal. In Limerick the mortality was "very small." In many places it is given at three in the hundred cases, in some places as high as six in the hundred. When deaths occurred, they were often sudden and unexpected,—more probable in the relapse than in the first onset. At Clonmel it was remarked that a certain blueness of the nose presaged death; in Fermanagh it was called the Black Fever, from the duskiness of the face. The report from Ballinrobe, Mayo, says that it was attended by rheumatic pains, which caused the patients to cry out when they stirred in bed[1]. It was mostly a fever of the first half of life, and more of the female sex than of the male. One says that it was commonest from five to fifteen years of age, another from ten to thirty years.

Relapsing fever was the most common fever of the famine years, in the cabins, workhouses and fever hospitals, in the country districts as well as the towns and cities. Dr Henry Kennedy says of Dublin: "Cases of genuine typhus were through the whole epidemic very rare, I mean comparatively speaking." But everywhere there was a certain admixture of typhus, and in some not unusual circumstances the typhus was peculiarly malignant or fatal—many times more fatal than the relapsing fever. The poor themselves do not appear to have suffered much from the more malignant typhus, unless in the gaols and workhouses. When the doors of the Cork workhouse were thrown open in December, 1846, five hundred were admitted pell mell in one week; the deaths in that workhouse were 757 in the month of March, 1847, and 3329 in the whole year. In the Ballinrobe workhouse, county Mayo, "men, women and children were huddled together in the same rooms (the probationary wards), eating, drinking, cooking, and sleeping in the same apartment in their clothes, without even straw to lie on or a blanket to cover them." Typhus at length appeared in that workhouse, said to have been brought in by a strolling beggar, and the physician, the master and the clerk died of it. Wherever the better-off classes caught fever, it was not relapsing but typhus, and a very fatal typhus. At Skibbereen the relapsing fever "was not propagated by contagion; but in persons so

---

[1] Pains resembling those of rheumatism were common in the fever of 1817–18 at Limerick.   Barker and Cheyne, I. 432.

C. II.

affected, when brought in contact with the more wealthy and better fed individuals, was capable of imparting fevers of different types[1]." There were many opportunities for such contact—in serving out food at the depôts, in superintending the gangs working on the roads, in attending the sessions, in visiting the sick. The crowds suffering from starvation, famine-fever or dysentery exhaled the most offensive smells, the smell of the relapsing fever and the anasarca being peculiar or distinguishable[2]. There appeared to be a scale of malignity in the fevers in an inverted order of the degree of misery. The most wretched had the mildest fever, the artizan class or cottagers had typhus fatal in the usual proportion, the classes living in comfort had typhus of a very fatal kind. This experience, however strange it may seem, was reported by medical observers everywhere with remarkable unanimity. One says that six or seven of the rich died in every ten attacks, others say one in three. Forty-eight medical men died in 1847 in Munster, most of them from fever; in Cavan county, seven medical men died of fever in twelve months, and three more had a narrow escape of death: two of the three physicians sent by the Board of Health to the coast of Connemara died of fever[3]. Many Catholic priests died as well as some of the Established Church clergy; and there were numerous fatalities in the families of the resident gentry, and among others who administered the relief. Yet a case of fever in a good house did not become a focus of contagion; the contagion came from direct contact with the crowds of starving poor, their clothes ragged and filthy, their bodies unwashed, and many of them suffering from dysentery. The greater fatality of fever among the richer classes had been a commonplace in Ireland since the epidemic of 1799–1801, and is remarked by the best writers[4]. At Loughrea, in Galway, Dr Lynch observed that "in the year 1840 the type of fever was very bad indeed, and

---

[1] Lamprey, u. s.

[2] Dr Kelly of Mullingar compared the smell of relapsing fever to that of burning musty straw. *Dub. Quart. Journ. Med.*, Aug. 1863, p. 341.

[3] Cusack and Stokes, *ibid.* IV. 134.

[4] Barker and Cheyne, Harty, and Rogan have been cited to this effect for earlier epidemics. Graves (*Clin. Med.* pp. 59–60) says: "In the epidemics of 1816, 1817, 1818 and 1819, it was found by accurate computation that the rate of mortality was much higher among the rich than among the poor. This was a startling fact, and a thousand different explanations of it were given at the time." He cites Fletcher (*Pathology*, p. 27) an Edinburgh observer, as follows: "The rich are less frequently affected with epidemic fevers than the poor, but more frequently die of them. Good fare keeps off diseases, but increases their mortality when they take place."

very many of the gentry were cut off by it." He reckoned that ordinarily one in six cases of fever among the richer class proved fatal, one in fifteen among the poor[1]. But in the great famine, six years after, the fever of the poor assumed the still milder type of relapsing, fatal perhaps to one in a hundred cases, or three in a hundred, while the fever which contact with them gave to those at the other extreme of well-being became a peculiarly malignant typhus, fatal to six or seven in ten cases, as Dr Pemberton of Ballinrobe found, or to three or four in ten cases, as many others found. Of course it was the peasantry who made up by far the greater part of the mortality in the years of famine; but they were cut off by various maladies, nondescript or definite, while the richer classes died, in connexion with the famine, of contagious typhus and here or there of contagious dysentery.

Even in the crowded workhouses and gaols, more deaths occurred from dysentery than from fever. But in some of the gaols great epidemics arose which cut off many of the poor by malignant infection. That was an old experience of the gaols, studied best in England in the 18th century; the worst fevers, or those most rapidly fatal, were caught by the prisoners newly brought to mix with others long habituated to their miserable condition. The gaols in Ireland during the famine were crowded to excess, not so much because the people gave way to lawlessness—their patience and obedience were matters of common complimentary remark—but because they committed petty thefts, broke windows, or the like, in order to obtain the shelter and rations of prisoners. The mortality in the gaols rose and fell as follows[2]:

Year	Deaths in gaol		Year	Deaths in gaol
1846	130		1849	1406
1847	1320		1850	692
1848	1292		1851	197

Most of the deaths in these larger totals came from two or three great prison epidemics in each of the series of years—at Tralee, Carrick-on-Shannon, Castlebar and Cork in 1847, at Galway in 1848, at Clonmel, Limerick, Cork and Galway in 1849, the highest mortality being 485 deaths in Galway county gaol in 1848. Descriptions remain of the state of the gaols at Tralee

[1] *Dub. Quart. Journ. Med. Sc.* N.S. VII. 388.
[2] *Census of Ireland,* 1851.

and Castlebar in 1847, from which it appears that they were frightfully overcrowded and filthy. Dr Dillon, of Castlebar, says that the county gaol there in March, 1847, had twice as many prisoners as it was built for, "those committed being in a state of nudity, filth and starvation." He expected an outbreak of typhus, and applied to the magistrates to increase the accommodation, which they declined to do. In due time, very bad maculated typhus broke out, of which the chaplain, matron and others of the staff died. This contagious fever is said to have proved fatal to forty per cent. of those attacked by it. The deaths for the year are returned at 83 in Castlebar gaol, those in Tralee gaol at 101, and in the gaol of Carrick-on-Shannon at 100.

No exact statistical details of the mortality in the great Irish famine of 1846–49 were kept. Ireland had then no systematic registration of deaths and of the causes of death, such as had existed in England since 1837. Information as to the mortality was got retrospectively once in ten years by means of the census, heads of families being required to fill in all the deaths, with causes, ages, years, seasons, &c., of the same, that had occurred in their families within the previous decennial period. This was, of course, a very untrustworthy method, more especially so for the famine years, when many thousands of families emigrated, leaving hardly a trace behind, many hamlets were wholly abandoned, and many parishes stripped of nearly half their inhabited houses. When a certain day in the year 1851 came round for the census papers to be filled up, a fourth part of the people were gone, and that fourth could have told more about the famine and the deaths than an equal number of those that remained. However, the Census Commissioners did their best with the defective, loose or erroneous data at their service. Much of the interest of the Irish Census of 1851 centered, indeed, in the Great Famine; and the two volumes of specially medical information compiled by Sir William Wilde, making Part V. of the Census Report, are a store of facts, statistical and historical, of which only a few can be given here[1].

---

[1] *The Census of Ireland of* 1851. Part V. Table of Deaths. 2 vols. Dublin, 1856. Upwards of two hundred pages are occupied with a chronological "Table of Cosmical Phenomena, Epizootics, Epiphitics, Famines and Pestilences in Ireland" from the earliest times. This retrospect, which is very replete but tedious and uncritical, is followed by a summary report of twenty pages on "The Last General Potato Failure, and the Great Famine and Pestilence of 1845–50," and by a long series of tabulated extracts from contemporary writings on all matters relating to the famine.

Table of Workhouses and Auxiliary Workhouses in Ireland during the Famine.

Year	No. of Workhouses	Numbers relieved	Numbers that died	Ratio of deaths One in
1846	129	250,822	14,662	17·11
1847	130	332,140	66,890	6·92
1848	131	610,463	45,482	13·4
1849	131	932,284	64,440	14·47
1850	163	805,702	46,721	17·74

During the ten years from 6 June, 1841, to 30 March, 1851, the deaths from the principal infective or "zymotic" diseases in the workhouses were as follows :

Dysentery	50,019	Measles	8,943
Diarrhoea	20,507	Cholera	6,716
Fevers	34,644	Smallpox	5,016

Besides the workhouses, there were during the famine 227 temporary fever hospitals, which received 450,807 persons from the beginning of 1847 to the end of 1850, of whom 47,302 died.

According to the Census returns, the deaths from the several causes connected with the famine were as follows in the respective years :

Year	Fever	Dysentery (with Diarrhoea)	Starvation
1845	7,249	—	—
1846	17,145	5,492	2,041
1847	57,095	25,757	6,058
1848	45,948	25,694[1]	} 9,395
1849	39,316	29,446[2]	
1850	23,545	19,224	—

According to this table, fever caused more deaths than dysentery. But there are reasons for thinking that the deaths from dysentery, anasarca and other slow effects of famine and bad food really made up more of the extra mortality of the famine-years than the sharp fever itself. In the returns from the workhouses, dysentery is actually credited with about one-half more deaths than fever. It is known that most of the mortality at the beginning of the famine, the winter of 1846–47, was from dysentery and allied chronic forms of sickness. Dysentery also followed the decline of the relapsing-fever epidemic of 1847–48. Dillon, of Castlebar, says that many, who had gone through the fever in the autumn of 1847, fell into dysentery in 1848, during which year it was very prevalent.

[1] Of this total, 18,430 deaths were from dysentery and 7,264 from diarrhoea.
[2] The increase in 1849 was doubtless owing to choleraic diarrhoea during the epidemic of Asiatic cholera, the deaths from dysentery being one-half of the total.

Mayne says that dysentery often attacked those recovering from fever, and proved fatal to them[1]. In the General Hospital of Belfast the fatality of fever-cases was 1 in 8, "but this included dysentery." Probably the same explanation should be given of the high rates of fatality in the Fever Hospital of Ennis, the chief centre of relief for the greatly distressed county of Clare: 1846, 1 in $12\frac{1}{2}$; 1847, 1 in $5\frac{3}{4}$; 1848, 1 in $5\frac{1}{2}$.

It will be noticed that some thousands of deaths were put down to starvation in the Census returns. Perhaps a more technical nosological term might have been found for a good many of these, such as anasarca or general dropsy. But even if physicians had made the returns, instead of the priests or relatives, they would have put many into a nondescript class, for which starvation was a sufficiently correct generic name. Scurvy was another disease of malnutrition which was far from rare during the famine; the deaths actually set down to that cause were some hundreds over the whole period.

The deaths from all causes in the decennial period covered by the Census of 1851 were 985,366. But these returns were made, as we have seen, on a population which had been reduced by a fourth part in the course of ten years, so that they fall considerably short of the reality. If the population of Ireland had multiplied at the same rate as that of England and Wales from 1841 to 1851, namely, 1·0036 per cent. per annum, it should have been 9,018,799 in the year 1851; but it was only 6,552,385. Emigration beyond the United Kingdom had averaged 61,242 persons per annum from the 30th of June, 1841, to the 31st December, 1845; next year, 1846, it rose to 105,955, in 1847 it was "more than doubled," in 1848 it was 178,159, in 1849, 214,425, in 1850 it was 209,054, and in 1851 it touched the maximum, 249,721. Nearly a million emigrated in the six years preceding the date of the Census, and there was besides a considerable migration to Liverpool, Glasgow, London and other towns of England and Scotland. It is probable that emigration accounts for two-thirds of the decrease of inhabitants revealed by the Census of 1851; but the extra mortality of the famine years, or the deaths over and above the ordinary deaths in Ireland during a decennial period, can hardly be estimated below half a million.

[1] R. Mayne, M.D., "Observations on the late Epidemic Dysentery in Dublin." *Dub. Quart. Journ. Med. Sc.* VII. 294. See also papers in *Dubl. Med. Press*, 1849.

Decrease of Typhus and Dysentery after 1849.

The potato famines of 1845–48 were a turning-point in the history of Ireland. From that time the population has steadily declined and the well-being of the people steadily improved. By the Census of 1871 the population was 5,386,708, by that of 1881 it was 5,144,983, by that of 1891 it was 4,704,750. Registration of births and deaths, which began in 1864, shows the following samples:

Year	Births	Deaths
1867	144,318	98,911
1871	151,665	88,720
1880	128,010	102,955
1888	109,557	85,892

The enormous amount of pauperism which followed the great famine was at length brought within limits: from 1866 to the present time it has been marked by a steady increase of out-door relief, and by some increase in the numbers within the Union Workhouses; the out-door paupers have increased from 10,163 on 1 Jan., 1866, to 53,638 on 1 Jan., 1881, the absolute number of indoor paupers having remained, on an average of good and bad years, somewhat steady in a declining population.

The public health has been undisturbed by great epidemics since the potato famine, although the effects of that calamity did not wholly cease until some years after. It is best estimated by the mean annual average of deaths among a thousand inhabitants, a ratio which has been low for the provinces of Connaught and Munster, and not excessive for the provinces of Ulster and Leinster. The following tables are of the death rates in two sample years, 1880 and 1889 respectively[1]:

	1880	1889
Connaught	15·3	12·4
Munster	19·5	15·1
Ulster	20·0	16·8
Leinster	23·3	18·3

Four healthiest counties:

1880		1889	
Mayo	14·5	Galway	11·8
Sligo	15·3	Kerry	12·1
Galway	15·6	Leitrim	12·1
Roscommon	15·8	Cavan	12·2

[1] 17th and 26th Reports of the Regr.-Genl. Ireland.

Four unhealthiest counties:

1880		1889	
Dublin co.	31·7	Dublin co.	24·5
Waterford co.	24·9	Antrim	21·2
Louth	22·6	Down	18·6
Antrim	21·9	Armagh	17·0

The higher death rates of some counties are chiefly owing to their greater urban populations. The health of the cottier districts is remarkably good, and is rarely if ever disturbed by any *morbus miseriae.* The cabins, except in a few remote parts, are more comfortable than they used to be, the diet is better, the clothing is better, the education of the children is better. The present happier lot of the Irish peasantry can be measured not unfairly by the statistics showing the decrease in the number of cabins of the lowest class, and the increase of dwellings in the higher classes.

The history of fever and dysentery in Ireland subsequently to the great epidemics of 1846–49 has few salient points. Dysentery, the old "country disease," has steadily declined to about a hundred deaths in the year, while the considerable mortality from diarrhoea, nearly two thousand deaths in a year, is nearly all from the cholera infantum or summer diarrhoea of children in the large towns. The history of the continued fevers is made complex by the modern identification of typhoid or enteric fever. According to the testimonies of several, it played but a small part in the epidemics of 1846–49, even in Dublin itself[1], and it can hardly be doubted that its recent increase in that city is not apparent but real. The following table from the year 1880 to the present time will show how the deaths from continued fever are now divided in the registration returns:

Year	Typhus	Simple continued	Enteric
1880	934	1073	1087
1881	859	774	813
1882	744	657	844
1883	810	593	853
1884	628	572	693
1885	505	443	716
1886	394	380	772
1887	405	385	740
1888	362	330	741
1889	359	250	968
1890	391	231	855
1891	266	183	859
1892	268	210	714

[1] Review of Murchison in *Dub. Quart. Journ. Med. Sc.*, Aug. and Nov. 1863,

This decline of typhus in a country where for many generations it seemed to be a national malady is a remarkable testimony to the influence of the changed conditions which have made typhus rare everywhere.

There are some interesting points in connexion with Irish typhus since 1849. After the subsidence of the great epidemic of relapsing and typhus fevers (1847–49), says Dr Dennis O'Connor, of Cork, "intermittent fever made its appearance, and, as long as it lasted, scarcely a case of continued fever was seen. As soon as the last cases of intermittent disappeared, the present epidemic broke out (1864–65), and still rages with much severity. This alternation of continued and intermittent fever is remarkable. Indeed it might have been observed that the fever of 1847 passed first into a remittent form, and gradually into the intermittent which prevailed more or less for ten years subsequently[1]." The same succession of relapsing fever by intermittent fever was observed after the epidemic of 1826 by Dr John O'Brien, of Dublin[2]. The epidemic of fever which Dr O'Connor describes for Cork in 1864–65, appeared in Dublin about the same time—the latter half of 1864. It was of the nature of typhus in both cities, cerebro-spinal in part, but probably not typhoid[3]. At Cork it had some peculiarities—a croupous-like exudation on the tongue, resembling thrush in the mouth, and a dark mottled rash (rubeola nigra), or fiery red spots on a dark red ill-defined base. "The true typhoid rash has been seen but seldom, and the petechiae of genuine typhus, so frequent in former epidemics, have been equally rare. The latter I attribute to the improved condition of our poor in good clothing and the ventilation of their dwellings." The intellect was little disturbed in this fever, there was usually a crisis about the fourteenth day, and there were no relapses. The sequelae were peculiar—"great nervous debility, leading to a semi-paralysed state of the limbs," congestion of the lungs, sometimes solidification, or gangrene or suppuration of them. It occurred at a time "when the food of the people is most abundant and of the best quality." There

---

pp. 169 and 339: "We are able, from extensive opportunities of observing the epidemic [of 1846–48] in Dublin, to verify the statement of Dr H. Kennedy as to the infrequency of enteric fever."

[1] *Dub. Quart. Journ. Med. Sc.* Nov. 1865, p. 285.

[2] See p. 273, *supra.*

[3] O'Connor, u. s. p. 286, "Typhoid has scarcely appeared in this locality, which cannot boast of the excellence of its sewerage."

had been three bad harvests in succession from 1860, but it may be inferred from a Dublin article of August, 1863, that no epidemic of typhus had arisen in Ireland down to that date, although there was much typhus in England, especially in Lancashire owing to the "cotton famine." When the epidemic did arise in Dublin, Cork, and doubtless elsewhere in Ireland, in the latter part of 1864, to continue throughout 1865, it was not connected with scarcity or distress among the common people. On the other hand, Dr Grimshaw, of Dublin, found that it was subject to influences of the weather, as if the infective principle had been a soil poison like that of plague, yellow fever, cholera, or enteric fever. Taking the Cork Street Fever Hospital for his study, he made out that there was a very close correspondence, from the 29th of May to the 31st of December, 1864, between the fluctuating pressure upon its accommodation and the periodic rises in the atmospheric moisture and heat, the crowd of patients being always greater when a high temperature coincided with a large rainfall[1]. One would not have been surprised to find some such law as that in enteric or typhoid fever, although a correspondence from day to day is subject to many sources of fallacy; but, by all accounts, the disease was typhus, the last of the considerable outbreaks of it in Ireland hitherto, and an outbreak that seemed to require, both at Cork and Dublin, the language of Sydenham's epidemic constitutions for its adequate description. For a good many years, the continued fever of Dublin has been chiefly enteric or typhoid. As late as 1862 a physician to the Fever Hospital, unconvinced by the method of Sir William Jenner, believed that he observed a transition from the old typhus into the new enteric: "The change at first seemed to be to the gastric type; to which was shortly added diarrhoea in nearly every instance; and this latter, again, occurring in a large number of cases which presented all the characters of typhus, including a dense crop of petechiae[2]." Assuming that there had been a mixture of cases of enteric and typhus fevers, the latter must have had diarrhoea among the symptoms, as they often had in special circumstances (as well as tympanitis). Since that time the species of typhus

---

[1] "On Atmospheric Conditions influencing the Prevalence of Typhus Fever." *Dub. Quart. Journ. Med. Sc.*, May, 1866, p. 309.

[2] H. Kennedy, M.D., "Further Observations on Typhus and Typhoid Fevers as seen in Dublin." *Ibid.*, Aug. 1862, p. 50.

has greatly declined, and the species of typhoid has considerably increased. The remodelling which Dublin has undergone, like all other old cities, explains the one fact. The notorious Liberties have been in great part rebuilt, and the conditions of typhus, as well as its actual fomites, to that extent removed. On the other hand, something has happened to encourage the soil poison of enteric fever. It is not easy to say what are the conditions that have favoured the enteric poison in modern towns; but there can be little doubt about the fact in general, or that Dublin and Belfast are among the best fields for the study of the problem[1].

[1] Nearly one-half of all the enteric fever deaths in Ulster and Leinster come respectively from Belfast and Dublin :

Year	Belfast	Dublin
1889	236	231
1890	190	168
1891	156	185

CHAPTER III.

INFLUENZAS AND EPIDEMIC AGUES.

EPIDEMIC agues are joined in the same chapter with influenzas for the reason that they can hardly be separated in the earlier part of the history. Until 1743 the name influenza was not used at all in this country. The thing itself can be identified clearly enough in certain instances from the earliest times. But there are periods, such as 1657–59, 1678–79, and 1727–29 when short waves of epidemic catarrhs or catarrhal fevers came in the midst of longer waves of epidemic agues, "hot agues," or intermittents, the whole being called by the people "the new disease," or "the new ague," while by physicians, such as Willis and Sydenham, they were taken to be the distinguishable constituent parts of one and the same epidemic constitution. The last period in which epidemic agues were so recognised and named in England was from 1780 to 1785 ; and in the midst of that also there occurred an epidemic catarrh—the "influenza" of the year 1782. It is possible that our own recent experience of a succession of influenzas, or strange fevers, from 1889 to 1893, in some respects the most remarkable in the whole history, would have seemed an equally composite group if they had fallen in the 17th century and had been described in the terminology of the time and according to the then doctrines or nosological methods. Without prejudice to the distinctness and unity of the influenza-type in all periods of the history, I am unable, after trying the matter in various ways, to do otherwise than take the epidemics of ague in chronological order along with the influenzas. As the history will require the frequent use of the name "ague," and, in due course, that of the name "influenza," it will be useful to examine at the outset their respective etymologies and the meanings that usage has given to them.

Originally the English name ague did not mean a paroxysmal or intermittent fever, or a fever with a long cold fit followed by a hot fit, or the malarial cachexia with sallowness, dropsy and enlarged spleen, or any other state of health arising from the endemic conditions which are known as malarial over so large a part of the globe in the tropical and sub-tropical zones. It meant simply *acuta*, the adjective of *febris acuta* made into a substantive. Thus Higden's reference in the *Polychronicon* (which is exactly in the words of Giraldus Cambrensis a century and a half before) to the *febris acuta* of Ireland is translated by Trevisa (14th cent.): "Men of that lond haue no feuere, but onliche the feuere agu, and that wel silde whanne"; and by an anonymous translator: "The dwellers of hit be not vexede with the axes excepte the scharpe axes, and that is but selde[1]." Again in the MS. English translation of the Latin essay on plague by the bishop of Aarhus, the acute fever which is described as the attendant or variant of bubo-plague proper (well known long after as the pestilential fever, a malignant form of typhus), is thus rendered:

"As we see a sege or prevy next to a chambre, or of any other particuler thyng which corrupteth the ayer in his substance and qualitee: whiche is a thing maye happe every daye. And therof cometh the ague of pestilence. And aboute the same many physicions be deceyved, not supposing this axes to be a pestilence...And suche infirmite sometime is an axes, sometime a postume or a swellyng—and that ys in many thinges."

The same use of ague is continued in the first native English book on fevers, Dr John Jones's 'Dyall of Agues,' which has chapters on plague as well as on pestilential fever and on all other fevers including intermittents. In Ireland the name of ague was applied until a comparatively late period to the indigenous typhus of the country, as if in literal translation of the *febris acuta* first spoken of by Giraldus in the 12th century. Ague in early English meant any sharp fever, and most commonly a continued fever. The special limitation to intermittents appears to have followed the revival of the study of the Graeco-Roman writers on medicine, Galen above all, in the sixteenth century. But Jones, who was freer than the more academical physicians of his time from classical influences, is shrewd enough to see that it was a mistake to transfer the experiences of Greece verbatim to England and to make them our standard of

---

[1] Higden's *Polychronicon*. Rolls Series, I. 332.

authority: he is speaking, however, not of intermittents but of the simple ephemeral fever, or inflammatory fever of one day:

> "Such as have the fever of heat or burning of the sun, sayeth Galen, theyr skin is drye and hot as that which is perched with the sun; of the which, in this orizon and countrye of oures, we have no great nede to entreate of, leaving it to the phisitions and inhabitantes that dwell nerer to the meridionall line and hoter regions, as Hispaine and Africke[1]."

At a later date, when the Hippocratic tradition had displaced the Galenic, Rogers of Cork, perhaps the earliest writer on fevers whose observations are essentially modern, has occasion thus to reflect upon the extreme deference of Sydenham to his Greek model: "Again we learn from Hippocrates that fevers in the warmer climates of Greece, at Naxos, Thasos or Paros, ran their course in certain periods of time, which no ways answers in regions removed at a farther distance from the sun,"—Rogers himself having had no experience of intermittents among all the fevers and dysenteries that he saw from 1708 to 1734, although Cork was surrounded by marshes[2].

At the time of the Latin translations of Greek medical writings by Linacre and Caius in the Tudor period, there were in this country actual experiences of strange fevers, which were interpreted according to the Greek teaching of quotidians, tertians and quartans, with their several bastard or hybrid or larval forms. These, as I have said, were certainly not the endemic fevers of malarious districts; they were, on the contrary, widely prevalent all over the country during one or more seasons in succession and more occasional for a few years longer; then there would be a clear interval of years, and again an universal epidemic of "the new fever," "the new acquaintance," "the new ague" or the like.

Sydenham, for example, has much to say of agues or intermittents prevalent in town and country for a series of years, and then disappearing for as long a period as thirteen years at a stretch. But he does not count these as the agues of the marsh; his single reference to the latter is in his essay on Hysteria, where he interpolates a remark that, if one spends two or three days in a locality of marshes and lakes, the blood is in the first instance impressed with a certain spirituous

[1] *Dyall of Agues.* London, [1564].
[2] *Essay on Epidemic Diseases.* Dublin, 1734.

miasma, which produces quartan ague, and that in turn is apt to be followed, especially in the more aged, by a permanent cachectic state[1]. If Sydenham had intended to bring all the intermittents of his experience into that class, he would not have left the paludal origin of them to a casual interpolated remark. On the other hand, he refers the epidemic agues, which occupy his pen so much, to emanations from the bowels of the earth, according to a theory of his friend Robert Boyle, applied by the latter to epidemical infections in general and to epidemic colds or influenzas in particular. Sydenham and his learned colleagues were not ignorant of the endemic agues of marshy localities, but they made little account of them in comparison with the aguish or intermittent fevers that came in epidemics all over England.

In admitting the reality of such agues, we must be careful not to ascribe them to such conditions as Talbor, the ague-curer, found in one village in Essex. We must be careful not to do so, because there are plausible reasons for doing so. The ground is much better drained now than formerly; there is less standing water, fewer marshes, a much smaller extent of water-logged soil. But the malarious parts of England have been tolerably well defined at all times; and at all times the greater part of the country was as little malarious as it is now. It is the frequent reference to agues in old medical writings that has led some modern authors to construct a picture of a marshy or water-logged England, for which there is no warrant. Cromwell died of a tertian ague which he caught at Hampton Court; therefore "the country round London in Cromwell's time" must needs have been "as marshy as the fens of Lincolnshire are now." The country round London was much the same then as now, or as in John Stow's time, or as in the medieval monk Fitzstephen's time, or as it has ever been since the last geological change. The ague of which Cromwell died in the autumn of 1658 was one of those which raged all over England from 1657 to 1659—so extensively that Morton, who was himself ill of the same for three months, says the country was "one vast hospital." Whatever was the cause of that great epidemic of "agues," and of others like it, we have no warrant to assume that "the country round London," or wherever else the epidemic

[1] *Dissert. Epistol.* § 93. Greenhill's ed. p. 378.

malady prevailed, was then as marshy as the fens of Lincoln-shire[1].

The other name in the title of this chapter, influenza, appeared comparatively late in the history. It is an Italian name, which is usually taken to mean the influence of the stars. It may have got that sense by popular usage, but the original etymology was probably different. As early as the year 1554 the Venetian ambassador in London called the sweating sick-ness of 1551 an *influsso*, which is the Italian form of *influxio*. The latter is the correct classical term for a humour, catarrh, or defluxion, the Latin *defluxio* itself having a more special limited meaning. It was not astrology, but humoral pathology, that brought in the words *influxio* and *influsso*; and I suspect that influenza grew out of the latter, but not out of the notion of an influence rained down by the heavenly bodies.

It was in 1743 that the Italian name of "influenza" first came to England[2], the rumour of a great epidemic, so called, at Rome and elsewhere in Italy having reached London a month or two before the disease itself. The epidemic of 1743 was soon over and the Italian name forgotten; so that when the same malady became common in 1762, some one with a good memory or a turn for history remarked that it resembled "the disease called influenza" nearly twenty years before. After the epidemic of 1782, the Italian name came into more general use, and from the beginning of the present century it became at once popular and vague. The great epidemics of it in 1833 and 1847 fixed its associations so closely with catarrh that an "influenza cold" became an admitted synonym for coryza or any common cold attended with sharp fever. Lastly, the series of epidemics

---

[1] One regrets to find the above mistake in the learned pages of Murchison (p. 8). The following by Dr Robert Williams (*Morbid Poisons*, II. 423) is absolutely erroneous: "In Sydenham's time, intermittent fever and dysentery were constantly endemic in London; and the mortality from the former cause alone averaged, in a comparatively small population, from one to two thousand persons annually." What Sydenham says is that dysentery was endemic in Ireland (on the authority of Boate, no doubt), that it was epidemic in London in the end of 1669 and in the three years following, and that for the space of ten years it had appeared quite sparingly (*quae per decennium jam parcius comparuerat*). As to intermittents, he says they were absent from London for thirteen years, from 1664 to 1677, except in sporadic or imported cases. In the London bills the deaths from "agues" are sometimes distinguished from "fevers," and are then seen to be only some dozen or twenty in two thousand.

[2] It is used in the Latin title of an Edinburgh graduation thesis, "De Catarrho epidemio, vel Influenza, prout in India occidentali sese ostendit," by J. Huggar, which is assigned in Häser's bibliography to the year 1703. Having been unable to find the thesis, I have not verified the date.

from 1889 to 1893 effectually broke the association with coryza or catarrh.

Before influenza became adopted as the common English name towards the end of last century, what were the names popularly given to the malady in this country? The earliest references to it are in the medieval Latin chronicles under the name of *tussis* or cough, or in some periphrasis. In the fifteenth century the English name was "mure" or "murre," which appears to be the same root as in murrain. Thus the St Albans Chronicle, under the year 1427, enters a certain "infirmitas rheumigata," which in English was called "mure"; and the obituary of the monks of Canterbury abbey has two deaths from "empemata, id est, tussis et le murra[1]." In the Tudor period there is no single distinctive name, unless it be "hot ague": in 1558 the name is "the new burning ague," in 1562 "the new acquaintance," in 1580 "the gentle correction," and at various times in the 17th century "the new disease," "the new ague," "the strange fever," "the new delight," "the jolly rant." Robert Boyle called one sudden outbreak "a great cold." Molyneux, of Dublin, mentions "a universal cold" in one year (1688), and "a universal transient fever" in another (1693). The earlier 18th century writers mostly use the word catarrh or catarrhal fever, either in Latin or in English, the popular names probably continuing fanciful as before, as for example Horace Walpole's "blue plagues." That which stands out most clearly in the English naming from the earliest times is the idea of something new or strange; but the newness or strangeness pertained quite as much to the agues as to the catarrhs. The notion of ague may be said to be uppermost in the 16th and 17th centuries, that of catarrh in the 18th and 19th; while our very latest experiences have once more brought a suggestion of ague to the front.

---

[1] *Annales Monastici* (St Albans), Rolls Series, No. 191, under the year 1427; *Hist. MSS. Commiss.* IX. pt. 1, p. 127, records of Canterbury Abbey.—An epidemic in Ireland a century before, in 1328, has been given by Sir W. R. Wilde, and by Dr Grimshaw following him, under the name of "murre," as if that had been its name at the time. The explanation seems to be that the contemporary Irish name *slaedan* was rendered by Macgeoghegan, in his translation of the Annals of Clonmacnoise, by the 15th century English term "murre." The "mure" of 1427 was a universal influenza; but the word was afterwards used for a common cold, along with poss, as in Gardiner's *Triall of Tabacco*, 1610, fol. 12 and 15: "stuffings in the head, murres and pose, coughs"; and "the poze, murre, horsenesse, cough" etc.

Retrospect of Influenzas and Epidemic Agues in the 16th and 17th centuries.

In the former volume of this history I have dealt with the various epidemics of "hot ague," "new disease" or the like down to the epidemic of 1657–59. It will be convenient to go over some of that ground again, with a view to distinguish, if possible, the catarrhal types from the aguish, and to illustrate the use of the word ague as applied to a universal epidemic. Two of the epidemic seasons in the 16th century, 1510 and 1539, are too vaguely recorded for our purpose; but I shall review briefly the seasons from 1557–58 onwards.

It is known from the general historians that there were two seasons of fever all over England in 1557 and 1558, of which the latter was the more deadly, the type according to Stow, being "quartan agues." In letters of the time the epidemic of 1557 is variously named: thus Margaret, Countess of Bedford, writes on 9 August from London to Sir W. Cecil that she "trusts the sickness that reigns here will not come to the camp [near St Quentin, where Francis, Earl of Bedford was]...As for the ague, I fear not my son." On the 18th of the same month, Sir Nicholas Bacon writes from Bedford to Cecil: "Your god-daughter, thanks be to God, is somewhat amended, her fits being more easy, but not delivered of any. It is a double tertian that holds her, and her nurse had a single, but it is gone clearly;" to which letter Lady Bacon adds a postscript about "little Nan, trusting for all this shrewd fever, to see her." On 21 September, it appears that the sickness had reached the English camp near St Quentin, for the Earl of Bedford writes: "Our general is sick of an ague, our pay very slack, and people grudge for want." As late as the 25th October the Countess of Bedford writes from London to Cecil that she "would not have him come yet without great occasions, as there reigns such sickness at London[1]."

Next year, 1558, the epidemic sickness returned in the summer and autumn, in a worse form than before. Stow calls it "quartan agues," which destroyed many old people and especially priests, so that a great number of parishes were unserved. Harrison, a canon of Windsor, says that a third part of the people did taste the general sickness. On the 6th September, sickness affected more than half the people in Southampton, Portsmouth, and the Isle of Wight. From the 20th October to the end of the year, no fewer than seven of the London aldermen died, a number hardly equalled in the first sweating sickness of 1485, and the queen (Mary) died of the lingering effects of an ague, which was doubtless the reigning sickness. On 17th October, the English commissioners being at Dunkirk to negotiate the surrender of Calais, one of them, Sir William Pickering, fell "very sore sick of this new burning ague: he has had four sore fits, and is brought very low, and in danger of his life if they continue as they have done." That year Dr Owen published *A Meet Diet for the New Ague,* and himself died of it in London on the 18th of October[2].

Fuller quaintly describes the ague of 1558 as "a dainty-mouthed disease, which, passing by poor people, fed generally on principal persons of greatest wealth and estate[3]." Roger Ascham wrote in 1562 to John

---

[1] *Cal. Cecil. MSS.* I. under the dates.
[2] Munk, *Roll of the College of Physicians,* I. 32.
[3] Cited in Southey's *Commonplace Book,* from Fuller's *Pisgah Sight,* p. 54.

Sturmius that, for four years past, or since 1558, "he was afflicted with continual agues, that no sooner had one left him but another presently followed; and that the state of his health was so impaired and broke by them that an hectic fever seized his whole body; and the physicians promised him some ease, but no solid remedy[1]." Thoresby, the Leeds antiquary of the end of the 17th century, found in the register of the parish of Rodwell, next to Leeds, a remarkable proof of the fatality of these agues, which fully bears out the general statements of Stow and Harrison. In 1557 the deaths in the register rose from 20 to 76, and in 1558, which the historians elsewhere say was the most fatal year, they rose to 124[2]. This was as severe as the sweating sickness of 1551, for example in the adjoining parish of Swillington, or in the parish of Ulverston, in Lancashire[3].

The English names of the epidemic sickness in the summers and autumns of 1557 and 1558 are all in the class of agues— "this new burning ague," "a strange fever," "divers strange and new sicknesses taking men and women in their heads, as strange agues and fevers," "quartan agues." One medical writer, Dr John Jones, says in a certain place that "quartans were reigning everywhere," and in another place, still referring to 1558, that he himself had the sickness near Southampton, that it was attended by a great sweat, and that it was the same disease as the sweating sickness of 1551. There were certainly two seasons of these agues, 1557 and 1558, the latter being the worst; and it is probable from Short's abstracts of a few parish registers in town and country that there was a third season of them in 1559. The year 1557 has been made an influenza year, perhaps because the Italian writers have emphasized catarrhal symptoms here or there in the epidemic of that year; while both the years 1557 and 1558 have been received into the chronology of epidemic or pandemic agues or malarial fevers[4]. There are perhaps a dozen English references in letters

[1] Southey, *Commonplace Book*, from Strype's *Memorials of Cranmer*, p. 284.
[2] Thoresby, *Ducatus Leodiensis*, ed. Whitaker, App. p. 152.
[3] Baines, *Lancashire*, II. 679: 39 deaths from 17 to 24 August, 1551, set down to "plague," i.e. sweat.
[4] Lest it may be supposed that there has been adequate discussion of the differences between epidemic agues and influenzas, I quote from Hirsch's *Handbuch der historisch-geographischen Pathologie* the passage in which these epidemics or pandemics of "malarial fever" are referred to: "These epidemics of malaria, which extend not unfrequently over large tracts of country, and sometimes even over whole divisions of the globe, forming true pandemics, correspond always in time with a considerable increase in the amount of sickness at the endemic malarious foci, whether near or distant; they either die out after lasting a few months, or they continue—and this applies particularly to the great pandemic outbreaks—for several years, with regular fluctuations depending on seasonal influences. On the very verge of the period to which the history of malarial epidemics can be traced back, we meet with a pandemic of that sort, in the years 1557 and 1558, which is said to have overrun all Europe (Palmarius, *De morbis contagiosis*. Paris, 1578, p. 322)...It is not until the years 1678-82 that we again meet with definite facts relating to an epidemic extending over a great part of Europe..." (Eng. Transl. I. 229.)

and chronicles to the sicknesses of those years, either to particular cases or to a general prevalence, but they do not enable us to distinguish a catarrhal type in 1557 from the aguish type which they assert for both 1557 and 1558.

Four years after, another very characteristic influenza was prevalent in Edinburgh.

> Randolph writes from Edinburgh to Cecil in the end of November, 1562: "Maye it please your Honer, immediately upon the Quene's (Mary's) arivall here, she fell acquainted with a new disease that is common in this towne, called here the newe acqayntance, which passed also throughe her whole courte, neither sparinge lordes, ladies nor damoysells, not so much as ether Frenche or English. It ys á plague in their heades that have yt, and a sorenes in their stomackes, with a great coughe, that remayneth with some longer, with others shorter tyme, as yt findeth apte bodies for the nature of the disease. The queen kept her bed six days. There was no appearance of danger, nor manie that die of the disease, excepte some olde folkes. My lord of Murraye is now presently in it, the lord of Lidingeton hathe had it, and I am ashamed to say that I have byne free of it, seinge it seketh acquayntance at all men's handes[1]."

It is not improbable that the interval between 1558 and 1562 may have been occupied with milder revivals of the original great epidemic, the one at Edinburgh counting in the series.

It appears from a Brabant almanack for the year 1561 that a sudden catarrhal epidemic was quite on the cards in those years: the astronomer foretells for the month of September, 1561: "Coughs innumerable, which shall show such power of contagion as to leave few persons unaffected, especially towards the end of the month[2]." There is an actual record from more

---

[1] *Queen Elizabeth and her Times.* Ed. Wright, 2 vols. Lond. 1838, I. 113. Sir W. Cecil writing from Westminster to Sir T. Smith on 29th December [1563] says: "The cold here hath so assayled us that the Queen's majestie hath been much troubled, and is yet not free from the same that I had in November, which they call a pooss, and now this Christmas, to keep her Majestie company, I have been newly so possessed with it as I could not see, but with somewhat ado I wryte this. We have had perpetuall frosts here sence the 16th of this month. Men doo now ordinarily pass over the Thamiss, which I thynk they did not since the 8th yere of the reign of King Henry the VIII." *Ibid.* I. 157. For "poss," see note p. 305.

[2] *Ephemer. Meteorol. anni* 1561 [for the latitude of Brabant]. Antwerp, 1561: "Tusses numero infinitae atque tanta contagionis vi praestabunt ut pauci immunes reliquant, praecipuè circa mensis finem." The almanacks of those times must have been constructed on the same principle as the weather forecasts of our own time—namely, that of using the experience of one year for the next, just as the weather of one day is an indication for the next. In 1575 Dr Richard Foster (who became president of the College of Physicians in 1601) issued an almanack in which he foretold "sweating fevers" for the month of July (*Ephemer. meteorol. ad ann.* 1575. Lond. 1575). Cogan says that Francis Keene, an astronomer, also prophesied the return of the sweating sickness in 1575, "wherein he erred not much, as there were many strange fevers and nervous sickness."

than one country (Italy, Barcelona, as well as Edinburgh) of such universal catarrhs and coughs a year later than the one foretold. The Italian writers assign the universal catarrhs and coughs to the autumn of 1562, the Barcelona writer to the winter solstice of that year, and the letter from Edinburgh to "the laste of November."

The next undoubted influenza, that of 1580, was compared abroad to the English sweat:

"In some places," says Boekel, "the sick fell into sweats, flowing more copiously in some than in others, so that a suspicion arose in the minds of some physicians of that English sweat which laid waste the human race so horribly in 1529;" and again, "the bodies were wonderfully attenuated in a short time as if by a malignant sudden colliquation, which made an end of the more solid parts, and took away all strength." The season of it was the summer.

The outbreak attracted much attention from its universality, and was described by many abroad.

Boekel says that it was of such fierceness "that in the space of six weeks it afflicted almost all the nations of Europe, of whom hardly the twentieth person was free of the disease, and anyone who was so became an object of wonder to others in the place...Its sudden ending after a month, as if it had been prohibited, was as marvellous as its sudden onset." It came up, he says, from Hungary and Pannonia and extended to Britain. The principal English account of this epidemic comes from Ireland[2]. In the month of August, 1580, during the war against the Desmonds, an English force had advanced some way through Kerry for the seizing of Tralee and Dingle; "but suddenlie such a sicknes came among the soldiers, which tooke them in the head, that at one instant there were above three hundred of them sicke. And for three daies they laie as dead stockes, looking still when they should die; but yet such was the good will of God that few died; for they all recovered. This sicknesse not long after came into England and was called the gentle correction."

This outbreak among the troops in Ireland is said to have been in August, before the sickness came to England. But it can be shown to have been at its height in London in the month of July. The year 1580 was almost free from plague in London; the weekly deaths are at a uniform low level (a good deal below the births) from January to December, except for the abrupt rise shown in the following table,—the kind of rise which we shall see from many other instances to be the infallible criterion of an influenza[3]:

[1] Johan Boekel, Συνοψις *novi morbi quem plerique medicorum catarrhum febrilem, vel febrem catarrhosam vocant, qui non solum Germaniam, sed paene universam Europam graviss. adflixit.* Helmstadtii, 1580.

[2] Hoker's "Irish historie...to the present year 1587," p. 165 a in Holinshed's *Chronicles.*

[3] This very moderate increase of the deaths in London in 1580 may be compared with the probably fabulous figures which Webster (I. 163) gives for continental cities the same year: Rome, 4000 deaths, Lübeck, 8000 deaths, Hamburg, 3000 deaths. I have given the weekly deaths and baptisms in London for five years, 1578–82, in my former volume, p. 341.

Weekly Deaths in London.

1580.

Week ending	Deaths by all causes	Dead of plague	Baptised
June 23	55	2	59
„ 30	47	4	57
July 7	77	4	65
„ 14	133	4	66
„ 21	146	3	61
„ 28	96	5	64
Aug. 4	78	5	73
„ 11	51	4	53
„ 18	49	1	72

As in 1557–58, the English references are to agues, both before and after the Gentle Correction of July–August, 1580. Cogan says that for a year or two after the Oxford gaol fever (1577) "the same kind of ague raged in a manner all over England and took away many of the strongest sort in their lustiest age, etc." And he seems to have the name "gentle correction" in mind when he says: "This kind of sickness is one of those rods, and the most common rod, wherewith it pleaseth God to brake his people for sin." Cogan's dates are indefinite. But there is a letter of the Earl of Arundel to Lord Burghley, 19th October, 1582, which shows that "hot ague" was epidemic as late as the second autumn after the influenza proper: "The air of my house in Sussex is so corrupt, even at this time of the year, as when I came away I left twenty-four sick of hot agues."

Two such epidemics in England as those of 1557–8 and 1580–82, of hot agues or strange fevers, taking the forms of simple tertian or double tertian or quartan or other of the classical types, would have made ague a familiar disease, and its name a household word. For not only were there two or more aguish seasons (usually the summer and autumn) in succession, but to judge by later experience there would have been desultory cases in the years following, and in many of the seizures acquired during the height of the epidemic, relapses or recurrences would have happened from time to time or lingering effects would have remained. Hence it is unnecessary to assume that the agues that we hear casual mention of had been acquired by residence in a malarious locality. They may have been, and most probably were, the agues of some epidemic prevalent in all parts of the country. These epidemics were the great opportunities of the ague-curers, as we shall see more fully in the sequel. It is to the bargaining of such an empiric with a patient that Clowes refers in 1579: "He did compound for fifteen pound to rid him within three fits of his ague, and to make him as whole as a fish of all diseases."

There were more sicknesses of that kind, perhaps not without

a sweating character, in the last ten years of the 16th century[1]. But they are indefinitely given as compared with earlier and later epidemics, and I shall pass to the next authentic instance.

The autumn of 1612 was undoubtedly a season of epidemic ague or "new disease" in England[2]. When Prince Henry, eldest son of James I., fell ill in November, in London, during the gaieties attending the betrothal of his sister the Princess Elizabeth to the Count Palatine of the Rhine, a letter-writer of the time said of his illness: "It is verily thought that the disease was no other than the ordinary ague that hath reigned and raged almost all over England since the latter end of summer[3]." The attack began in the end of October. The spirited and popular prince had been leading the gaieties in place of his father, who could not stand the fatigue, and was "seized by a fever that came upon him at first with a looseness, but hath continued a quotidian ever since Wednesday last [before the 4th of November], and with more violence than it began, so that on Saturday he was let blood by advice of most physicians, though Butler, of Cambridge, was loth to consent. The blood proved foul: and that afternoon he grew very sick.......I cannot learn that he had either speech or perfect memory after Wednesday night, but lay, as it were, drawing on till Friday between eight and nine of the evening that he departed. The greatest fault is laid on Turquet, who was so forward to give him a purge the day after he sickened, and so dispersed the disease, as Butler says, into all parts; whereas if he had tarried till three or four fits had been passed, they might the better have judged of the nature of it; or if, instead of purging, he had let him blood before it was so much corrupted, there had been more probability." At the dissection, the spleen was found "very black, the head full of clear water and all the veins of the head full of clotted blood. Butler had the advantage, who maintained that his head would be found full of water, and Turquet that his brains would be found overflown and as it were drowned in blood[4]." Butler, it appears, was "a drunken sot." When King James asked him what he thought of the prince's case, he replied "in his dudgeon manner" with a tag of verse from Virgil ending with "et plurima mortis imago." The Princess Elizabeth could not be admitted to see her brother "because his disease was doubted to be contagious[5]." It was at least epidemic, for in the same week alderman Sir Harry Row and Sir George Carey, master of the wards, died "of this new disease[6]." The earliest reference to it that I find is the death, previous to 11 September, of Sir Michael Hicks at his house Rackholt in Essex, "of a burning ague," which came, as was thought, by his

---

[1] There is a curious reference to "the sweat" in Shakespeare's *Measure for Measure*, Act I. scene 2, where the bawd, in an aside, says: "Thus, what with the war, what with the sweat, what with the gallows, and what with poverty, I am custom-shrunk." It is known that Shakespeare adapted and condensed his play from Whetstone's *Promus and Cassandra*, printed in 1578, who took it from an Italian romance. But Whetstone's dialogue, which is pointless and verbose beside Shakespeare's, gives an entirely different speech to the bawd at the same place in the action, making no reference to "the sweat." The date of *Measure for Measure* is not certain; but it seems to belong to the earlier period of Shakespeare's work, when he was adapting old plays most freely. Whatever its date, the war, the sweat, the gallows and poverty are evidently topical allusions pointed enough for the audience to have taken up.

[2] The year 1610 is mentioned by Short as a season of universal catarrhal fever abroad; but that epidemic is not in the modern chronologies of influenza.

[3] Chamberlain to Carleton in *Court and Times of James I.* I.

[4] Same to same 4 Nov. 1612. *Ibid.* I. p. 201.

[5] *Court and Times of James I.* I. p. 206.   [6] *Ibid.* p. 208.

often going into the water this last summer, he being a man of years[1]; but much more probably was a case of "the ordinary ague that hath reigned and raged almost all over England since the latter end of summer." The next year was still more unhealthy, to judge by samples of parish registers; agues are mentioned also in letters; thus, one going on 25 March, 1613, to visit Sir Henry Savile, found him "in a fit, an ague having caught hold of him[2]."

The winter of 1613-14 was marked by most disastrous floods in Romney Marsh, in Lincolnshire, in the Isle of Ely, and about Wisbech, and most of all in Norfolk[3]; but the malarious conditions so brought about, being subsequent to, were not conceivably the cause of, the epidemics of ague in the autumn of 1612 and 1613, which made so great an excess of burials over christenings in the parish registers.

A curious record remains of an aguish sickness in a child, which had begun about January, 1614. On 18 March, of that year, the dowager Countess of Arundel wrote from Sutton, near Guildford, to her son Earl Thomas, who was making the grand tour to Rome and elsewhere with his wife, and had left the children to the care of their grandmother: " Your two elder boys be very well and merry, but my swett Will[m.] continueth his tersion agu still. This day we expect his twelfth fitt. I assur myselfe teeth be the chefe cause. I look for so spedy ending of it, he is so well and merry on his good days, and so strong as I never saw old nor yonge bear it so well. I thank Jesu he hath not any touch of the infirmity of the head, but onely his choler and flushe apareth, but he is as lively as can be but in the time of his fits onely, which continueth some eight hours[4]."

The epidemic of ague or "new disease," which began to rage all over England in the end of the summer, 1612, had probably recurred in the years following, down to 1616. There is not a trace of plague during those years in any known record; and yet they are among the most unhealthy years in Short's abstracts of town and country parish registers[5].

The first half of the 17th century is a period which is almost a blank in the conventional annals of "influenza" in Europe. But that period, which was the period of the Thirty Years' War, had many widespread sicknesses. I do not wish to claim these as influenzas, or to contend that they were infections equivalent thereto in diffusiveness. We may, however, find a place for them in this context; for they were certainly as mysterious as any epidemics admitted into the canon of influenzas. So far as concerns Britain, the first was the epidemic ague, or "new disease," of 1612 and 1613, probably recurring until 1616. The second was the universal spotted fever of 1623 and 1624, of which I have given an account in the chapter on typhus. That was followed by the plague of 1625, and that again by a harvest ague in the country in the end of the same year. The next epidemic ague or "general sickness, called the new disease," fell mostly in England upon the two years 1638 and 1639. It was

---

[1] *Court and Times of James I.* p. 197.
[3] *Ibid.* Letter of 25 Nov. 1613.
[4] *Cal. Coke MSS.* I. 83.
[2] *Ibid.* p. 237.

in part a harvest ague, "a malignant fever raging so fiercely about harvest that there appeared scarce hands enough to take in the corn[1]"; but it was also a winter disease. I pass over the war-typhus of 1643, to which the name of "new disease" was also given, and the widespread fever of the year following. In 1651 we hear again of a strange ague, which "first broke out by the seaside in Cheshire, Lancashire and North Wales," eighty or a hundred being sick of it at once in small villages. Whitmore, who saw this epidemic in Cheshire, identified it with the Protean disease which he described in 1657–58, and hazarded the theory that the former was a diluted or "more remiss" infection carried by the wind from Ireland, where the plague was then raging, in Dublin, Galway, Limerick and other places, after their sieges or occupations by the army of the Commonwealth.

Thus in the first half of the 17th century we have more or less full evidence of epidemics of "new disease" in 1612–13, 1623–24, 1625, 1638–9, 1643–4 and 1651, not one of which was an influenza as we understand the term[2].

We come at length to the years 1657–59, in the course of which one catarrhal epidemic, or perhaps two, did prevail for a few weeks. The hot agues or "new disease" had been raging all over the country from the summer of 1657; then in April, 1658, there came suddenly universal coughs and catarrhs, "as if a blast from the stars"; they ceased, and the hot agues dragged on through the summer and autumn. A letter from London, 26 October, 1658, says: "A world of sickness in all countries round about London: London is now held to be the wholesomest place," and adds that "there is a great death of coach-horses almost in every place, and it is come into our fields[3]." It was after this, in the spring of 1659, if Whitmore has made no mistake in his dates, that coughs and catarrhs "universally infested London, scarce leaving a family where any store were, without some being ill of this distemper." The details have been

[1] Graunt, *Obs. upon the Bills of Mortality*, 1662.
[2] Robert Boyle did not attach much importance to the name of "new disease." "The term *new disease*," he says, "is much abused by the vulgar, who are wont to give that title to almost every fever that, in autumn especially, varies a little in its symptoms or other circumstances from the fever of the foregoing year or season." (Boyle's *Works*. 6 vols. 1772, v. 66.) But it was the name commonly given to the epidemics of catarrhal fever among others, and it does not appear, when the history is examined closely, that it was ever given except to some epidemic separated by several years from the last of the kind.
[3] Sir R. Leveson's Letters. *Hist. MSS. Commiss.* v. 146.

given fully in the former volume[1]. I wish merely to remark here that the two catarrhal epidemics, or influenzas proper, in two successive springs, were sharply defined episodes in the midst of a period of epidemic agues, and that the "new disease" as a whole, during the two or three years that it lasted, had such an effect in the way of ill health and mortality that it was afterwards viewed as a "little plague" worthy of being set in comparison with the Great Plague of 1665.

Willis does not say that the epidemic agues lasted after 1658, perhaps because his essay was printed early in 1659; but Whitmore, whose preface is dated November, 1659, says, without distinguishing the hot ague from the catarrhal fever but speaking of them both as one Protean malady: "it now begins again, seizing on all sorts of people of different nature, which shows that it is epidemic." Sydenham does not appear upon the scene until 1661; but when his epidemic constitutions do begin, it is with intermittents or agues, which lasted, according to him, until 1664. Perhaps if Sydenham's experience had extended back to 1657 he would have made his aguish constitution to begin with that year, and to go on continuously until 1664. At all events it does not appear that the year 1660 was a clear interval between Willis's and Whitmore's period of 1657–59, and Sydenham's period of 1661–64; for it so happens that John Evelyn has left the following note of his own illness:

"From 17 February to 5 April [1660] I was detained in bed with a kind of double tertian, the cruell effects of the spleene and other distempers, in that extremity that my physicians, Drs Wetherburn, Needham and Claude were in great doubts of my recovery." Towards the decline of his sickness he had a relapse, but on the 14th April "I was able to go into the country, which I did to my sweete and native aire at Wooton." On the 9th of May he was still so weak as to be unable to accompany Lord Berkeley to Breda with the address inviting Charles II. to assume the crown.

Sydenham makes the "constitution" which began for him in 1661 to decline gradually, and to end definitely in 1664, after which he finds intermittents wholly absent for thirteen years, or until 1677. This clear interval will make a convenient break in the chronology, whereat we may bring in the popular and professional notions of ague then current, and the popular practice in that disease by empirics.

[1] Pp. 568–577.

The Ague-Curers of the 17th Century.

It is to be observed that all the respectable writers of the profession speak of agues or intermittents as epidemic over the country for a definite period, and as disappearing thereafter for years together. At the same time they say little or nothing of the endemic malarious fevers of marshy localities. Further, it appears that the professed ague-curers, although they would wish to represent ague as a perennial disease, are really basing upon the same experiences of occasional epidemics which Willis, Whitmore and Sydenham recorded as occasional. The best instance of this is the 'Pyretologia' by Drage of Hitchin. It was published for practice in 1665, being designed to show forth the author's skill as an ague-curer[1]. When we examine its generalities closely, we find that they all come from the sickly season of 1657, the first of those described by Willis.

The great autumnal epidemic of that year (and the following), which we know from other sources to have been reckoned a "little plague," he describes as "a malignant sickness," which was followed in the winter by quartans. He himself escaped the autumnal fever but he incurred the quartan later in the year. In his own case, while the original paroxysm of this ague was still going on, a new one arose towards evening, and again, on the following day, a new paroxysm gathered vigour and supplanted the old, becoming the substantive paroxysm. Many of those who died of the quartan in 1657 had either the paroxysms duplicated, or a total want of them, or, in another passage, "the quartan which followed the autumnal disease of heterogeneous quality in 1657, cut off divers old people, the fever being erratic, duplicated or triplicated." It was a bad sign when the quartan became doubled or trebled; regularity of the paroxysm was a sign of a good recovery. The symptoms of a quartan are various; but it is not easy to pronounce that these all are the symptoms of an intermittent fever, or the prodromal signs thereof, unless intermittent fevers be epidemic at the time. He gives the case of a civil and pious priest who had a tedious quartan from being struck with lightning; he was confined to bed for two years, with loss of hearing, but, strangely enough, retaining the use of his eyes; sometimes he was vexed with convulsions, sometimes with quartan fever. The "plebs medicorum" say that a quartan fever comes of melancholy, a tertian of choler, a quotidian of putrefied pituitous matter. The "plebs plebis" think that the cause is wind or flatus, and that they get rid of the ague by belching. In his own case he observed that if he drank more cold ale than usual, he was seized with distension in the loins and with palpitation, and belched up "flatus and crass vapours infected with the quality of a quartan." He knew a man who, in the fourth or fifth month of a quartan, drank wine too freely, so that the paroxysms came every day, and that violently; after a week he had an especially severe paroxysm, and then no more for three weeks, when the fever returned under the type of an exquisite quartan. One case, which he mentions twice, led him to doubt whether quartans were not catching: a

[1] Πυρετολογια *sive Gulielmi Dragei Hitchensis* Ιατρου και Φιλοσοφου *Observationes ab Experientia de Febribus Intermittentibus.* Londini, 1665.

certain girl suffering from a quartan asked her father, who was skilled in the art, to open a vein; her parent declared that during the blooding the morbid smell of the flowing blood reached his nostrils, so that he was seized of his daughter's fever at the proper time of her paroxysms, having three or four ague fits in due order; meanwhile the girl was free from the paroxysms for a whole week, but no longer. The singular nature of quartans is further brought out in the fact that papules, pustules and exanthems breaking out on the skin were quite common in the quartan fever which followed the malignant epidemic of the autumn of 1657. "In the fevers hardly any heat is perceived; and so the unskilled vulgar say 'This is an ague' (Hoc est anglicè *Ague*), and 'This is fever and ague' (Et hoc est febris et anglicè *Ague*) when cold and heat are mixed equally or combined regularly." Peruvian bark does not evacuate the morbific matter unless by chance it provokes vomiting; cases treated by it often relapse, and are not well in the intervals. Bark does not occur in his own prescriptions; but he had cured many with "pentaphyllum." He knew several physicians in the epidemic of quartans in 1657 who trusted to narcotics entirely.

Drage must have had a real experience of aguish distempers of one kind or another during the sickly seasons of 1657–59. But it is clear from the essays or advertisements of empirics that agues were discovered in many forms of sickness that were neither intermittent fevers nor fevers of any distinctive type. One of these practitioners in the time of Charles I. claims to be "the king's majesty's servant in ordinary[1]"; which is not incredible, as Sir Robert Talbor, whom Charles II. deigned to honour, was an ague-curer of the same class.

"An ague, which hitherto amongst all sorts hath been accounted the physitian's shame, both for definition and cure (thus farre hath ignorance prevailed), but that the contrary is manifest appeareth sufficiently by this following definition: and shall be cured whether *tertian*, *quartern* or *quotidian*, by me Aaron Streater, physitian of Arts in Oxford, approved by Authority, the King's Majesties servant in ordinary, and dwelling against the Temple, three houses up in Chancerie Lane, next house to the Golden Anchor." An ague, he goes on, is either interpolate (intermittent) or continual; it is either engendered of a melancholic humour or it is a splenetic effect; the liver is obstructed by abundance of choler proceeding from a salt rheum that cometh from the brain" etc. Agues are to be dreaded most for their remote effects: "Say not therefore, 'It is but an ague, but a feaver; I shall wear it out.' Dally not with this disease;" and he adds a case to show what people may come to if they neglect an ague at the beginning: "Being carried downe from London to South-hampton by Master Thomas Mason,— September 1640, word was brought me of a Mayd dead, 16 years of age: and being requested to see what disease she dyed of, I took my chirurgion with me and went. And after section or search, I found as followeth: a gallon and a half of green water in the belly, that stunk worse than carrion; under the lyver an impostume as bigg as my fist, full of green black corrupted matter, and the lyver black and rot. The spleen and kidneys wholly decayed, and the place as black as soot; the bowels they were fretted, ulcerated and rotten. In the chesse was two great handfuls of black burnt blood in dust or powder; the heart was all sound, but not a drop of blood in it; nor one spoonfull in the whole body.

---

[1] His tract is dated 1641.

Here was an Annatomy indeed, skinne and bone; and I verily beleeve that there was no braine left, but that she lived while that was moyst: the sent was so ill, and I not well, that I forbore to search it.

God that knowes the secrets of all hearts knowes this is a truth, and nothing else here written. Arthur Fauset, chirurgion at Southampton, was the man I employed to cut her up, as many there can witness that were present.

And what of all this, may some say? Why this. An eight weeks' ague in the neglect of it breeds all these diseases, and finally death."

Let us take next the advertisement of an apothecary a generation after, who professed to cure Kentish agues,—" the description and cure of Kentish and all other agues...and humbly showing (in a measure) the author's judgment why so many are not cured, with advice in relation thereunto, whether it be Quotidian, Tertian or Quartan, simple, double or triple[1]." Before the Fire of London he had practised in Mark Lane, but after his house was destroyed he removed to Kent, attending Maidstone market every Thursday, and residing at Rochester, a city which, " besides being subject to diseases in common with others, hath two diseases more epidemical, namely, the Scurvey for one but the Ague in special." The symptoms of scurvy, as he gives them, cover perhaps the one moiety of disease, and those of ague the other.

Agues are of two sorts, curable and incurable; the curable are those that come in a common way of Providence, the incurable those that are sent more immediately from God in the way of special judgment, as instances adduced from Scripture show. What is an ague? Some think it is a strange thing, they know not what; the more ignorant think it is an evil spirit, but coming they know not whence. Agues have their seat in the humours either within the vessels or without them; those residing within are continual quotidians, continual tertians, continual quartans; those without are intermittent ditto. (This distinction of within and without the vessels is traditional, and is found in Jones's *Dyall of Agues* as well as in Dutch medical books a century later.) The paroxysms of the intermittents are really the uprising of the Archaeus [of van Helmont], or spirit, to oppose the rottenness of the humours. A quartan is harder to cure than any other ague; part of its cure is an old 14th-century rule of letting blood in the plague; "let blood in the left hand in the vein between the ring finger and the little finger, which said thing to my knowledge was done about sixteen years ago [to say nothing of three hundred years ago] by the empiric Parker in this country, with very good success and to his great honour and worldly advancement." This ague-curer says little of Peruvian bark; his specific is the powder of Riverius, "the preparation of which, as well as some of the powder itself is lately and providentially come to my hands." Three doses cost not above five shillings, "and I never yet gave more in the most inveterate of these diseases...My opinion is that he that will not freely part with a crown out of his pocket to be eased of such a disease in his body deserves to keep it."

[1] By Nicholas Sudell, licentiate in physick and student in chimistry. London, 1669.

The most celebrated ague-curer of the Restoration period was Sir Robert Talbor, who thus describes the high motives that made him a specialist[1]:

"When I first began the study and practice of Physick, amongst other distempers incident to humane bodies I met with a quartan ague, a disease that seemed to me the *ne plus ultra* of physic, being commonly called Ludibrium et Opprobrium Medicorum, folly and derision of my profession, did so exasperate my spirit that I was resolved to do what study or industry could perform to find out a certain method for the cure of this unruly distemper...I considered there was no other way to satisfy my desire but by that good old way, observation and experiment. To this purpose I planted myself in Essex near to the seaside, in a place where agues are the epidemical diseases, where you will find but few persons but either are, or have been afflicted with a tedious quartan. In this place I lived some years, making the best use of my time I could for the improving my knowledge."

Talbor's first chapter is a fluent account of how agues are produced by "obstructions" of the spleen. This was a matter of theoretical pathology which an empiric could make a show with as well as another. But the empiric betrays himself as soon as he comes to practice. The enlarged spleen of repeated agues, or of the malarial cachexia, is commonly known as the ague-cake. There is no doubt that much of the unhappiness of the aguish habit resides in the ague-cake, and that one of the best pieces of treatment is to apply counter-irritants or the actual cautery to the left side, against which the enlarged spleen presses as a cake-like mass. Talbor, however, desired to free the patient from his "ague-cake" altogether:

"I have observed these in four patients: two were cast out the stomach by nature, and the other two by emetic medicines. One of them was like a clotted piece of phlegm, about the bigness of a walnut, pliable like glue or wax, weighing about half an ounce; another about the bigness of the yolk of a pullet's egg, and like it in colour, but stiffer, weighing about five drachms; the other two of a dark colour, more tough, about the like bigness, and heavier. It is a general observation amongst them that their ague comes away when they see those ague-cakes[2]."

Having followed this "good old way of observation and experiment" for several years among the residents of the Essex

[1] Πυρετολογια. *A rational account of the Cause and Cure of Agues, with their signs, Diagnostick and Prognostick. Also some Specified Medicines prescribed for the Cure of all sorts of Agues, &c. Whereunto is added a short account of the Cause and Cure of Feavers and the Griping in the Guts.* Authore Rto. Talbor, Pyretiatro. Londini, 1672.

[2] Sir Thomas Watson (*Practice of Physic*, I. 725) has a story which shows how long these fancies, encouraged by quacks, may linger: "A coachman by whose side I sat while travelling from Broadstairs to Margate was speaking of the rarity of ague in that part of the Isle of Thanet. His father, he said, once had the complaint, and a fit came on while he was on a visit to him, the coachman, at Ramsgate. The son administered to his suffering parent a glass of brandy; whereupon 'he threw the agy off his stomach; and it looked for all the world like a lump of jelly.'"

marshes, Talbor came to London, and set up his sign next
door to Gray's Inn Gate in Holborn.   In 1672 (14th July) he
issued a small work with a Greek title—the quacks were fond
of the Greek character on their title-pages—" Πυρετολογια, a
rational account of the cause and cure of agues, with their
signs : whereunto is added a short account of the cause and
cure of feavers."   He made a bid also for practice in "scurvy,"
a disease of landsmen in those times which was more a bogey
than ague itself—"a strange monster acting its part upon the
stage of this little world in various shapes, counterfeiting the
guise of most other diseases...sometimes it is couchant, other
times rampant, so alternately chronic and acute."

Most of the agues which Talbor professed to have met with
in London in those years must have been equally factitious :
for Sydenham, who makes more of "intermittents" than other
writers of repute, was of opinion that, for thirteen years from
1664 to 1677, fevers of that type had not been seen in London,
except some sporadic cases or cases in which the attack had
begun in the country.   But the air was then full of talk and
controversy about Peruvian bark, or Jesuits' powder (*pulvis
patrum*), or "the cortex," which was cried up as a specific in
agues by some, and cried down by others.   Talbor had seized
upon this specific, and claimed to have an original way of
administering it, whereby its success was assured.   We get a
glimpse of his practice from Dr Philip Guide, a Frenchman who
came to London and practised for many years as a member of
the College of Physicians[1].   Talbor had cured the daughter of
Lady Mordaunt of an ague, and the cure had reached the ears
of Charles II.   One of the French princesses having been long
afflicted with a quartan ague,

"The king commanded Mr Talbor to take a turn at Paris, and as a mark
of distinction he honoured him with the title of knight.   He succeeded
wonderfully.   But he could not cure Lady Mordaunt's daughter a second
time, whom he had cured once before at London, by whom he gained most of
his reputation."   He tried for two months, but did not relieve the symptoms.
Dr Guide was called in, and being asked to give his opinion of the ague that
the young lady was afflicted with, "after some inquiry I found her distemper
was complicated and quite different from the ague, which made me lay the
thought of the ague aside, and apply myself wholly to the complicated
disease, which I effectually cured in twelve days, together with her ague,
without having any further need of the infallible specific of Sir Robert
Talbor."

[1] Philip Guide, M.D., *A Kind Warning, &c.*   Lond. 1710.

The Peruvian Bark Controversy.

It can hardly be doubted that the conflicting opinions as to the benefit of Peruvian bark in ague, which have been often cited in disparagement of medicine and as an example of its intolerance, arose from the indiscriminate use of it in "agues" diagnosed as such by quacks and pushing practitioners. The bark had been brought first to Spain in 1632 and had been tried medicinally in 1639[1]. It was under the powerful patronage of the Jesuits, especially of Cardinal de Lugo, and most of it at that time found its way to Rome, the centre of a malarious district. In 1652 it failed to cure a "double quartan" in an Austrian archduke, and thereafter fell into some disrepute. A violent controversy on its specific use in agues arose in the Netherlands; it had failed in every case at Brussels, it had not failed in a single case at Delft. Meanwhile it remained very dear, sixty florins having been paid at Brussels in 1658 for as much as would make twenty doses, to be sent to Paris. The London 'Mercurius Politicus' of the week 9–16 December, 1658, contained an advertisement[2] that a supply of it had been brought over by James Thompson, merchant of Antwerp, and was to be had either at his own lodgings at the Black Spotted Eagle in the Old Bailey or at Mr John Crook's, bookseller, at the sign of the Ship in St Paul's Churchyard. The London physicians such as Prujean and Brady countenanced it, and Willis, in reprinting his essay on Fevers in 1660, spoke of it as coming into daily use. Sydenham, whose publisher was the same Crook at the sign of the Ship, made a brief reference to it in the first edition (1666) of his *Observationes Medicae*, in the section upon the epidemic constitution of intermittents during the years 1661–64. He admits that the bark could keep down fermentation for the time being; but the *materies* which the fermentation would have dissipated if it had been allowed its way, will remain in the system and quickly renew its power. He had known a quartan continue for several years under the use of bark. It had even killed some patients when given immediately before the paroxysm. Prudently and cautiously given, in the decline of such fevers, it had been sometimes

[1] The best summary of the "history of the use of Peruvian bark" is by Sir George Baker, in *Trans. Col. Phys.* III. (1785), 173.
[2] Cited by Baker, *l.c.* p. 190.

useful and had stopped the paroxysms altogether, especially if the aguish fits were occurring at a season when the malady was less epidemical. But it is clear that Sydenham in 1666 inclined strongly to non-interference with the natural depuratory action of the fever upon the *materies* of the disease. His teaching that the cortex, while it kept down the fermentation of the blood for a time, left the dregs of the fever behind, was thus popularly stated some years after by Roger North in relating the fatal illness of his brother the Lord Keeper Guilford in the summer of 1685[1].

The fever of Lord Guilford was not an intermittent at all, but a "burning acute fever without any notable remissions and no intermissions," a case of the epidemic typhus of that and the succeeding year, elsewhere described. The treatment was first in the hands of Dr Masters, pupil and successor of Dr Willis, whose cardinal doctrine of fevers was that they were a natural fermentation of the blood. He ordered phlebotomy. Next Dr Short, of another school, was sent for: "So to work with his cortex to take it off: and it was so done; but his lordship continued to have his headache and want of sleep. He gave him quieting potions, as they called them, which were opiates to make him sleep; but he ranted and renounced them as his greatest tormentors, saying 'that they thought all was well if he did not kick off the clothes and his servant had his natural rest; but all that while he had axes and hammers and fireworks in his head, which he could not bear.' All these were very bad signs; but yet he seemed to mend considerably; and no wonder, his fever being taken off by the cortex. And it is now found that, without there be an intermission of the fever, the cortex doth but ingraft the venom to shoot out again more perniciously." The Lord Keeper's illness dragged on, and at length the physicians "found he had a lent fever which was growing up out of the dregs which the cortex had left; and if it were not taken off, they knew he would soon perish. So they plied him with new doses of the same under the name of cordial powders, whereof the quantity he took is scarce credible; but they would not touch his fever any more than so much powder of port. And still he grew worse and worse. At length the doctors threw up[2]."

Sydenham having indicated in his edition of 1666 that bark was dangerous when given immediately before a paroxysm, but that it was sometimes useful in the decline of the fever, and that its benefits were greatest in those desultory agues which appeared at, or continued into, a season when agues had become less epidemical, he proceeded in his third edition of 1675 to enlarge these indications for giving bark in ague. He begins, as Talbor had begun in his essay of 1672, and as the empiric Streater had in his advertisement of 1641, by calling quartans the *opprobrium medicorum,* and he then lays down precisely how

---

[1] *Lives of the Norths.* New ed. by Jessopp. Lond. 1890, III. 188.
[2] He fell into a kind of decline and died at his country house on 5 September, Dr Radcliffe having been summoned from London without avail.

bark was to be given in those obstinate fevers, as well as in tertians of the aged or feeble: namely, after the fever had exhausted itself *suo Marte*, in the intervals between two paroxysms, an ounce of bark (in two ounces of syrup of roses) to be taken in the course of the two free days, a fourth part at a time morning and evening. The dosage may have been borrowed from Talbor, as Sir George Baker alleges[1]; it matters little for anyone's fame. Sydenham, however, in a letter of October, 1677, thus claimed to have been independent of Talbor so far as concerned the directions for giving bark which he inserted in his edition of 1675 :

"I have had but few trials, but I am sure that an ounce of bark, given between the two fits, cures; which the physicians in London not being pleased to take notice of in my book, or not believing me, have given an opportunity to a fellow that was but an apothecary's man, to go away with all the practice on *agues*, by which he has gotten an estate in two months, and brought great reproach on the faculty[2]."

Talbor was patronised by Charles II., who caused him to be made one of his physicians. On 2 May, 1678, a few months after the date of Sydenham's letter, Lord Arlington wrote to the president of the College of Physicians[3]: "His Majesty, having received great satisfaction in the abilities and success of Dr Talbor for the cure of agues, has caused him to be admitted and sworn one of his physicians." Next year, 1679, the king had an attack of the reigning ague, and a recurrence of it in 1680. It is probably to the occasion of one or other of these attacks that an undated letter belongs from the Marquis of Worcester to the marchioness : "The physicians came to the Council to acquaint them that they intend to give the king the Jesuit's powder five or six times before he goes to Newmarket, which they agreed to. He looks well, eats two meals of meat a day, as he used to do[4]." Evelyn has preserved a story told him by the Marquis of Normanby, which probably relates to the same aguish attack of Charles II.[5]:

[1] Baker, *l.c.*, "Had not physicians been taught by a man whom they, both abroad and at home, vilified as an ignorant empiric, we might at this day have had a powerful instrument in our hands without knowing how to use it in the most effectual manner." This was written at a time when physicians spoke of "throwing in the bark"—throwing it in "with a shovel," as an Edinburgh professor used to say.
[2] John Barker, M.D., of Sarum, and afterwards physician to the forces, says in 1742 (in his essay on the epidemic fever of 1741, u. s. p. 112) that he had Sydenham's letter in manuscript before him, and that it was written in October, 1677.
[3] Cited by Baker, *Trans. Col. Phys.* III. 208.
[4] Beaufort MSS. *Histor. MSS. Com.* XII. App. 9. p. 85.
[5] Evelyn's *Diary*, under the date of 29 Nov. 1694.

"The physicians would not give the *quinquina* to the king, at a time when, in a dangerous ague, it was the only thing that could cure him (out of envy, because it had been brought into vogue by Mr Tudor [Talbor] an apothecary), till Dr Short, to whom the king sent to know his opinion of it privately, sent word to the king that it was the only thing which could save his life, and then the king enjoined his physicians to give it to him, which they did, and he recovered. Being asked by this lord [Normanby] why they would not prescribe it, Dr Lower said it would spoil their practice, or some such expression."

What Dr Lower was most likely to have said was, that it went against his principles to give bark in fevers. He was a physiologist, in the sense of an anatomist, the pupil of Willis at Oxford and his successor in practice in London. It was the teaching of Willis that blood was like the juice of vegetables, particularly the juice of the grape, in respect of fermenting, just as it was like milk in respect of curdling. Fever was a sudden access of fermentation, apt to arise in spring and autumn, from internal or constitutional occasions, as well as to come at any time by infection; by this febrile ferment, ebullition or commotion, the blood was purged of certain impurities, comparable to the lees of wine, which were removed from the body in the sweat, the urine or other critical evacuation. Jesuit's bark was believed to check fermentation, or, in the later phrase of Pringle and others, it was antiseptic; and it was probably because he thought it would check the natural defaecating action of the blood in an ague that Lower refused to prescribe it. Sydenham was more tentative, pliant, empirical. He cavilled at Willis's doctrine of the ebullition or fermentation of the blood without actually rejecting it; for he held practically the same view of the salutary or depuratory nature of fever, which was indeed the Hippocratic view of it. Accordingly in his first reference to bark, in 1666, he sustains the objection to it, that it interfered with a natural depuratory action; and it was only in following the lead of Talbor, a more empirical person than himself, that Sydenham overcame his doctrinal scruples. Dr Short, to whom Charles II. sent privately for advice, was of Sydenham's party; soon after that occasion, the latter dedicated to Short his 'Tractate on Gout and Dropsy' (1683). It was Short who "went to work with his cortex" upon the Lord Keeper in 1685, after Dr Masters, of the school of Willis, had tried his hand with phlebotomy. The king's experiences, a few months before the Lord Keeper's death, had been just the same, and with the same result: the deathbed of Charles II., it is well known, was

the scene of ecclesiastical rivalries; but the physicians at the bedside of the king had their rivalries too.

On Monday the 2nd of February, at eight in the morning, the king had a seizure of some kind in his bed-chamber, which was currently said to have been an "apoplectic fit[1]," although there is nothing said of paralysis. A letter of the 3rd February[2] says the king "was seized in his chair and bed-chamber with a surprising convulsion fit which lasted three hours." Dr King, an expert operator who had assisted Lower in the delicate operation before the Royal Society on 23 November, 1667, of transfusing blood from one body to another, happened to be at hand, and, at once drawing his lancet, bled the king. His promptitude in action, which probably left him little time for diagnosis, was much applauded, and the Privy Council voted him a reward of a thousand pounds, which Burnet says he never received.

"This rescued his Majesty for the instant," says Evelyn, (who came up from Wooton on hearing the news, and is probably correct in his narrative), "but it was only a short reprieve. He still complained, and was relapsing, often fainting, with sometimes epileptic symptoms, till Wednesday, for which he was cupp'd, let blood in both jugulars, had both vomit and purges, which so reliev'd him that on Thursday hopes of recovery were signified in the public Gazette; but that day, about noone, the physitians thought him feverish. This they seem'd glad of, as being more easily allay'd and methodically dealt with than his former fits; so as they prescribed the famous Jesuit's powder: but it made him worse, and some very able doctors who were present did not think it a fever, but the effect of his frequent bleeding and other sharp operations us'd by them about his head, so that probably the powder might stop the circulation, and renew his former fits, which now made him very weake. Thus he pass'd Thursday night with greate difficulty, when, complaining of a paine in his side, they drew 12 ounces more of blood from him; this was by 6 in the morning on Friday, and it gave him reliefe; but it did not continue, for being now in much paine, and struggling for breath, he lay dozing, and after some conflicts, the physitians despairing of him, he gave up the ghost at halfe an houre after eleven in the morning, being 6 Feb. 1685, in the 36th yeare of his reigne, and 54th of his age....Thus died King Charles II. of a vigorous and robust constitution, and in all appearance promising a long life[3]."

Whether the bark would have saved him if the aguish nature of the paroxysms (such as he had in 1679 and again in 1680) had been clear from the first, may be doubted. But his chances of recovery were certainly made worse by the halting

[1] Evelyn; Luttrell, I. 327.
[2] *Hist. MSS. Com.* v. 186. Sutherland correspondence.
[3] *The Diary of John Evelyn,* under the date 4 Feb. 1685.

and stumbling diagnosis, (according to Evelyn)—now apoplexy, now epilepsy, now fever[1].

The true value of cinchona bark in medicine was not seen until much that was vague in the use of the term "ague" had been swept away. In the last great epidemic period of agues in this country, as we shall see, from 1780 to 1786, bark was found, for some reason, to be ineffective. It is not in the treatment of epidemic agues, but of agues in malarious countries, that the benefits of Jesuits' bark have been from first to last most obvious.

The practice in so-called agues was long in the hands of empirics, who, like their class in general, made business out of ignorant or lax diagnosis. I shall add here what remains to be said of specialist ague-curers in later times. They are heard of in London in the Queen Anne period, and as late as 1745.

Swift writes in his Journal to Stella, 25 December, 1710, from Bury Street, St James's: "I tell you a good pun: a fellow hard by pretends to cure agues, and has set out a sign, and spells it *egoes*; a gentleman and I observing it, he said, 'How does that fellow pretend to cure agues?' I said, I did not know, but I was sure it was not by a *spell*. That is admirable." In 1745, Simon Mason, of Cambridge, published by subscription and dedicated to Dr Mead an essay, *The Nature of an Intermitting Fever and Ague considered* (Lond. 1745), in which he has the following on "charm-doctors":—"When one of these poor wretches apply to a doctor of this stamp, he enquires how many fits they have had; he then chalks so many strokes upon a heater as they tell him they have had fits, and useth some other delusions to strengthen the conceit of the patient" (p. 167). Francis Fisher, who had been upper hostler in a livery stable in Crutched Friars near forty years, "told me he seldom missed a week without several ague patients applying to him, and he cured great numbers by a charm they wore in their bosoms" (p. 239). Another, who kept a public-house near St George's Fields, Southwark, sold "febrifuge ale" at a shilling a pint. It was a small ale brewed without hops, but with bark, serpentery, rhubarb and cochineal mixed in the brewing. The receipt was given him by an old doctor who was a prisoner in the King's Bench. His customers came in the morning fasting, and drank their shilling's worth after the publican had given them faith by a cordial grip of the hand. "By this means," he told Mason, "I got a good trade to my house, and a comfortable maintenance too."

We may now return to the actual history of the epidemic fevers upon which the Peruvian bark was first tried on a large scale in England. The "intermittent" constitution which began in 1677 and lasted year after year until 1781 or even longer was

---

[1] The popular imagination at the time appears to have been most impressed by Dr King's promptitude in whipping out his lancet. Roger North must have had it incorrectly in his mind when he wrote: "About the time of the death of Charles II., it grew a fashion to let blood frequently, out of an opinion that it would have saved his life if done in time."

a very remarkable one. It was called at the time the new fever, or the new ague, and it had at least one short interlude of influenza or epidemic catarrhal fever in the winter of 1679, just as the last epidemic of the kind, in 1657–59, had at least one, and probably two, short and swift epidemic catarrhs in spring. But before we come to that epidemic of 1678–81, there falls to be noticed an epidemic in the month of November, 1675, which has always been counted among the influenzas proper. After giving the particulars of it from Sydenham and from the London bills of mortality, I shall show from Sydenham and the bills of mortality that there was an exactly similar epidemic in the month of November, 1679, which has not been admitted into the conventional list of influenzas. Thereafter I shall proceed to the epidemic constitution of 1678–81 as a whole, which has been reckoned among the epidemic agues or malarious epidemics.

The Influenza of 1675.

The first that we hear of the universal cold of 1675 is an entry which Evelyn makes in his diary under 15 October: "I got an extreme cold, such as was afterwards so epidemical as not only to afflict us in this island, but was rife over all Europe, like a plague. It was after an exceeding dry summer and autumn." It was not until November that the epidemic cold made an impression upon the death-rate in London; the deaths mounted up from 275 in the week ending 2 November, to 420 and 625 in the two weeks following, and thereafter gradually declined to an ordinary level. Part of the excess, but by no means the greater part of it, was set down under fevers, as the following section from the weekly bills of the year will show :

1675

Week Ending	Fever	Smallpox	Griping in the Guts	All causes
Nov. 2	42	9	29	275
9	60	12	42	420
16	130	13	43	625
23	99	2	28	413
30	61	6	29	349
Dec. 7	54	7	25	308
14	43	5	12	266

This shows the characteristic rise and fall of an epidemic

catarrh both in the article of fever deaths and in the column of deaths from all causes. The other excessive articles besides fever in the two worst weeks are also characteristic of influenza mortality:

	Week ending 9 Nov.	Week ending 16 Nov.
Consumption	68	99
Aged	40	67
Tissick	10	35

Sydenham's account bears out the figures[1]. At the end of October, he says, the mild, warm weather turned to cold, while catarrhs and coughs became more frequent than at any time within his memory. They lasted until the end of November, when they ceased suddenly. Afterwards he gives a special chapter to the "Epidemic Coughs of the year 1675, with Pleurisies and Pneumonias supervening." The epidemic spared, he says, hardly anyone of whatever age or temperament; it went through whole families at once. A fever which he calls *febris comatosa* had been raging far and wide since the beginning of July, with which in the autumn dysenteric and diarrhoeal disorders were mingled (it was an exceedingly dry season). This constitution held the mastery all the autumn, affecting now the head, now the bowels, until the end of October, when catarrhs and coughs became universal and continued for a month. Sydenham's view of the sequence of events was his usual one, namely, that one constitution, by change of season, passed by transition into another. Whatever the constitution of "comatose" fevers may have been, which prevailed "far and near," it has left no trace upon the bills of mortality in London, which are remarkably low until the beginning of November. But as soon as the epidemic of coughs begins, the weekly deaths mount up in an unmistakeable manner, so that for two or three weeks in November, the mortality is nearly double that of the weeks preceding or following.

The "severe cold and violent cough," of 1675, says Thoresby of Leeds[2], who was then a boy, "too young or unobservant to

[1] *Obs. Med.* 3rd ed. 1675, v. 5.
[2] Ralph Thoresby, *Ducatus Leodiensis*, ed. Whitaker, App. p. 151. Brand, *Hist. of Newcastle*, under the year 1675, says that "the jolly rant" caused 724 deaths in that town, the authority given being Jabez Cay, M.D., who left his papers to Thoresby. The number given is probably the mortality from all causes.

make such remarks as might be of use," was known in the north of England "profanely" by the name of the "jolly rant." Thoresby well remembered that it affected all manner of persons, and that so universally that it was impossible, owing to the coughing, to hear distinctly an entire sentence of a sermon. He gives December as the month of it in Leeds, and says that it affected York, Hull, and Halifax, as well as the counties of Westmoreland, Durham, and Northumberland. In Scotland also we find a trace of a strange epidemic sickness. It was the time of the persecution of the Covenanters, whose preachers moved hither and thither among the farm-houses. One of them, John Blackadder, was at the Cow-hill in the parish of Livingstown in August, 1675. He came in one evening from the fields very melancholy, and in reply to questions, he said he was afraid of a very dangerous infectious mist to go through the land that night. He desired the family to close doors and windows, and keep them closed as long as they might, and to take notice where the mist stood thickest and longest, for there they would see the effects saddest. "And it remained longest upon that town called the Craigs, being within their sight, and only a few families; and within four months thereafter, thirty corpses went out of that place[1]." The prophecy was fulfilled within four months, which would bring us to the date of the influenza, although the mortality for a small place is somewhat excessive.

The Influenza of 1679.

For the sake of comparison, I pass at once to an epidemic of coughs and colds in the month of November, 1679, which Sydenham has chronicled, but no one except Cullen[2] has thought of including among the influenzas. It produced the characteristic effect of influenza on the London weekly bills, and it came in the midst of epidemic agues, just as the epidemic catarrhs of 1658 and 1659 had done. The following rise and fall are just as distinctive of an influenza as on the last occasion in 1675:

---

[1] Patrick Walker's *Life of Cargill*, pp. 29, 30.
[2] *Synopsis Nosologiae.* 3rd ed. Edin. 1780, ii. 173.

1679

Week ending	Fever	Smallpox	Griping of the Guts	All causes
Nov. 11	50	18	34	328
18	89	27	39	541
25	126	21	55	764
Dec. 2	82	27	38	457
9	63	12	38	388

Sydenham's account[1] of this remarkable November outburst of sickness in London, written within a few weeks of its occurrence, is almost exactly a repetition of his language concerning the epidemic coughs of November, 1675. The prevailing intermittent fevers, he says, gave place to a new epidemic depending upon a manifest crasis of the air. The new epidemic was one of coughs, which were so much more general than at the same season in other years that in nearly every family they affected nearly every person. In some cases of the cough, the aid of a physician was hardly needed; but in others the chest was so shaken by the violent convulsive cough as to bring on vomiting, and the head was affected with vertigo. For the first few days the cough was almost dry, and so purely paroxysmal as to remind Sydenham of the whooping-cough of children. Everyone was surprised, he says, at the frequency of these coughs in this season. His own suggestion was that the rains of October[2] had filled the blood with crude and watery particles, that the first access of cold had checked transpiration through the skin, and that Nature had contrived to eliminate this serous colluvies either by the branches of the "vena arteriosa" or (as some will have it) by the glands of the trachea, and to explode it by the aid of a cough. Phlebotomy and purging were the best cures; diaphoretics he considered less safe, and he ascribed to their abuse the fever into which some fell, and the pleurisies which were apt to attack patients with great violence during the subsidence of the epidemic catarrh.

The Epidemic Agues of 1678–80.

The other English writer on the epidemic constitution of 1678–79 is Dr Christopher Morley[3]. Like Sydenham, he is

---

[1] *Epist. respons. ad R. Brady*, § 42.
[2] Luttrell (*Diary*, I. 23) enters under Oct. 1629: "About the middle of this month vast great rains fell which have been very prejudiciall to many persons."
[3] Christopher Love Morley, M.D., *De Morbo Epidemico tam hujus quam superioris Anni, id est 1678 et 1679 Narratio*. Preface dated London, 31 Dec. 1679.

occupied almost exclusively with the epidemic agues; but he also records the extraordinary rise of the mortality in London for a few weeks in the last months of the year, and the causes thereof, although it did not occur to him to count that as a separate part of "the new disease," still less as the principal part, which it really was in London so far as concerned the death-rate. Dating his preface from London, the 31st of December, 1679, he says in the text: "Within the very days of my present writing, it happens that as many as four hundred deaths more than usual have taken place in a fortnight," the excessive mortality having been due to "coryza, bronchitis, catarrh, cough and fever," which were the effects of "most pernicious destillations."

I shall now go back to the beginning of the epidemic constitution in the midst of which this November interlude occurred, and I shall follow it season after season to the end, so as to set forth in historical prominence that which was regarded at the time as "the new disease." When Sydenham returned to London in the autumn of 1677, after six months' rest from practice, he was told by his professional friends that intermittents were being seen here and there (after a clear interval of thirteen years), being more frequent in the country than in the city. In the letter of October, 1677, cited above, he speaks of Talbor having made a fortune in two months by his cures of agues with bark.

The first particular notice of the "new fever" occurs in a London letter of 23 February, 16⅞: "Lady Katherin Brudenhall has been in great danger of death by the new feaver[1]." A severe aguish illness of Roger North, fully described in his 'Autobiography,' was probably another instance of the reigning malady; it came upon him in the hot weather of 1678, while he was residing with his brother, Lord Guilford, at Hammersmith[2]. In the autumn of 1678, the "new fever" came more into notice. On the 8th of September, a letter was brought to Evelyn in church, from Mr Godolphin (afterwards celebrated as the minister of William III.), to say that his wife was exceedingly ill and to ask Evelyn's prayers and assistance. Evelyn and his wife took boat at once to Whitehall, and found the young and much-beloved Mrs Godolphin "attacqu'd with the new fever then reigning this excessive hot autumn, and which was so violent that it was not thought she could last many hours." She died next day, in her twenty-ninth year; but, as she had been brought to bed of a son six days before, her fever may have been more from puerperal causes than from "the new fever then reigning." Other known cases of ague the next season were those of Sir James Moore, his majesty's engineer, who, in August, 1679, coming from Portsmouth "was seized with an ague, and had two or three violent fits, which carried him off[3];" and of the king, Charles II., who was congratulated on his recovery

[1] Lady Chaworth to Lord Roos, *Calendar of the Belvoir MSS.* II. 47.
[2] *Lives of the Norths.* Ed. cit. III. 143.
[3] Luttrell's *Historical Relation.* Oxford, 1857, I. 19.

by the lord mayor and aldermen, on 15 September, and had a recurrence of
the aguish attack ("two or three fits") on 15 May, 1680[1]. There are also
references to the agues of 1679 in the country, in the letters of Lady
North[2].

Sydenham wrote his account of this epidemic of intermittents
in compliance with a request from Dr Brady, Master of Gonville
and Caius College, Cambridge, that he would continue the
method of his 'Observationes Medicae' into the years following,
and in particular give an account of his method of administering
bark. He occupied most of his space with treatment; but he
gives here and there the following epidemiological details. The
agues were mostly tertians, or quotidians, or duplex forms of these,
whereas on a former occasion they had been mostly quartans;
after two or three intermissions they were apt to become
continual fevers. The agues, which had occurred in the spring
of 1678, became more common in the summer and autumn,
when they raged so extensively that no other disease deserved
the name of epidemic so much. In winter smallpox took the
lead; but early in July, 1679, the agues began again, and so
increased day by day that in August they were raging excessively and destroying many. It was in August that the king
had his "great cold" at Windsor, which afterwards changed to
an ague. Sydenham then comes to the November interlude of
epidemic catarrhs, which was followed by "a fever without cough"
(*non penitus deleta, sed manente adhuc in sanguine, malae crasis
impressione*), lasting to the beginning of 1680. As that year
wore on, the intermittent fevers began again, and continued
more or less until 1685, becoming indeed less common in
London, and less severe, than in the first four years of the
constitution, but in other places, now here, now there, not less so
than at first[3].

[1] Luttrell, *loc. cit.* I. 20, 21, 44.
[2] On 16 March, the illness of "little Frank...hath made me suspect some kind of
aguish distemper; but, if it be, it is so little that we neither perceive coming nor
going." On 7 July, another child is recovered of her feverish distemper. On
5 October, "all my little ones are very well, but some of my servants have quartan
agues." *Lives of the Norths*, Letters of Anne, Lady North.
[3] An authentic case of these lingering epidemic agues was that of John Evelyn in
the beginning of 1683. On 7th February, 1687, he writes: "Having had several
violent fits of an ague, recourse was had to bathing my legs in milk up to the knees,
made as hot as I could endure it; and sitting so in a deep churn or vessel, covered
with blankets, and drinking carduus posset, then going to bed and sweating. I not
only missed that expected fit, but had no more, only continued weak that I could not
go to church till Ash Wednesday, which I had not missed, I think, so long in twenty
years"—in fact, since his "double tertian" in 1660, which kept him in bed from
17th February to 5th April.

I have kept to the last the special account of this epidemic written by Morley at the end of the second year of it, namely, in December, 1679. He had been a witness of this fever, first at Leyden in the autumn of 1678, and next in England in the autumn of 1679, and he made it the subject of a treatise at the request of an eminent physician in London. It was not so severe by half in England as in Holland, but the English made a great deal more of it, calling it the New Disease, the New Ague, the New Fever, the New Ague Fever, and, in Derbyshire sarcastically, the New Delight. In Holland they called it neither new nor old, neither intermittent nor continued, nor a conjunction of both, but simply *morbus epidemicus*, or *febris epidemica*. His master at Leyden, Professor Lucas Schacht, taught very decidedly that it was of a scorbutic nature, and as early as the month of June, 1678, had prophesied the arrival of such an epidemic fever because "tertians were becoming more and more scorbutic," just as they had done before the great epidemic of fever in Holland in 1669. Morley claims, however, that the fever of 1678 was in some respects different from that of 1669, as well as from that of the year immediately preceding, 1677, when "an incredible multitude of people all over Belgium, and in every city and town, fell sick." The Dutch, it appears, called these occasional outbreaks simply "the epidemic fever," neither intermittent nor continued; and certainly that of 1669, which is sometimes counted among the epidemic agues, was a very remarkable "ague." (See Chapter I. p. 19.)

The epidemic fever of 1678, wherever it may have been bred or engendered, was prevalent in England at the same time as in Holland—in an exceedingly hot and dry autumn. The most constant symptoms, says Morley (and he writes both for Holland[1] in 1678 and for the country districts of England in the autumn of the following year), were nausea, severe vomiting, incredible tightness about the breast, weight in all the limbs, weariness, giddiness, vigils, thirst, restless tossing, and languor remaining after the disease was gone. Among the more remarkable symptoms were the following: Many had aphthae of the mouth, some twice or thrice, some being endangered by the severity and closeness of the patches of thrush. In some there

[1] Ralph Thoresby caught it at Rotterdam, suffered from it, in the tertian form, for several weeks of October and November, 1678, and brought it home with him to Leeds. He gives a good account of the illness in his *Diary* (2 vols. Lond. 1830).

occurred bleeding from the nose, or from piles, stranguary, etc. Round worms were observed, issuing both by the mouth and anus. In some few there were spots on the skin, but hardly ever petechiae or tumours near the ears. It affected all classes equally, all ages and both sexes. Some said it was easier to children than to adults, but others denied this. Some said it was more pernicious in the country than in the towns. In Leyden, the deaths never exceeded 150 in the week, being about twenty in a week above the ordinary level. More died from the coughs, anginas, peripneumonies and pleurisies that followed, than from the disease itself. Schacht says that the wind for nearly two years had been steadily from the North, or veering to the East or West. The Leyden faculty, and the Dutch generally, did not think the disease a malignant one; it was very freely called so, however, in England, the chorus being led by empirics and illiterate persons: "Ac indicio est," says Morley, "libellus perexiguus nostra lingua ab Empirico conscriptus de hoc morbo." This seems to refer to the tract by one Simpson, which I shall notice briefly[1].

Simpson styles himself a Doctor of Physic, and denies that he is an empiric. One sign of his affinity to that order, however, is that he objects to the orthodox treatment—emetics, drenches, a too cooling regimen, and purges, while he thinks blood-letting of doubtful utility. The symptoms were chills at the outset, pains in the head and back (in some with shaking), then intense burning heat, thirst, profuse immoderate sweats and great debility, a general lassitude, dulness, and stupor which in many were followed by delirium and a comatose state. Sometimes the fever simulated a quotidian, sometimes a tertian. He calls it "this new fever so grassant in city and country" and says that in many it assumed "the guise of a morbus cholera, known by the much vomitings or often retchings to vomit; and in others under the livery of the gripes with looseness, or, in some, looseness without gripes." This choleraic tendency concurring with other usual causes from the late season of fruit-eating etc., had swelled the bills of mortality. The morbus cholera and the gripes were to the new fever "like the circumjoviales that move in the same sphere with (but at some distance from) their master-planet."

The meaning of all this is obvious on turning to the London weekly bills of mortality. In the months of August and September for three years in succession, 1678–80, the deaths from "griping in the guts" and from "convulsions" rose greatly. These were, indeed, three successive seasons of fatal diarrhœa, mostly infantile, as I shall show in the chapter on that disease.

[1] *The History of this present Fever, with its two products, the Morbus Cholera and the Gripes.* By W. Simpson, Doctor in Physick. London, 1678.

The following extracts from the London weekly bills of mortality show how "fevers," as well as other diseases, contributed to the great rise in the autumns of 1678, 1679, and 1680.

Autumnal London Mortality in 1678.

1678

Week ending	Fever	Smallpox	Griping in Guts	All causes
Aug. 20	77	31	87	459
27	79	37	130	510
Sept. 3	82	37	121	530
10	103	27	164	621
17	82	23	178	580
24	83	20	152	528
Oct. 1	82	25	117	485
8	77	27	106	456

Summer and Autumnal London Mortality in 1679.

1679

Week ending	Fever	Smallpox	Griping in Guts	All causes
July 22	42	55	101	442
29	60	50	134	565
Aug. 5	78	63	143	531
12	62	43	161	579
19	55	64	149	545
26	68	53	112	514
Sept. 2	96	40	97	466
9	92	47	75	471
16	85	50	87	462

(For the Influenza weeks, see former Table.)

Autumnal London Mortality in 1680.

1680

Week ending	Fever	Smallpox	Griping in Guts	All causes
Aug. 10	70	17	108	427
17	90	6	132	494
24	98	17	127	552
31	140	18	228	816
Sept. 7	101	14	215	671
14	94	13	173	635
21	106	9	175	628
28	130	9	159	615
Oct. 5	125	16	138	597
12	121	10	94	530
19	109	14	68	488
26	93	5	58	407
Nov. 2	77	10	53	396

The last of the three autumnal seasons, 1680, is one of the few in the bills with high deaths from fever along with high

deaths from choleraic disease; and that excess of fever mortality may have been due in part to the ague epidemic, then in its third season.

The following extracts from Short's summation of parish registers show the great excess of burials over baptisms in various parts of England during the years of the aguish epidemic constitution.

Country Parishes.

Year	Registers examined	Sickly parishes	Baptisms in do.	Burials in do.
1678	136	17	312	527
1679	137	44	800	1203
1680	137	54	1093	1649
1681	137	41	679	1156
1682	140	30	632	975

Market Towns.

Year	Registers examined	Sickly parishes	Baptisms in do.	Burials in do.
1678	22	5	578	789
1679	23	7	877	1371
1680	24	7	946	1494
1681	24	9	945	1333
1682	25	9	795	1092
1683	25	8	1109	1398
1684	25	8	865	1243
1685	25	4	741	1191

The Influenza of 1688.

The seasons continued, according to Sydenham, to produce epidemic agues until 1685, when the constitution radically changed to one of pestilential fevers, affecting many in all ranks of society and reaching a height in 1686. Sydenham records nothing beyond that date, having shortly after fallen into ill health and ceased to write or even to practise. One would wish to have known what he made of the "new distemper" in the summer of 1688, for it was a sudden universal fever and yet not a catarrh or a "great cold." It is thus referred to in a letter of the month of June, from Belvoir, Rutlandshire[1]: "The man that dos the picturs in inemaled is gon up to London for a weke ...I wish the man dos not get this new distemper and die before he comes agane." On turning to the London weekly bills of

[1] *Cal. Belvoir MSS.* II. 120. June, 1688. Bridget Noel to the Countess of Rutland.

mortality we find in the first weeks of June the characteristic rise of one of those sudden epidemic fevers or new diseases, of which the earliest with recorded figures was the "gentle correction" of July, 1580. The following are the weekly London figures corresponding to the "new distemper" of 1688:

Weekly London Mortalities.

1688

Week ending	Fevers	All causes
May 29	58	368
June 5	76	518
12	101	559
19	65	435
26	66	437

The contemporary London notice of this "influenza" comes from Dr Walter Harris, who mentioned it in a book written the year after[1]:

"From the middle of the month of May in the year 1688, for some weeks, a slight sort of fever became epidemical. It affected the joints of the patients with slight pains, and they complained of a pain in their heads, especially in the fore-part, and of a sort of giddiness. It was more rife than any that I ever observed before, from any cause whatsoever, or in any time of the year. A great many whole families were taken at once with this fever, so that hardly one out of a great number escaped this general storm. Now this so epidemical or febrile insult seemed plainly to me to depend upon the variety of the season of the year, the most intense heat of some days being suddenly changed to cold...Never were so many people sick together: never did so few of them die. They recovered under almost any regimen,--almost everyone of them."

It will be seen, however, that the bills rose very considerably for four weeks, and that, too, in the healthiest season of the year.

A somewhat fuller account of its symptoms is given by Molyneux for Dublin[2]. He had been informed by a learned physician from London that it had been as general there as in Dublin, which we know to have been the case from Harris's account. Both Molyneux and Harris call it a slight fever, without mentioning catarrhal symptoms. The spring months immediately preceding had been remarkable for drought.

At Dublin this "short sort of fever" was first observed about the beginning of July, or some six weeks later than in London. "It so universally seized all sorts of men whatever, that I then made an estimate not above one in fifteen escaped. It began, as generally fevers do, with a chilness and

[1] Walter Harris, M.D., *De morbis acutis infantum.* Lond. 1689. English transl. by Cockburn, 1693, p. 88.

[2] "Historical Account of the late General Coughs and Colds, with some Observations on other Epidemical Distempers." *Phil. Trans.* XVIII. (1694), p. 109.

shivering all over, like that of an ague, but not so violent, which soon broke out into a dry burning heat, with great uneasiness that commonly confined them to their beds, where they passed the ensuing night very restless; they commonly complained likewise of giddiness, and a dull pain in their heads, chiefly about the eyes, with unsettled pains in their limbs, and about the small of their back, a soreness all over their flesh, a loss of appetite, with a nausea or aptness to vomit, an unusual ill taste in their mouths, yet little or no thirst. And though these symptoms were very violent for a time, yet they did not continue long: for after the second day of the distemper the patient, usually of himself, fell into a sweat (unless 'twas prevented by letting blood, which, however beneficial in other fevers, I found manifestly retarded the progress of this): and if the sweat was encouraged for five or six hours by laying on more cloaths, or taking some sudorifick medicine, most of the disorders before mentioned would entirely disappear or at least very much abate. The giddiness of their head and want of appetite would often continue some days afterwards, but with the use of the open fresh air they certainly in four or five days at farthest recovered these likewise and were perfectly well. So transient and favourable was this disease that it seldom required the help of a physician; and of a thousand that were seized with it, I believe scarce one dyed. By the middle of August following, it wholly disappeared, so that it had run its full course through all sorts of people in seven weeks time...This fever spread itself all over England; whether it extended farther I did not learn."

This short fever of men was preceded by a slight but universal horse-cold[1].

The Influenza of 1693.

Molyneux considered the strange transient fever of the summer of 1688 to have been the most universal fever that perhaps had ever appeared, and he thought the universal catarrh of five years' later date (1693) to have been "the most universal cold." We have thus a means of contrasting in the descriptions of the same author a universal slight fever and a universal catarrh, which happened within five years of each other, and were neither of them called at the time by the name of influenza, —a name not known in Britain until half a century later. Before coming to Molyneux's description, it should be said that the London bills of mortality bear no decided trace of an influenza in the end of the year 1693, the following being the highest weekly mortalities nearest to the date given for the epidemic at Dublin[2]:

[1] "'Twas very remarkable that in England as well as this kingdom a short time before the general fever, a slight disease, but very universal, seized the horses too: in them it showed itself by a great defluxion of rheum from their noses; and I was assured by a judicious man, an officer in the army of Ireland, which was then drawn out and encamped on the Curragh of Kildare, there were not ten horses in a regiment that had not this disease." Molyneux, u. s.
[2] Evelyn says nothing of a great epidemic cold in this season, but makes the following remarks on the weather: "Oct. 31. A very wet and uncomfortable season.

London Weekly Mortalities.

1693

Week ending	Fever	All causes
October 10	43	353
17	62	353
24	53	384
31	69	457
November 7	68	455
14	48	365

Molyneux's account of the flying epidemic of 1693 is as follows[1]:

"The coughs and colds that lately so universally prevailed gave us a most extraordinary instance how liable at certain times our bodies are, however differing in constitution, age and way of living, to be affected much in the same manner by a spreading evil...'Twas about the beginning of November last, 1693, after a constant course of moderately warm weather for the season, upon some snow falling in the mountains and country about the town [Dublin], that of a sudden it grew extremely cold, and soon after succeeded some few days of very hard frost, whereupon rheums of all kinds, such as violent coughs that chiefly affected in the night, great defluxion of thin rheum at the nose and eyes, immoderate discharge of the saliva by spitting, hoarseness in the voice, sore throats, with some trouble in swallowing, whesings, stuffings and soreness in the breast, a dull heaviness and stoppage in the head, with such like disorders, the usual effects of cold, seized great numbers of all sorts of people in Dublin.

"Some were more violently affected, so as to be confined awhile to their beds; those complained of feverish symptoms, as shiverings and chilness all over them, that made several returns, pains in many parts of their body, severe head-aches, chiefly about their foreheads, so as any noise was very troublesome: great weakness in their eyes, that the least light was offensive; a perfect decay of all appetite; foul turbid urine, with a brick-coloured sediment at the bottom; great uneasiness and tossing in their beds at night. Yet these disorders, though they very much frightened both the sick and their friends, usually without help of remedy would abate of themselves, and terminate in universal sweats, that constantly relieved...When the cold was moderate, it usually was over in eight or ten days; but with those in whom it rose to a greater height, it continued a fortnight, three weeks, and sometimes a month. One way or other it universally affected all kinds of men; those in the country as well as city; those that were much abroad in the open air, and those that stay'd much within doors, or even kept close in their chambers; those that were robust and hardy, as well as those that were weak and tender—men, women and children of all ranks and conditions...Not one in thirty, I may safely say, escaped it. In the space of four or five weeks it had its rise, growth, and decay; and though from first to last it seized such incredible numbers of all sorts of men, I cannot learn that any one truly dyed of it, unless such whose strength was before spent by some tedious fit of sickness, or laboured under some heavier disease complicated with it. .It spread itself all over England in the same manner it did here, particularly it seized them at London and Oxford as universally and with the same symptoms as it seized us in Dublin; but with this observable difference that

Nov. 12. The season continued very wet, as it had nearly all the summer, if one might call it summer, in which there was no fruit, but corn was very plentiful."

[1] Molyneux, *Phil. Trans.* XVIII. (1694), p. 105.

it appeared three or four weeks sooner in London, that is, about the beginning of October...Nor was its progress, as I am credibly informed, bounded by these Islands for it spread still further and reached the Continent, where it infested the northern parts of France (as about Paris) Flanders, Holland, and the rest of the United Provinces with more violence and no less frequency than it did in these countries."

Yet no other writer, English or foreign, appears to have mentioned it. Its existence rests on the authority of Molyneux alone, according to the above very circumstantial narrative.

The Influenza of 1712.

There were so many fevers from 1693 to the end of the century that it is not easy to distinguish epidemic agues or catarrhs among them. If we follow the continental writers, it is not until 1709 and 1712 that there is any concurrence of testimony for such widespread maladies. Evelyn, however, says that in the remarkably dry and fine months of February and March, 1705, "agues and smallpox prevail much in every place" (21st February). The very general coughs and catarrhs of 1709 seem to have been really caused by the severity of the memorable hard winter, the frost having begun in October, 1708 and lasted until March, 1709. The evidences of a truly epidemic infectious catarrh or influenza all over Europe in 1709 are scanty and ambiguous. It is probably to this "universal cold" that Molyneux refers under the year 1708[1]; but English writers have not otherwise mentioned an epidemic in 1709.

The next, in 1712, was a "new ague" of the kind without catarrhal symptoms, like that of 1688. One German writer called it the "Galanterie-Krankheit," another the "Mode-Krankheit," and it was about the same time that the French name "la grippe" came into use. These names all mean "the disease *a la mode*" or the reigning fashion[2]; they remind one of the earlier "trousse galante" and "coqueluche" (a kind of bonnet), and of the "grande gorre" of 1494. It appears to have made little or no impression on the mortality, and would hardly have been noticed but for its wide prevalence. In

---

[1] "An universal cold that appeared in 1708, and was immediately preceded by a very sudden transition from heat to cold in Dublin and its vicinity." Molyneux's *Memoirs*.

[2] *La Grippe* may, of course, be taken literally to mean seizure; but the common use of the word seems to have been figurative for some fancy that seized many at once and became the fashion.

England it was the subject of a brief essay by Dr John Turner under the title of "Febris Britannica Anni 1712[1]"—a certain epidemic fever, of the milder kind, fatal to none, but prevalent far and wide and leaving very few families untouched. It was marked by aching and heaviness of the head, burning or lancinating pains in the back, pains in the joints like those of rheumatism, loss of appetite, vomiting, pains of the stomach and intestines. The venom though not sharp, acted quickly. Turner ascribed it to malign vapours from the interior of the earth (*malignos terrae matris halitus*). Its season in England, as in Germany, was probably the summer or autumn. Turner begins his discourse with a reference to the plague in the East of Europe, which, he says, had been kept out of England by quarantine, to the murrain which was then raging in Italy (and appeared in England in 1714), and to fevers of a bad type which had traversed all France during the past spring, invading noble houses and even the royal palace. Having begun his discourse thus, he ends it by remarking that the slight British fever did not, in his opinion, forebode a plague to follow. It may have been a recurrence of this epidemic next year that Mead speaks of under the name of the "Dunkirk rant" (supposed to have been brought over from Dunkirk by returning troops after the Peace of Utrecht) in September, 1713; it was, he says, a mild fever, which began with pains in the head and went off easily in large sweats after a day's confinement[2]. The weekly bills of mortality in London are no help to us to fix the date of the one or more slight fevers or influenzas about 1712–13. The great fever-years of the period were 1710 and 1714; but the fever was typhus, probably mixed with relapsing fever, according to the evidence in another chapter. Even compared with the universal fever or influenza of 1688, that of 1712 must have been unimportant; for the former sent up the London mortality considerably, whereas there is no characteristic rise to be found in any month of 1712 or 1713.

---

[1] Joannes Turner, M.D., *De Febre Britannica Anni* 1712. Lond. 1713, pp. 3, 4.
[2] Mead, *Short Discourse concerning Pestilential Contagion.* Lond. 1720, p. 8. But Short, who wrote in 1749, places the "Dunkirk rant" under the year 1710: (*Air, Weather, &c.* I. 455).—"March 1, began and reigned two months an epidemic which missed few, and raged fatally like a plague in France and the Low Countries, and was brought by disbanded soldiers into England, namely a catarrhous fever called the Dunkirk rant or Dunkirk ague...It lasted eight, ten, or twelve days. Its symptoms were a severe, short, dry cough, quick pulse, great pain of the head and over the whole body, moderate thirst, and sweating. Diuretics were the cure."

Either to this period, or to the undoubted aguish years 1727–28, belongs a curious statement as to "burning agues, fevers never before heard of to be universal and mortal," in Scotland, the same having been a "sad stroke and great distress upon many families and persons." The authority is Patrick Walker, who traces these hitherto unheard of troubles to the Union of the Crowns (1707)[1].

On other and perhaps better authority, it does appear that Scotland before that period was reputed to be remarkably free from agues; and it is probable that the universal and mortal burning agues some time between 1707 and 1728, had come in one of those strange epidemic visitations, just as the agues of 1780–84 did. It would be erroneous to conclude from such references to ague that Scotland had ever been a malarious country. Robert Boyle refers in two places to the rarity of agues in Scotland in the time of Charles II.; the Duke of York, he says[2], on his return out of Scotland, 1680, mentioned that agues were very unfrequent in that country, "which yet that year were very rife over almost all England"—to wit, the epidemic of 1678–80. Again, agues, especially quartans, are rare in many parts of Scotland, "insomuch that a learned physician answered me that in divers years practice he met not with above three or four[3]." However, Sir Robert Sibbald, while he admits the rarity of quartans, does allege that quotidians, tertians and the anomalous forms occurred, that agues might be epidemic in the spring, with different symptoms from year to year, and that certain malignant fevers, not called agues, were wont to rage in the autumn[4].

Epidemic Agues and Influenzas, 1727–29.

The contemporary annalist of epidemics in England is Wintringham, of York, who enters remittents and intermittents almost every year from 1717 to the end of his first series of

[1] "The effects and evidences of God's displeasure appearing more and more against us since the incorporating union [1707], mingling ourselves with the people of these abominations, making ourselves liable to their judgments, of which we are deeply sharing; particularly in that sad stroke and great distress upon many families and persons, of the burning agues, fevers never heard of before in Scotland to be universal and mortal." *Life and Death of Alexander Peden.* 3rd ed. 1728. *Biog. Presb.* I. 140.
[2] Boyle's *Works.* Ed. 1772, v. 725.
[3] *Ibid.* v. 49.
[4] *Scotia Illustrata.* Edin. 1684. Lib. II. "De Morbis," p. 52.

annals in 1726; but none of his entries points very clearly to an epidemic of ague[1]. It is not until the very unwholesome years 1727–29 that we hear of intermittent fevers being prevalent everywhere, with one or more true influenzas or epidemic catarrhs interpolated among them. To show how unhealthy England was in general, I give a table compiled from Short's abstracts of the parish registers, showing the proportion of parishes, urban and rural, with excess of burials over christenings :

Country Parishes.

Year	Registers examined	Registers showing high death-rate	Births in ditto	Deaths in ditto
1727	180	55	1091	1368
1728	180	80	1536	2429
1729	178	62	1442	2015
1730	176	39	1022	1302

Market Towns.

Year	Registers examined	Registers showing high death-rate	Births in ditto	Deaths in ditto
1727	33	19	2441	3606
1728	34	23	2355	4972
1729	36	27	3494	6673
1730	36	16	2529	3445

It is clear from the accounts by Huxham, Wintringham, Hillary, and Warren, of Bury St Edmunds[2], that much of the excessive sickness in 1727–29 was aguish, although much of it, and probably the most fatal part of it, was the low putrid fever so often mentioned after the first quarter of the 18th century. At Norwich, where the burials for three years, 1727–29, were nearly double the registered baptisms, many were carried off, says Blomefield, "by fevers and agues, and the contagion was general." In Ireland also, a country rarely touched by true agues, Rutty enters intermittent fever as very frequent in May, 1728; and again, in the spring of 1729: "Intermittent fevers were epidemic in April; and some of the petechial kind. Nor was this altogether peculiar to us; for at that same time we were informed that intermittent and other fevers were frequent

---

[1] *Commentar. Nosolog.* Lond. 1727.
[2] *The Method and Manner of curing the late raging Fevers, and of the danger, uncertainty and unwholesomeness of the Jesuit's bark.* Dated 6 Dec. 1728: "You see that intermitting fevers, when they come to be chronical (and you may see it almost everywhere) make room for a great many distempers, and those very difficult to cure." p. 49.

in the neighbourhood of Gloucester and London; and very mortal in the country places, but less in the cities."

In the midst of this epidemic constitution of agues and other fevers there occurred one or more horse-colds, and one or more epidemic catarrhs of mankind. The most definitely marked or best recorded of these was the influenza of 1729.

The universal cold or catarrh of 1729 fell upon London in October and November, and upon York, Plymouth and Dublin about the same time. It prevailed in various parts of Europe until March, 1730, its incidence upon Italy being entirely after the New Year. The rise in the London deaths was characteristic: the level was high when the epidemic began, but the epidemic nearly doubled the already high mortality during the worst week and trebled the deaths from "fever."

London Weekly Mortalities.

1729

Week ending		Fever	All causes
October	21	88	564
	28	118	603
November	4	213	908
	11	267	993
	18	166	783
	25	124	635

The high mortalities of the weeks following may be taken as due to the sequelae of the epidemic (pneumonias, pleurisies, malignant fevers) and are indeed so explained in one contemporary account :

Week ending		Fever	All causes
December	2	92	678
	9	132	779
	16	116	707
	23	123	710
	30	109	628

The influenza of October and November, 1729, was the occasion of a London essay[1], which appears to treat solely of the epidemic catarrh and its after-effects, and not of the two years' previous sicknesses, which are the subject of another essay, by Strother, written before the influenza began. London, says

---

[1] *An Enquiry into the Causes of the Present Epidemical Diseases, viz. Fevers, Coughs, Asthmas, Rheumatisms, Defluxions, &c.* By the author of "The Family Companion for Health." London, 1729, pp. 6, 7.

this author, as well as Bath, and foreign parts, have been on a sudden seized universally with the disorders named in his title (fevers, coughs, asthmas, rheumatisms, defluxions etc.). These had come in the course of an unusually warm and wet, or relaxing, winter; "we have for some time past dwelt in fogs, our air has been hazy, our streets loaden with rain, and our bodies surrounded with water." So many different symptoms attend the "New Disease" that a volume, he says, would not suffice to describe them, but he thus summarizes them:

Sudden pain in the head, heaviness or drowsiness, and anon their noses began to run; they coughed or wheezed, and grew hoarse; they felt an oppression and load on their breasts, and turned vapourish, either because they apprehended ill consequences, or because their spirits were oppressed with a load of humours. The victims of the epidemic, he says again, were very subject to vapours; they are, upon the least fatigue or emotion of mind, dispirited, and flag upon every emergency. Among other symptoms were, quick pulse, thirst, loss of appetite and vertigo: the mouth and jaws hot, rough and dry, the thrush raising blisters thereon; the throat hoarse; a fierce brutal cough, which weakens by bringing on profuse sweats; the urine, muddy and white, "if they who are seized have been old asthmaticks."

He speaks of cases that had proved suddenly fatal and says that all who died of "epidemical catarrhs" had been found to have polypuses in their hearts. If reference be made to the Table, it will be seen that the high mortality continued in London for at least a month after the epidemic had passed through its ordinary course of rise, maximum and decline; and it is probably to that post-epidemic mortality that the author refers in the following passages:

"Numbers, as appears by our late bills, are taken with malignant fevers, or malignant pleurisies or with pleuritic fevers....Whosoever, then, would prevent a defluxion from turning into a fever, or from anything yet worse, if worse can be, must keep warm and observe a diluting regimen so long as till their water subsides and the symptoms are vanquished...I am convinced by experience that many poor creatures have perished under these late epidemical fevers, from the fatal mistake of never retiring from their usual employments till they have rivetted a fever upon them, and till they have neglected twelve or fourteen days of their precious time." This was fully endorsed by Huxham for the influenza of 1733: "Morbus raro lethalis, quem tamen, multi, vel ob ipsam frequentiam, temeri spernentes, seras dedére poenas stultitiae, asthmatici, hectici, tabidi."

Hillary's account for Ripon is very brief[1]:

"The season continuing very wet, and the wind generally in the southern points, about the middle of November [1729] an epidemical cough seized

[1] "Variations of the weather and Epid. Diseases, 1726-34 at Ripon." Appendix to *Essay on the Smallpox.* Lond. 1740, p. 35.

almost everybody, few escaping it, for it was universally felt over the kingdom; they had it in London and Newcastle two or three weeks before we had it about Ripon."

Wintringham, of York, says the epidemic in the early winter of 1729 was "a febricula with slight rigors, lassitude, almost incessant cough, pain in the head, hoarseness, difficulty in breathing, and attended with some deaths among feeble persons, from pleuritic and pulmonary affections[1]." There was a tradition at Exeter as late as 1775 that two thousand were seized in one night in the epidemic of 1729. Huxham, of Plymouth, says of the epidemic in November:

"A cartarrhal febricula, with incessant cough, slight dyspepsia, anorexia, languor, and rheumatic pains, is raging everywhere. When it is more vehement than usual, it passes into bastard pleurisy or peripneumony; but for the most part it is easily got rid of by letting blood and by emetics." In December, the coughs and catarrhal fever continued, while mania was more frequent than usual, and in January, 1730, the cartarrhal fever still infested some persons.

Rutty, of Dublin, merely says: "In November raged an universal epidemic catarrh, scarce sparing any one family. It visited London before us[2]."

These references to the unusual catarrhal febricula in November, 1729, are all that occur in the epidemiographic records kept by some four British writers who recorded the weather and prevalent diseases of those years. The epidemic catarrh made a slight impression upon them beside some other epidemics, and hardly a greater impression than another of the same kind, which seems to have occurred in the beginning of 1728. Thus, Rutty says, under November, 1727: "In Staffordshire and Shropshire their horses were suddenly seized with a cough and weakness. In December, it was in Dublin and remote parts of Ireland; some bled at the nose." On December 25th, he enters: "The horses growing better, a cough and sore throat seized mankind in Dublin[3]." Huxham, for Devonshire, under Oct.–Nov. 1727 confirms this: "a vehement cough in horses, which lasted to the end of December; the greater number at length recovered from it." He does not say in that context

---

[1] *Comment. Nosol.* p. 142.

[2] This epidemic appears to have made a much greater impression in Italy. The *Political State of Great Britain* for 1730, p. 172, under the date of 12th January, N.S. speaks of "the influenza, a strange and universal sickness and lingering distemper," as causing thirty deaths a day in the public hospital of Milan, as well as fatalities at Rome, Bologna, Ferrara and Leghorn, including the deaths of two cardinals.

[3] *Chronological History*, p. 10.

that an epidemic cough followed among men, as Rutty does say for Dublin; but in a subsequent note upon horse-colds, he says: "In 1728 and 1733 it [the precedence of the horse-cold] was most manifest; in which years a most severe cough seized almost all the horses, one or two months earlier than men." From which it would appear that the influenza of Nov.-Dec. 1729, was not the only one during the aguish years 1727–29.

In the weekly London bills the other series of mortalities that look most like those of an influenza are in the month of February, 1728 (748, 889, 850 and 927 in four successive weeks, being more than double the average).

The Influenza of 1733.

The next influenza was three years after that of 1729—in January, 1733. In London, it raised the weekly deaths for a couple of weeks to a far greater height than the preceding had done. Also the purely catarrhal symptoms of running from the eyes and nose are more prominent in the accounts for 1733 than for the influenza of 1729. The first notice of it comes from Edinburgh. The horses having been "attacked with running of the nose and coughs towards the end of October and beginning of November," the same symptoms began suddenly among men on the 17th December, 1732[1]. By the 25th the epidemic was general in Edinburgh, very few escaping, and it continued in that city until the middle of January, 1733. In a great many it began with a running of lymph at the eyes and nose, which continued for a day. Generally the patients were inclined to sweat, and some had profuse sweats. It was noted as remarkable that the prisoners in the gaol escaped; also the boys in Heriot's Hospital, as well as the inhabitants of houses near to that charity. The Edinburgh deaths rose as in the following table; the bulk of these extra burials are said to have been at the public charges, the epidemic having swept away a great number of poor, old, and consumptive people:

[1] *Edinburgh Medical Essays and Observations*, II. p. 22, Art. 2. "An Account of the Diseases that were most frequent last year in Edinburgh" (June, 1832 to May, 1833): There had been tertian agues throughout the month of June, 1732, and from August to October an epidemic in the suburbs and villages near Edinburgh, of a slow fever, having symptoms like the "comatose" fever of Sydenham, or the remittent of children.

Buried in November, 1732	89
„ „ December, 1732	109
„ „ January, 1733	214
„ „ February, 1733	135

Hillary[1] fixes the date of its beginning at Leeds on 3 February, one week later than at York, three weeks later than at Newcastle, or than in London and the south of England generally. At Leeds in three days' time about one-third part of the people were seized with chills, catarrh, violent cough, sneezing and coryza; the epidemic lasted five or six weeks in the town and country near. Dr John Arbuthnot, who was then living in Dover Street, is clear that the outbreak in London was later than in Edinburgh, which indeed appears also from the paragraph in the *Gentleman's Magazine*, dated Wednesday the 11th January, and from a comparison of the dates of highest mortalities in London (p. 349) and Edinburgh. It was in Saxony from the 15th November to the 29th of that month, and in Holland before it broke out in England. But it had begun in New England in the middle of October, and had broken out soon after in Barbados, Jamaica, Mexico and Peru. Its outbreak in Paris was at the beginning of February, 1733, and at Naples in March. The symptoms, says Arbuthnot, were uniform in every place—small rigors, pains in the back, a thin defluxion occasioning sneezing, a cough with expectoration. In France the fever ended after several days in miliary eruptions, in Holland often in imposthumations of the throat. In some, the cough outlasted the fever six weeks or two months. The horses were seized with the catarrh before mankind[2].

The account of the influenza of 1733 in London in the *Gentleman's Magazine* is under the date of 11 January: "About this time coughs and colds began to grow so rife that scarce a family escaped them, which carried off a good many, both old and young. The distemper discovered itself by a shivering in the limbs, a pain in the head, and a difficulty of breathing. The remedies prescribed were various, but especially bleeding, drinking cold water, small broths, and such thin liquids as dilute the blood[3]."

Huxham says that it was in Cornwall and the west of Devon in February, 1733, and that at Plymouth, on the 10th of that

---

[1] *Op. cit.* p. 47.
[2] John Arbuthnot, M.D., *Essay concerning the Effects of Air on Human Bodies.* London, 1733, p. 193. His remarks upon the "hysteric" maladies that were common after the wave of influenza in Jan.–Feb. 1733, are referred to in the chapter on Continued Fevers, along with the corresponding information from Hillary, of Ripon.
[3] *Gent. Magaz.* 1733, Jan. p. 43.

month, some were suddenly seized: "the day after they fell down in multitudes, and on the 18th or 20th of March, scarce anyone had escaped it."

It began with slight shivering, followed by transient erratic heats, head-ache, violent sneezing, flying pains in the back and chest, violent cough, a running of thin sharp mucus from the nose and mouth. A slight fever followed, with the pulse quick, but not hard or tense. The urine was thick and whitish, the sediment yellowish-white, seldom red. Several had racking pain in the head, many had singing in the ears and pain in the meatus auditorius, where sometimes an abscess formed: exulcerations and swelling of the fauces were likewise very common. The sick were in general much given to sweating, which, when it broke out of its own accord and was very plentiful, continuing without striking in again, did often in the space of two or three days carry off the fever. The disorder in other cases terminated with a discharge of bilious matter by stool, and sometimes by the breaking forth of fiery pimples. It was rarely fatal, and then mostly to infants and old worn out people. Generally it went off about the fourth day, leaving a troublesome cough often of long duration, "and such dejection of strength as one would hardly have suspected from the shortness of the time." The cough in all was very vehement, hardly to be subdued by anodynes: and it was so protracted in some as to throw them into consumption, which carried them off within a month or two[1].

Huxham is unusually full on the coughs and anginas of horses for several months before the influenza of men. In August, 1732, coughs were troubling some horses; in September, a coughing angina (called "the strangles") everywhere among horses which almost suffocates most of them; in October the disease of horses is raging at its worst; and in December it is still among them.

The Influenza of 1737.

After several years, unhealthy in other ways, the influenza came again in the autumn of 1737. In Devonshire, according to Huxham, the horses began to suffer from cough and angina, and some of them to die, as early as January, 1737, the epizootic being mentioned again in February, but not subsequently. The same observer says the influenza began at Plymouth in November and lasted to the end of December, 1737, seizing almost everyone, and proving much more severe than the epidemic catarrhal febricula of 1733[2]. In London it must have begun in the end of August, to judge by the characteristic rise in the weekly bills, and in the item of "fevers" more especially; and

[1] Huxham, *Obs. de aere et morbis epidemicis*, 1728–52, *Plymuthi factae.*
[2] *De Aere, &c.* pp. 3, 136–8.

although the deaths kept high for a longer period than in 1733, yet no single week of 1737 had much more than half the highest weekly mortality of the preceding influenza season.

London Weekly Mortalities.

1733				1737			
Week ending	Fevers	All causes		Week ending	Fevers	All causes	
January 16	69	531		August 30	117	611	
23	83	783		September 6	161	720	
30	243	1588		13	201	837	
February 6	170	1166		20	229	861	
13	110	628		27	167	770	
20	66	591		October 4	143	687	
				11	114	551	

In Dublin the worst week's mortality in 1737, in the month of October, was 144, whereas in the influenza of 1733 the highest weekly bill had been only 98[1]. Hardly any particulars of the influenza of 1737 remain, although it appears to have been widely diffused, being recorded for Barbados and New England. The only source of English information is Huxham of Plymouth, who mentions some symptoms which should serve to characterize this outbreak, namely : violent swelling of the face, the parotids and maxillary glands, followed by an immense discharge of an exceedingly acrid pituita from the mouth and nose; toothache and, in some, hemicrania ; "in multitudes," wandering rheumatic pains; in others violent sciatics; in some griping of the bowels. Huxham makes one interesting statement: "This catarrhal fever has prevailed more or less for several winters past;" or, in other words, the interval between the severe influenza of 1733 and the milder influenza of 1737 was not altogether clear of the disease. He adds that it put on various forms, according to the different constitutions of those it attacked.

The Influenza of 1743.

Six years after, in 1743, came another influenza, which presents some interesting points. A writer in the *Gentleman's Magazine* for May, 1743, says that the epidemic began in September last in Saxony, that it progressed to Milan, Genoa, and Venice, and to Florence and Rome, where it was called the Influenza ; in February last (1743) no fewer than 80,000 were

[1] Rutty, *Chronol. Hist. of Diseases in Dublin.* Lond. 1770.

sick of it [? in Rome] and 500 buried in one day. At Messina it was suspected to be the forerunner of a plague—which did, indeed, ensue. It is now (May) in Spain, depopulating whole villages. The outbreak in Italy is authenticated by many notices collected by Corradi, Brescia having had the epidemic in October, 1742, Milan and Venice in November, Bologna in December, Rome, Pisa, Leghorn, Florence and Genoa in January, 1743, Naples and the Sicilian towns in February. The English troops, in cantonments near Brussels, were little touched by it when it reached that capital about the end of February, but, strangely enough, "many who in the preceding autumn had been seized with intermittents then relapsed[1]."

In London the epidemic appears to have begun in the end of March, and had trebled the deaths in the week ending 12th April; by the beginning of May it was practically over.

London Weekly Mortalities.

1743

Week ending	Fevers	All causes
March 29	94	579
April 5	189	1013
12	300	1448
19	223	1026
26	115	629
May 3	82	537

The familiar view of the influenza in London is given in a letter by Horace Walpole from Arlington Street, 25 March, 1743[2]:

"We have had loads of sunshine all the winter: and within these ten days nothing but snows, north-east winds and *blue plagues*. The last ships have brought over all your epidemic distempers; not a family in London has scaped under five or six ill; many people have been forced to hire new labourers. Guernier, the apothecary, took two new apprentices, and yet could not drug all his patients. It is a cold and fever. I had one of the worst, and was blooded on Saturday and Sunday, but it is quite gone; my father was blooded last night; his is but slight. The physicians say there has been nothing like it since the year thirty-three, and then not so bad [the bill of mortality almost the same]; in short our army abroad would shudder to see what streams of blood have been let out! Nobody has died of it [as yet, but later some 1000 in a week above the usual bill] but old Mr Eyres of Chelsea, through obstinacy of not bleeding; and his ancient Grace of York; Wilcox of Rochester succeeds him, who is fit for nothing in the world but to die of this cold too."

[1] Pringle, *Diseases of the Army*, p. 16.
[2] *Letters of Horace Walpole*, ed. Cunningham, I. 235.

The account in the *Gentleman's Magazine* confirms the vast shedding of blood: "In the last two months it visited almost every family in the city; so that the surgeons and all the phlebotomists had full employment. Bleeding, sweating and blistering were the remedies usually prescribed. All over the island it cut off old people. At Greenwich upwards of twenty hospital men and boys were buried in a night[1]." In Edinburgh, as in London, the weekly burials were trebled. On Sunday, May 6th, fifty sick persons were prayed for in the Edinburgh churches, and in the preceding week there had been seventy burials in the Greyfriars, being three times the usual number[2]. It reached Dublin in May, proving milder and less fatal than in London (perhaps that is why the writer in the *Gentleman's Magazine* says it did not visit Ireland at all); it visited, also, the remote parts of Ulster and Munster, scarce sparing a family[3].

It had reached Plymouth in the end of April. Huxham, who is again the chief witness to its symptoms, says that it was much less severe there than in the south of Europe or even than in London.

Innumerable persons were seized at once with a wandering kind of shiver and heaviness in the head; presently also came on a pain therein, as well as in the joints and back; several, however, were troubled with a universal lassitude. Immediately there ensued a very great and acrid defluxion from the eyes, nostrils and fauces, and very often falling upon the lungs, which occasioned almost perpetual sneezings, and commonly a violent cough. The tongue looked as if rubbed with cream. The eyes were slightly inflamed; and, being violently painful in the bottom of the orbit, shunned the light. The greater part of the sick had easy, equal and kindly sweats the second or third day, which, with the large spitting, gave relief. Great loss of strength, however, remained. Frequently towards the end of this "feveret," several red angry pustules broke out: often, likewise, a sudden, nay a profuse, diarrhoea with violent griping. In many cases Huxham was astonished at the vast sediment (yellowish white), which the urine threw down, "than which there could not be a more favourable symptom[4]." One remarkable feature of the epidemic of 1743 was recalled by W. Watson in a letter to Huxham on the epidemic of 1762: "In the disorder of 1743 the skin was very frequently inflamed when the fever ran high; and it afterwards peeled off in most parts of the body[5]."

---

[1] *Gent. Magaz.* XIII. May 1743, p. 272.

[2] R. Chambers, *Domestic Annals of Scotland*, III. 610.

[3] Rutty, u. s. under the year 1743. In an earlier passage, he says that the influenza of 1743 raised the Dublin weekly bills to a highest point of 67, so that it must have been very slight in that city.

[4] Huxham, *Obs. de aere etc.*, 2nd ed. 3 vols. Lond. 1752–70, II. 99.

[5] W. Watson, *Phil. Trans.* LII. 646.

Some Localized Influenzas and Horse-colds.

For the space of nineteen years, from 1743 to 1762, there occurred no universal cold common to all the countries of Europe; the convergence of positive testimony, which is so remarkable on many occasions from the 16th century onwards, is found on no occasion during that interval. And yet the period is not wanting in instructive notices of epidemic catarrh, which I shall take from English writings only. British troops occupied Minorca during some of those years, and the epidemics of the island were carefully noted by Cleghorn. Under the year 1748 he writes:

"About the 20th April there appeared suddenly a catarrhal fever, which for three weeks raged so universally that almost everybody in the island was seized with it. This disease exactly resembled that which was so epidemical in the year 1733. For in most part of the sick the feverish symptoms went off with a plentiful sweat in two or three days; while the cough and expectoration continued sometime longer. In a few athletic persons, who were not blooded in time, it terminated in a fatal pleurisy or phrensy[1]."

Another English epidemiographist, Hillary, who had begun his records at Ripon, was in those years resident in Barbados; and in that island, as in Minorca, we hear of unmistakeable universal colds, although none of them at the same time as the one recorded by Cleghorn. The Barbados annalist records a general catarrhous fever in September, 1752[2], and a recurrence of the same in the end of December, lasting until February 1753 (catarrh and coryza, cough, hoarseness, a great defluxion of rheum, some having fever with it). As it ceased in February, 1753, a slow nervous fever began, and continued epidemic for eighteen months, until September, 1784, when it totally disappeared, and was not seen again so long as Hillary remained in the island (1758). In 1755 there was another epidemic catarrhal fever, first in February and again in the end of the year. In the earlier outbreak, few escaped having more or less of it, the symptoms being cold ague for a few hours, followed by a hot fever with great pain in the head, or pains in the back and all

---

[1] Cleghorn, *Observations on the Epidemical Diseases in Minorca*, 1744-49, p. 132.
[2] This influenza was observed in the North American Colonies. It is noteworthy that Huxham, of Plymouth, records under October, 1752, that hundreds of people at once had cough, sore throat, defluxions from the nose, eyes and mouth, attended with a slight fever, and more or less of a rash, several having a great flux of the belly.— *On Ulcerous Sore Throat*, 1757, p. 13.

over the body, which lasted two or three days, or longer, and then went off in some by a critical sweat. In the October outbreak it affected children mostly. Once more, in 1757, the same catarrhous fever returned, with almost the same circumstances[1]. That year there was a universal catarrh in North America.

Not less remarkable than the epidemic catarrhal fever in Minorca in 1748, or those in Barbados in 1752–3, 1755 and 1757, was the epidemic of 1758 in Scotland[2]. It was first noticed with east winds from the 16th to 20th September, several children having taken fever like a cold. In the last week of September thirty out of sixty boys at the Grammar School of Dalkeith were seized with it in two or three days. In October it became more general, among old and young, and increased till about the 24th, when it began to abate. In Edinburgh not one in six or seven escaped. It was in most parts of Scotland in October—Kirkaldy, St Andrews, Perthshire (where many died of it), Ayrshire, Glasgow, Aberdeenshire, Rossshire (end of October). A gentleman told Dr Whytt that in the Carse of Gowrie, in September, "before this disease was perceived, the horses were observed to be more than usually affected with a cold and a cough."

The symptoms in Scotland were of the Protean kind of "influenza": there might be fever with no cold; or a coryzal attack with little or no fever; or some had bleeding at the nose for several days, which might be profuse; or the soreness and pains in the bones might be in all parts of the body, or confined to the cheekbones, teeth and sides of the head. Others had a fever without any distinctive concomitant, but a cough when the fever subsided[3]. One of Whytt's patients, a lady aged thirty, had been feverish for four days, when a scarlet rash

---

[1] W. Hillary, M.D., *Obs. on...Epid. Diseases in Barbadoes.* Lond. 1760.

[2] It is not described for England, unless a reference by Bisset for Cleveland, Yorkshire, should apply to it. Short says, under the year 1758 (*Increase and Decrease of Mankind in England, &c.* 1767): A healthy year in general, "only in the harvest was a very sickly mortal time among the poor, of a putrid slow fever, which carried off many. An epidemic catarrh broke out in November, and made a sudden sweep over the whole kingdom." Barker, of Coleshill, says, in his *Putrid Constitution of 1777* (Birmingham, 1779, p. 49): "In the remarkable intermittents of 1758 or 9... the early and consequently injudicious use of the bark was attended with such fatal effects that a few doses only sometimes totally oppressed the head, brought on a most rapid delirium, and cut off persons in half-an-hour."

[3] Robert Whytt, M.D., "On the Epidemic Disorder of 1758 in Edinburgh and other parts of the South of Scotland." *Med. Obs. and Inq. by a Society of Physicians,* 6 vols. Lond. II. (1762), p. 187. With notices by Millar, of Kelso, and Alves, of Inverness.

appeared, but did not come fully out; the fall of the pulse and fever coincided with the beginning of a troublesome tickling cough, "so that the cough might be said to have been truly critical." Those who exposed themselves too soon frequently relapsed. Few died of the disease, except some old people. "In some parts of the country, when the disease was not taken care of in the beginning, as being attended with no alarming symptoms, it assumed the form of a slow fever, which sometimes proved mortal."

The year after the localised influenza of Scotland there was an epidemic of the same kind in Peru and Bolivia, that year, 1759, being one in which no universal fever or catarrh is reported from any other country. It extended from south to north, along the coast as well as over the high table-lands of Bolivia and the sierra region of Peru, invading, among others, the populous towns of Chuquisaca, Potosi, La Paz, Cuzco and Lima. In five or six days hardly one inhabitant of a place had escaped it, although some had it very slightly. As it was swift in its attack, so it was soon over, lasting about a month in each place. Its symptoms were great dizziness and heaviness of the head (vertigo and gravedo), feebleness of all the senses, deafness, strong pains over all the body, moderate fever, weariness, great prostration, complete loss of appetite, bleeding from the mouth and nostrils (this had been noted in Scotland the year before), and a long convalescence. Dogs shared the disorder, and might have been seen lying stretched out in the streets, unable to stand. It will be observed that the symptoms given do not include catarrh[1].

Before we come to the next general influenza in Britain, that of 1762, there are some facts to be mentioned as to agues and horse-colds in the interval since 1743. In Rutty's Dublin chronology, agues are entered as prevalent in 1745. In 1750, about the middle or end of December, the most epidemic and universally spreading disease among horses that anyone living remembered made its appearance in Dublin, and in Ulster and Munster almost as soon. It had been in England in November, and was like that which preceded the universal catarrhs of mankind in 1737 and 1743. In 1751, irregular agues were

[1] Archibald Smith, M.D., "Notices of the Epidemics of 1719–20 and 1759 in Peru," &c. from the Medical Gazette of Lima, on the authority of Don Antonio de Ulloa. *Trans. Epid. Soc.* II. pt. 1, p. 134.

frequent in March, as were also tumours of the face, jaws and throat. Agues also continued to be frequent in April, both in Dublin and in several parts of the country. In December, 1751, and January, 1752, there was another horse-cold, the same as a twelvemonth before. In 1754 the spring agues were frequent in Kilkenny and Carlow, though rare in Dublin. In 1757, "intermittent fevers, which had not appeared since April, 1746," came in the end of February. In 1760, a great catarrh among horses became general in Dublin in April. Coughs and tumours about the fauces and throat, with a slight fever, often occurred in March; and regular intermittents, tertians or quotidians, were more frequent than for some years past. These, according to Sims, of Tyrone, abated after 1762, so that he had not seen an intermittent since 1764 until the date of his writing, 1773.

The horse-cold of 1760 was observed in London in January. The *Annual Register* says under date 27 Jan.: "A distemper which rages amongst horses makes great havock in and about town. Near a hundred died in one week." In a letter a day later (28 Jan.) Horace Walpole writes: "All the horses in town are laid up with sore throats and colds, and are so hoarse you cannot hear them speak....I have had a nervous fever these six or seven weeks every night, and have taken bark enough to have made a rind for Daphne[1]." This same horse-cold is reported from the Cleveland district of Yorkshire: "In February, [1760] horses were invaded by the most epidemic cold or catarrh that has ever happened in the remembrance of the oldest men living[2]." The same authority for Cleveland says that intermittents were frequent and obstinate in the spring of 1760.

Among these miscellanies of the history may be mentioned an outbreak of "violent pleuritic fever or peripneumene" in the spring of 1747, which was fatal to a comparatively large number in the parish of George Ham, North Devon. Thirteen died of it from the 20th to the 31st March, four in April, four in May, and one in June, "most of them in four or five days after the first seizure." The same family names recur in the list[3].

[1] Horace Walpole's *Letters*, ed. Cunningham, III. 281.
[2] C. Bisset, *Essay on the Medical Constitution of Great Britain*, 1 *Jan.* 1758, *to Midsummer* 1760. Lond. 1762, p. 279.
[3] Extract from the parish register printed by Dr G. B. Longstaff in an appendix to his *Studies in Statistics*. Lond. 1891, p. 443.

23—2

The Influenza of 1762.

The universal slight fever or catarrhal fever of 1762 was, in London, much less mortal than those of 1733 and 1743.

London Weekly Mortalities.

1762

Week ending	Fevers	All causes
May 4	72	467
11	104	626
18	159	750
25	162	659
June 1	121	516
8	85	504

It began in London about the 4th of April, and by the 24th of that month "pervaded the whole city far and wide, scarcely sparing anyone." It was in Edinburgh by the beginning of May, and in Dublin about the same time, but did not reach some parts of Cumberland until the end of June. Short, who was then living at Rotherham, says that it "continued most of the summer[1]." It had the usual variety of symptoms in the individual cases, of which only a few need be again particularized. Where the fever was sharp, it usually remitted during the day, having its exacerbation in the night. Sometimes it proved periodical, and of the tertian type: "it usually returned every night with an aggravation of the feverish symptoms" (Rutty). Perspiration was a constant symptom; the tongue was as if covered with cream (Baker repeats this figure of Huxham's in 1743). "Depression of mind and failure of strength were in all cases much greater than was proportionate to the amount of disease. A great number of those affected were very slowly restored to health, languishing for months, and some even for a whole year with cough and feverishness—relics of the disease which it was difficult to shake off. Some, after struggling long with impaired health, fell victims to pulmonary consumption. In some there were pains in all the joints and in the head, with lassitude and vehement fever, but with little signs of catarrh." Rutty, of Dublin, says that in some a measly efflorescence or a red rash was seen, attended by violent itching[2]. Among

---

[1] *Increase and Decrease of Mankind in England &c.* London, 1767.
[2] Rutty, *op. cit.* p. 275. Compare Watson, *supra*, p. 351.

labourers in the country, the pestilence was so violent as to destroy many within four days, from complications of pneumonia, pleurisy and angina. Sometimes it took the form of a slow fever, "and approximated to that form of malady which the ancients denominated 'cardiac'[1]."

The mortality is said to have varied much. White, of Manchester, declared that fewer died there than in ordinary while the epidemic lasted. On the other hand Offley, of Norwich, said there were more victims there than by the epidemic of 1733 "or by the more severe visitation called influenza in 1743"—the two visitations which were incomparably the worst in the whole history, according to the London bills. Baker says that it infested cities and the larger towns crowded with inhabitants earlier than the surrounding villages, and is inclined to think that it was mostly brought by persons coming from London[2].

The progress of this epidemic over Europe had been peculiar. It was seen in the end of February, 1762, at Breslau, where the deaths rose from 30 or 40 in a week to 150. It was in Vienna at the end of March, and in North Germany about the same time as in England—April and May. There were at that time British troops in Bremen, among whom the epidemic appeared shortly after the 10th April[3].

"It looked at first as if they were going to have agues, but soon they were attacked with a cough and a difficulty of breathing and pain of the breast, with a headache, and pains all over the body, especially in the limbs. The first nights they commonly had profuse sweats. In several it had the appearance of a remitting fever for the two or three first days." The cough in many was convulsive. The epidemic seized most of the people in the town of Bremen: very few of the British escaped, but none of them died, except one or two, from a complication of drunkenness and pneumonia.

It is said to have been nowhere in France except in Strasburg and the rest of Alsace, in June. Baker says, "Whilst

[1] G. Baker, *De Catarrho et de Dysenteria Londinensi epidemicis,* 1762, Lond. 1764; W. Watson, "Some remarks upon the Catarrhal Disorder which was very frequent in London in May 1762, and upon the Dysentery which prevailed in the following autumn." *Phil. Trans.* LII. (1762), p. 646.

[2] Professor Alexander Monro, *primus,* of Edinburgh, describes his own attack in a letter to his son, Dr Donald Monro, 11 June, 1766 (*Works of Alex. Monro, M.D. with Life.* Edin. 1781, p. 306): "My case is this: in May, 1762, I had the epidemic influenza, which affected principally the parts in the pelvis; for I had a difficulty and sharp pain in making water and going to stool. My belly has never since been in a regular way, passing sometimes for several days nothing but bloody mucus, and that with considerable tenesmus" &c. Dysentery was epidemic in 1762 as well as influenza.

[3] Donald Monro, M.D., *Diseases of the British Military Hospitals in Germany, &c.* Lond. 1764, p. 137.

it raged everywhere else, it did not reach Paris or its vicinity, a fact which I learned from trustworthy persons." On board British ships of war in the Mediterranean it occurred in July. Its severity appears to have varied greatly in different cities of the same country. Rutty, for Ireland, agrees with Baker, for England, that it was more fatal in the country than in the towns.

The Influenza of 1767.

The next influenza, that of 1767, was so unimportant that its existence in England would hardly have been known but for Dr Heberden's paper, "The Epidemical Cold in June and July 1767[1]." Those few who were affected by a cold in London early in June observed that it differed from a common cold, and resembled the epidemical cold of the year 1762, on account of the great languor, feverishness, and loss of appetite. It became more common, was at its height in the last week of June or beginning of July, and before the end of July had entirely ceased. It was less epidemical and far less dangerous than the cold of 1762, so much so that the London bills of mortality hardly witness at all to its existence. The attack began with several chills; then came a troublesome and almost unceasing cough, very acute pains in the head, back, and abdomen under the left ribs, occasioning want of sleep. Many of the symptoms hung upon several for at least a week, and sometimes lasted a month. The fever might be great enough to bring on deliriousness, yet had plain remissions and intermissions. The same disorder was reported to be common about the same time in many other parts of England, and more fatal than it was in London. Heberden did not anticipate from it the lingering effects in the individual, for months or years, which marked so many of the cases in 1762[2].

[1] *Med. Trans. published by the College of Physicians in London*, I. 437. Heberden's paper was read at the College, Aug. 11, 1767.

[2] The nearest approach to Heberden's London influenza of 1767 is an epidemic that Sims observed in Tyrone in the autumn of 1767; a season remarkable for measles and acute rheumatism. At the same time that the acute rheumatism prevailed, a fever showed itself, like it; the patients for two or three days were languid, chilly, with pains in the bones, headache, stupor, dry tongue, costiveness. It was marked by remissions, was by no means mortal, and usually ended by a sweat from the 14th to the 17th day, followed by a copious deposit in the urine. James Sims, *Obs. on Epidemic Disorders*, Lond. 1773, p. 84.

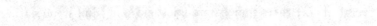

The Influenza of 1775.

Heberden invited physicians in the provinces to send in accounts of the epidemic of June and July, 1767, but no one seems to have responded. However, the next epidemic catarrh, of November and December, 1775, was made the subject of many communications from all parts of Britain, in response to a circular drawn up by Dr John Fothergill. This was a distinctly catarrhal epidemic, running of the nose and eyes, cough and (or) diarrhoea, being commonly noted.

At Northampton some had "a severe pain in one side of the face, affecting the teeth and ears, and returning periodically at certain hours in the evening, or about midnight, attended with vertigo, delirium and limpid urine during the exacerbation. Some whose cases were complicated with the above symptoms had a general rash, but without its proving critical...Many of those who escaped the catarrh have been more or less sensible of giddiness, or pains in the head or face," with limpid urine, etc., as if they had a full attack[1]. The epidemic began in London about the 20th October, and made a slight impression upon the bills of mortality in some weeks of November and December[2]. Grant says that it lasted nearly five months in London, having been attended by the same "comatose" fever which Sydenham associated with the epidemic catarrh of 1675. The fatalities in Grant's practice occurred late in the epidemic :

"On the 23rd December [1775] I had lost one patient, and soon after two others; all died comatous, owing, as I then imagined, to the remains of the comatose fever of Sydenham, which had raged all the autumn, was complicated with the catarrhous fever, and continued by the wet, warm uncommon weather for the season of the year; and I still [1782] am of opinion that this complication is the reason why the epidemic catarrh of 1775 proved much more fatal than it did in 1782—a fact known to all of us[3].'

---

[1] Anthony Fothergill, *Mem. Med. Soc.* III. 30. This paper is not included in John Fothergill's series. There is also a separate Dublin essay, *Advice to the People upon the Epidemic Catarrhal Fever of Oct. Nov. Dec.* 1775. By a Physician.

[2] I have not found the weekly bills for this year in London; but the following averages, taken from the four-weekly or five-weekly totals in the *Gentleman's Magazine*, will show how slight the rise was :

1775.	October	weekly average	323 births	345 deaths
	November	,,	,, 334	,, 447 ,,
	December	,,	,, 369	,, 449 ,,

[3] W. Grant, M.D., *Observations on the late Influenza as it appeared at London in* 1775 *and* 1782. Lond. 1782. Also, by the same, *A Short Account of the Present Epidemic Cough and Fever, in a letter &c.* First printed at Bath, and afterwards at London, 1776.

A Liverpool writer also says that the catarrh of 1782 "distinguished by the same title," was a much slighter complaint than the "influenza" of 1775. The latter, however, was a summer epidemic, and was naturally less complicated with pneumonia and bronchitis, whatever the "comatose" fever of 1775 may have been. Grant's statement that the influenza of 1775 lasted five months in London is borne out by the Foundling Hospital records: on 11 November, there were 16 in the Infirmary with "epidemic fever and cough," next week 22 with "fevers, coughs and colds," and so on week by week under the same names until the 9th of March, 1776[1]. At Dorchester it was general after 10th November; about the same time it was in Exeter, where within a week it seized all the inmates, but two children, in the Devon and Exeter Hospital, to the number of 173 persons. The middle of November is also the date of its decided outbreak at Birmingham, at Worcester, and at Chester, where Howard found the prisoners suffering from it. At York in the north, as at Blandford in the south, it is claimed to have begun earlier than in London. At Lancaster it was not seen until three weeks after the accounts of its prevalence in London began to come in, but only three days after it was first heard of in Liverpool. At Aberdeen it was fully a month later than in London. It did not visit Fraserburgh, though there was a putrid fever there very fatal at that time[2].

In many cases the disease assumed the type of an intermittent towards its decline, but bark was not useful (Fothergill, Ash, while Baker says that bark did good when the fever was spent). All the observers agree both as to its slight fatality and its universality. At Chester it attacked 73 out of 97 affluent persons, neighbours in the Abbey Square; at the Cross, inhabited by people in trade, 109 had the disease out of 144; in the House

---

[1] MS. Infirmary Book.

[2] The reports collected by Dr John Fothergill (*Med. Obs. and Inquir.* VI. 340) were by himself, and by Pringle, Baker, Heberden and Reynolds, of London; Cuming, of Dorchester; Glass, of Exeter (long account): Ash, of Birmingham; White, of York; Haygarth, of Chester; Pulteney, of Blandford; Thomson, of Worcester; Skene, of Aberdeen; and Campbell, of Lancaster. The papers of this collective inquiry, as well as the two collections in 1782, the collection of Simmonds in 1788, that of Beddoes in 1803 (in a digest) and the Report of the Provincial Medical Association in 1837, together with some other extracts from books or papers, were brought together in a volume, without much editing, by Dr Theophilus Thompson, under the title of *The Annals of Influenza in Great Britain from 1510 to 1837.* London, 1852. This has been reprinted and brought down to date by Dr Symes Thompson, 1891.

of Industry, not one escaped out of 175 ; it attacked people in the country rather later than in the town, and less generally, but it was in villages and even in solitary houses.

The unusual prevalence of catarrh among horses (and dogs) is asserted by John Fothergill ("during this time"), Cuming ("after the middle of August very generally in Yorkshire"), Glass (in September), Haygarth (in North Wales, about August and September), Pulteney ("before we heard of it among the human race"). The fullest statement is by Dr Anthony Fothergill, of Northampton:

"This distemper prevailed some time among horses before it attacked the human species. The cough harassed them severely and rendered them unfit for work, though few died. About the same time also it infested the canine species and with great fatality, especially hounds. An experienced huntsman informed me that it ran through whole packs in many parts of England and that several dogs died[1]."

The progress of influenza from other countries towards Britain was so much a matter of rumour or vague statement in the earlier periods that it has not seemed worth while to make a point of it under each epidemic. It happens, however, that there is good evidence of the line of progress of the epidemic of 1775. The afterwards celebrated Professor Gregory, of Edinburgh, encountered it in Italy in the autumn, and followed it all the way home to Scotland. He saw it successively in Genoa, in the south of France, in the north of France, in London, and last of all in Edinburgh, where he himself at length fell ill with it, several of his travelling companions having taken it in Italy two or three months before. In his lectures long after (as reported by Christison, who heard them about 1817) he traced the influenza of 1775 from south to north: "It appears to have broken out somewhere on the north and west coast of Africa, whence it spread not only north into Europe, but likewise eastward to Arabia, Egypt, Syria, Palestine, Asia Minor, Hindostan, China, and was ascertained to have spread over the whole immense empire of the Chinese. From China it returned westward by a northern route through the extensive dominions of Russia and from that country it was sent again over Europe in 1782[2]."

[1] *Mem. Med. Soc.* III. 34
[2] *Life of Sir Robert Christison*, 2 vols. Edin. 1885, vol. I. (Autobiography), p. 82.

The Influenza of 1782.

Seven years after, in the early summer of 1782, there came another swift and brief wave of catarrhal fevers over England, Scotland and Ireland, in the midst of a great "constitution" of epidemic agues which continued for several years. This was the occasion when the Italian name of "influenza" was formally adopted by the College of Physicians. Perhaps the first appearance of the name in English was in an account of the epidemic in Italy in 1729, given by a London periodical devoted to political news from foreign countries, and called, "The Political State of Great Britain[1]." In 1743 the news of the Italian epidemic under its native name reached London before the infection itself, the Italian name being frequently given to it while it lasted that season in England. When the next epidemic came, in 1762, it was not called the influenza as a matter of course, but was compared to the disease in 1743 "called the influenza." In the epidemic of 1775, "influenza" came more into use, and in 1782 it was the name usually given to the epidemic malady. The adoption of this name put an end at length to the ambiguity between epidemic agues and influenzas, leaving the curious correspondences between them in time and place, or the nosological affinities between them, as interesting as ever.

As late as the very fatal aguish years 1727–29, there was no clear separation of the epidemic agues from the influenzas, of which latter there were two or more, the one in the end of 1729 being easy to identify. In the great aguish constitution of 1678–81, Sydenham distinguished the epidemic coughs and catarrhs in Nov. 1679; but Morley made no such distinction, describing the whole series of agues for two seasons (and he might have done so for two seasons more) as the "new fever," "new ague," or "new delight," as in Derbyshire, without a suspicion that the universal coughs, catarrhs and fevers in November, 1679, were something nosologically distinct, which the future would identify as "influenza." In like manner Whitmore, in the great aguish period immediately preceding, that of 1658–59, had described the "new disease" as one single Proteus. In the still earlier epidemic seasons of 1557–58 and 1580–82, everything was "ague," although we now discover influenza mixed therewith.

---

[1] For the year 1730, under the date 12 January, p. 172.

I do not say that this inclusive naming was the better scien-
tifically; nor do I uphold Willis and Sydenham in their teaching
that the intermittent constitution passed into the catarrhal, in
1658 and 1679 respectively. But it is necessary to bear in mind
the matter of fact, namely, that those agues, amidst which the
"great colds" occurred, were epidemic agues, and not the
endemic fevers of malarious places; and I have now to show
that the "influenza" of 1782 was in like manner a brief episode
in the midst of several successive seasons of agues, which were
as much "new" or "strange" as any of those in the earlier
history. Whether the epidemic agues of 1780–85 were the last
of the kind in Britain had better be left an open question until
our most recent and most strange experiences in 1890–93 are
read in the light of history.

The influenza of 1782 was a very definite incident of a few
weeks—*teres atque rotundus*. It is easily discoverable in the
weekly bills of mortality in London to have fallen in the month
of June :

London Weekly Mortalities.

1782

Week ending	Fevers	All causes
May 21	45	336
28	49	390
June 4	57	385
11	121	560
18	110	473
25	89	434
July 2	49	296

The sudden rise and fall of the deaths and the height reached
are much the same as in other such epidemics in the summer—
the "gentle correction" of 1580, the "transient slight fever" of
1688, and the epidemic catarrh of 1762. On the other hand the
epidemics of autumn, winter or spring in 1729, 1733, 1737 and
1743 were far more severe, while the winter epidemics of 1675
and 1679 had figures almost the same as the summer epidemics.

The influenza of 1782 was not remarkable, whether in its
fatality or in its characters; but it received far more attention
than any that had preceded it. Two collective inquiries were
held upon it, one by a Society for promoting Medical
Knowledge[1], the other by a committee of the College of

[1] "An Account of the Epidemic Catarrh of the Year 1782; compiled at the request
of a Society for promoting Medical Knowledge." By Edward Gray, M.D., F.R.S.,
Medical Communications, I. (1784), p. 1.

Physicians of London[1], many physicians all over England, Scotland and Ireland contributing to one or other. There were also three or more separate essays[2].

The epidemic appeared in 1782 at Newcastle in the end of April, and raged there all May and part of June. In London it appeared between the 12th and 18th of May, in the Eastern Counties about the middle of May, in Surrey and at Portsmouth, Oxford and Edinburgh, also about the third week of May, but not in Musselburgh until the 9th or 10th of June. It was at Chester on the 26th of May, at Plymouth on the 30th, at Ipswich, Yarmouth, York, Liverpool and Glasgow in the first week of June. In Northumberland it was raging in July, and did not cease until the third week of August. In Scotland it was at a height in July, during the haymaking[3]. The most curious fact in its incidence comes from North Devon; it was prevalent in Barnstaple at the usual time, the month of June; but the neighbouring town of Torrington was not then affected by it, having previously gone through the epidemic, it is said, from a date as early as the 24th of March[4]. In all places it spread quickly, affecting from three-fourths to four-fifths of the adult inhabitants, but children not so much. At Christ's Hospital, London, only fourteen out of seven hundred boys had it. Wherever it attacked children, it did so mildly. It lasted under six weeks in each place that it came to. There were some strange attacks of it in London in September, "two months after the late epidemical catarrh had entirely disappeared from England." The king's ships 'Convert' and 'Lizard' arrived in the Thames from the West Indies in September. Their crews were perfectly healthy till they reached Gravesend, where they took on board three custom-house officers; and in a very few hours after that the influenza began to make its appearance. Hardly a man in either ship

---

[1] "An Account of the Epidemic Disease called the _Influenza_, of the Year 1782, collected from the observations of several physicians in London and in the Country; by a Committee of the Fellows of the Royal College of Physicians in London." _Medical Transactions published by the Coll. of Phys. in London_, III. (1785), p. 54. Read at the College, June 25, 1783.

[2] John Clark, M.D., _On the Influenza at Newcastle._ Dated 26 May, 1782; Arthur Broughton, _The Influenza or Epid. Catarrh in Bristol in 1782._ London, 1782; W. Falconer, _Account of the Influenza at Bath in May–June,_ 1782. Bath, 1782.

[3] Gregory, cited by Christison, _Life &c._ I. 84: "I have been told of the haymakers attempting to struggle with the sense of fatigue, but being obliged in a few minutes to lay down their scythes and stretch themselves on the field."

[4] Gray, u. s. p. 107.

escaped it ; and many both of the officers and common seamen had it in a severe degree[1].   Others who came to London from the West Indies in merchantmen in the end of September were attacked by influenza in their lodgings in the beginning of October[2].   To this epidemic belong also the strange experiences of the Channel Fleet in its two divisions under Howe and Kempenfelt ; but I postpone for the present the whole question of influenza at sea.

Gray thus sums up the great variety of symptoms as related by his numerous correspondents :

Chilliness and shivering, sometimes succeeded by a hot fit, the alternation continuing for some hours ; languor and lassitude, sneezing, discharge from the nose and eyes, pain in the head (particularly between or over the eyes), cough, sometimes dry, sometimes accompanied with expectoration, inflammation in one or both eyes, oppression and tightness about the praecordia, difficulty of breathing, pain in the breast or side, pain in the loins, neck, shoulders or limbs, sense of heat or soreness in the throat and trachea, hoarseness, bleeding from the nose, spitting of blood and loss of smell and taste, nausea, flatulence.   Also watery blisters about the upper parts of the body, and swellings in the face and other parts, attended with considerable soreness, apparently erysipelatous.   In some the catarrhal symptoms were very slight, or entirely wanting, the disorder in those cases being like a common fever.

The committee of the College of Physicians said that "the universal and almost pathognomonic symptom was a distressing pain and sense of constriction in the forehead, temples, and sometimes in the whole face, accompanied with a sense of soreness about the cheek-bones under the muscles," reminding one of the *fierro chuto* or "iron cap" of the South American epidemic in 1719.   Sometimes no catarrhous affection followed these strange head pains.   The languor of body and depression of spirits were thought to be more protracted than in 1762, but the fatalities at the time were fewer than in the earlier epidemic, and there were fewer consumptions following.   Sweating, also, was said by some to be less remarkable than in 1762 ; but Carmichael Smyth said : "The late influenza [1782] might very properly have been named the sweating sickness, as sweating was the natural and spontaneous solution of it[3]."   One distinctive

---

[1] *The London Medical Journal*, III. (1783), 318.
[2] College of Physicians' Report : "A family which came in the Leeward Islands fleet in the end of September, 1782, was attacked by it in the beginning of October. This family afterwards told the physician who attended them that several of their acquaintances, who came over in the same fleet with them, had been attacked at the same time and in the same manner as themselves."
[3] He had another experience not quite the rule : "Children and old people either escaped this influenza entirely, or were affected in a slight manner."

thing in the epidemic of 1762 was missed by most in 1782, namely, the peculiar constriction of the breast, with heat and soreness of the trachea, as if excoriated; but Hamilton describes that very thing for 1782 in Bedfordshire[1]. As in other epidemics of the kind, especially those which have been least catarrhal, there were hardly two cases quite the same.

The Epidemic Agues of 1780–85.

Let us now take up the strange history of epidemic agues for two or three years preceding and following the influenza of June, 1782. Sir George Baker begins his account of them thus[2]: "The predominance of certain diseases observable in some years, and the total or partial disappearance of the same in other years, constitute a subject worthy of our contemplation."

These agues were first noticed in London in the spring and autumn of 1780, but they infested various parts of England a little earlier. In the more inland counties the agues were "often attended with peculiarities extraordinary and alarming. For the cold fit was accompanied by spasm and stiffness of the whole body, the jaws being fixed, the eyes staring and the pulse very small and weak." When the hot fit came on the spasms abated, and ceased in the sweating stage; but sometimes the spasm was accompanied by delirium, both lasting to the very end of the paroxysm. Even in the intermissions a convulsive twitching of the extremities continued to such a degree that it was not possible to distinguish the motion of the artery at the wrist. "This fever had every kind of variety, and whether at its first accession it were a quotidian, a tertian or a quartan, it was very apt to change from one type to another. Sometimes it returned two days successively, and missed the third day; and sometimes it became continual. I am not informed that any died of this fever whilst it intermitted. It is, however, certain that many country people whose illness had at its beginning put on the appearance of intermission, becoming delirious, sank under it in four or five days."

Reynolds, another London physician, in a letter to Sir George Baker confirms all that the latter says of these singular epidemic agues: "No two cases resembled each other except in very few circumstances[3]"—the remark commonly made about the influenza itself. If these descriptions of the epidemic ague had not been given by physicians living as late as 1782, and altogether modern in their methods, we might have

---

[1] R. Hamilton, M.D., "Some Remarks on the Influenza in Spring, 1782," *Mem. Med. Soc.* II. 422. This author had some difficulty in deciding where the influenza ended and the epidemic ague began.

[2] *Trans. Col. Phys.* "On the late Intermittent Fevers," III. 141. Read at the College, 10 Jan., 1785.

[3] *Ibid.* p. 168.

supposed that they were confusing influenzas with agues, or using the latter term inexactly. "The ague with a hundred names" is the striking phrase of Abraham Holland, in his poem on the plague of 1625. Whitmore, describing the fatal epidemic ague (with an episode of influenza) in 1658–59, does not say that it had a hundred names, but that it assumed a hundred shapes, "which render it such a hocus-pocus to the amazed and perplexed people, they being held after most strange and diverse ways with it....So prodigious in its alterations that it seems to outvie even Proteus himself[1]."

As farther showing the anomalous character of these epidemic agues, or their difference from the endemic, Baker adds :—

"It is a remarkable fact, and well attested, that in many places, whilst the inhabitants of the high grounds were harassed by this fever, in its worst form, those of the subjacent valleys were not affected by it. The people of Boston and of the neighbouring villages in the midst of the Fens were in general healthy at a time when fever was epidemic in the more elevated situations of Lincolnshire." Women were nearly exempt, but few male labourers in the fields escaped it.

Baker heard from all parts that the same constitution continued through 1781 and 1782 ; and that since that time, though it seemingly abated, yet agues had been much more prevalent than usual, and had even been frequent in places where before that period they were uncommon. They were very noticeable in London from 1781 to 1785, not least so during the very severe cold of the winter and spring of 1783–84. We hear of great numbers attacked at Hampstead with common inter-mittents in February and the following months of 1781, during which time even the measles, in the greater number of cases, "ended in very troublesome intermittents[2]"—just as they were apt to end often in troublesome coughs.

The annals of Barker, of Coleshill, are full of references to agues, among other fevers, from 1780 onwards. Under 1781 he writes :—

"This spring that very peculiar, irregular, dangerous and obstinate disease, the burning, or as the people in Kent properly enough called it, the Plague-ague, made its appearance, became very epidemical in the eastern part of the kingdom, and raged in Leicestershire, the lower part of Northamptonshire, Bedfordshire, and in the fens throughout the year...This

---

[1] *Febris Anomala, or the New Disease.* Lond. 1659, p. 1.
[2] "Remarks on the Treatment of Intermittents, as they occurred at Hampstead in the Spring of 1781." By Thomas Hayes, Surgeon. *Lond. Med. Journ.* II. 267.

strongly pestilential disease had such an effect upon them that the complexion of their faces continued for a time as white as paper, and they went abroad more like walking corpses than living subjects."

As many as five persons in an evening were buried from it in some large towns in Northamptonshire; and about Boston it was so general and grievous that out of forty labourers hired for work in harvest, half of them, it was said, would be laid up in three days[1]. In 1783 the "pestilential agues" were as bad in Northamptonshire and eastern parts as the year before. A Liverpool writer says:

"In the autumn of 1782 the quartan ague was very prevalent on the opposite snore of the river in Cheshire: it was universal in the neighbourhood of Hoylake, where many died of it. Yet it was scarcely heard of in Liverpool, although from the uncommon wetness of the season it prevailed throughout the kingdom[2]."

On October 25, 1783, a correspondent of the *Gentleman's Magazine* offered an explanation of the "present epidemic disorder, which has so long ravaged this country, and that in the most healthy situations of it," namely, "the putrescent air caused by the number of enclosures, and the many inland cuts made for navigation[3]." Next year, 1784, appears to have been the principal season of epidemic agues on both sides of the Severn valley, one practitioner at Bridgenorth making them the subject of a special essay[4].

It was at this time that Fowler brought into use his solution of arsenic as a substitute for bark in agues, the latter having notably failed in the epidemics since 1780.

Baker says: "The distinguishing character of this fever was its obstinate resistance to the Peruvian bark; nor, indeed, was the prevalence of the disease more observable than the inefficacy of the remedy:" in that respect the epidemic agues had belied the experience with bark in ordinary agues. Again, it is

---

[1] *Epidemicks* (1777-95), pp. 58, 72, 75, &c. Barker's annals from 1779 to 1786 are full of references to agues, "bad burning fevers" and the like, but are on the whole too confused to be of much use for history. See the Boston bills under Small-pox.

[2] W. Moss, *Familiar Medical Survey of Liverpool.* Liverpool, 1784, p. 117. This writer's object is to show that Liverpool escaped most of the epidemic diseases that troubled other places, including typhus fever. As to the influenzas he says: "The influenza of 1775, so universal and very fatal in many parts, was less fatal here; and also that much slighter complaint, distinguished by the same title, which appeared in the spring of 1783."

[3] *Gent. Magaz.* LIII. pt. 2, p. 920. Letter dated from "Pontoon."

[4] William Coley, *Account of the late Epidemic Ague in the neighbourhood of Bridgenorth, Shropshire, in 1784...to which are added some observations on a Dysentery that prevailed at the same time.* Lond. 1785.

singular that bark had failed most, and arsenic been especially
useful in those parts of England where ordinary malarious
agues were never seen. One practitioner in Dorset laid in a
large stock of arsenic, wherewith he "hardly ever failed to stop
the fits soon [1]." Another, at Painswick, in Gloucestershire, used
it successfully in two hundred cases of epidemic agues from
1784 onwards. He gives the following account of these unusual
agues at Painswick:

"This town, which is situated on the side of a hill, and is remarkable for
the purity of its air, is very populous. In the year 1784 the epidemic ague,
that prevailed in many parts of the kingdom, made its appearance in this
place, and has continued till the present time [Nov. 1787], although
previously to that period the disease was hardly ever seen here, unless a
stranger came with it for the recovery of his health, on account of the
healthy situation of the place. I+ affected whole families, and appeared to be
most violent in spring and autumn. In the summer of 1786 it was followed
by a fever of the kind called typhus, or low nervous fever, which not
unfrequently degenerated into a putrid fever and proved very fatal[2]." In
May, 1785, at a general inoculation of smallpox, "many had been afflicted
with intermittents of several months' duration attended with anasarcous
swellings[3]."

It will be seen from the following table of cases treated at
the Newcastle Dispensary, under the direction of Dr John
Clark, during twelve years from 1 October, 1777, to 1 September,
1789, that influenza makes the smallest show among them,
being far surpassed by the intermittent fevers and dysenteries,
while all three together are greatly exceeded by the perennial
typhus fever:

	Cases treated
Putrid fever	1920
Intermitting fever	313
Epidemic dysentery in 1783 and 1785	329
Influenza of 1782	53

In Scotland, also, agues became epidemic about the year
1780. There is no reason to suppose that their prevalence in
these years was less exceptional there than in England and
Ireland. It will be seen, indeed, from the following table
compiled from the books of the Kelso Dispensary that the only
years of their considerable prevalence were the same as the
years of epidemic ague in England.

---

[1] Baker, u. s.
[2] "An Account of the Effects of Arsenic in Intermittents." By J. C. Jenner,
surgeon at Painswick, Gloucestershire. *Lond. Med. Journ.* IX. (1788), p. 47.
[3] *Ibid.* VII. (1786), p. 163.

C. II.

Kelso Dispensary[1].

Year	All cases	Cases of Ague	Year	All cases	Cases of Ague
1777	302	17	1792	570	16
1778	306	33	1793	666	19
1779	460	70	1794	447	9
1780	675	161	1795	513	23
1781	510	103	1796	355	12
1782	440	61	1797	318	9
1783	510	73	1798	415	7
1784	459	40	1799	558	2
1785	573	62	1800	665	4
1786	563	48	1801	433	9
1787	525	24	1802	377	5
1788	577	25	1803	308	2
1789	546	48	1804	422	5
1790	640	18	1805	469	0
1791	715	13	1806	318	1

It was doubtless the recollection of these epidemic agues that led the parish ministers who wrote in the 'Statistical Account of Scotland' from 1791 to 1799 to remark upon a supposed progressive decline of endemic ague, which they set down to drainage of the land[2]. It is probable, however, that each tradition of ague in Scotland dated from one of its epidemic periods; it has been shown, indeed, in the foregoing that Scotland in the end of the 17th century was reputed tolerably free from ague, and that the severe agues previous to 1728, which belonged to the epidemical kind, were thought to be something new.

The Influenza of 1788.

According to Barker, of Coleshill, who kept systematic notes of the epidemic maladies from year to year, there were several recurrences of the influenza of 1782[3]. But there is only one of

---

[1] Table compiled by Dr Mackenzie, and printed by Christison, *Trans. Soc. Sc. Assoc.* Edin. Meeting, 1863, p. 97. Christison pointed out very fairly the difficulties in the way of accepting the drainage-theory for the decline of ague (p. 98), but he had not realized the fact that the disease used to come in epidemics at long intervals.

[2] e.g. parish of Dron, Perthshire (IX. 468): "The return of spring and autumn never failed to bring along with them this fatal disease [ague], and frequently laid aside many of the labouring hands at a time when their work was of the greatest consequence and necessity." That had now ceased, owing to drainage. See also Cramond parish, I. 224, and Arngask, Perthshire, I. 415.

[3] The following extracts are from Barker's book, *Epidemicks*, Birmingham [1795]:
1782. Influenza in the latter end of spring. Nine out of ten in Lichfield and other towns had violent defluxions of the nose, throat and lungs, bringing on violent sneezings, soreness of the throat, coughs, &c. attended with a pestilential fever, of which many were relieved by perspiration...Some had swelled faces, and violent pains

these seasons, the summer of 1788, that other English writers have singled out as a time of influenza. It was undoubtedly of a very mild type, producing hardly any effect upon the bills of mortality; but it attracted the notice of several. Dr Simmons, the editor of the *London Medical Journal,* became the recorder of it, collecting reports from various parts, as others had done in 1782. He himself treated 160 cases at the Westminster General Dispensary, and 65 more elsewhere. It was most prevalent in London from the second to the fourth week of July, but the mortalities for those weeks show no abrupt rise. It was at Chatham, Dover, Plymouth and Bath about the same time, at Manchester in the beginning of August, in Cornwall in the middle of August, and at Montrose about the end of August, or perhaps most certainly in October. On 5 August, a physician at York wrote: "We have not had the slightest appearance of a catarrh in our city or neighbourhood during the year." The epidemic was undoubtedly a partial one in Britain, and so slight as to have made little impression where it did occur. It is said to have been very general at Warsaw in April or May, at Vienna in April (20,000 cases before the 20th), at Munich in June, at Paris in the end of August and still continuing on the 24th October, at Geneva on the 10th October. Its most constant symptom in England was pain in the fore-part of the head, with vertigo; next most constant was a pain at the pit of the stomach and along the breast-bone; cough was wanting in perhaps a third of the cases and was always slight, diarrhoea was somewhat general, running from the eyes exceptional, sore-throat in perhaps one-sixth of the cases[1]. At Plymouth where it was seen earliest and clearest among the

in the teeth...Some, giddiness and violent headaches, accompanied with a slow fever, and even loss of memory...By its running through whole families it appeared also to be communicable by infection.

1783. The influenza also began to appear again; and those who had coughs last year began now to be afflicted with them again, the disorder at length frequently ending in a consumption. Also dogs in this year and the next had running at the eyes and a loss of the use of their hind legs, which in the end killed most of those that were seized with it. Horses also suffered.

1786. In the middle of this season the influenza returned, and colds and coughs were epidemical.

1788 [spring]. A species of influenza of the pestilential kind, akin to that of 1782, has almost constantly returned in spring and autumn since that time...[summer] A species of influenza, as in the spring, and it is also at Edinburgh,

1789 [spring]. Influenza returned. Even dogs affected.

1791. Influenza very bad, especially in London.

[1] Samuel Foart Simmons, M.D., F.R.S., "Of the Epidemic Catarrh of the year 1788." *Lond. Med. Journ.* IX. (1788), p. 335.

regiment of artillery and in the guardships, the symptoms were pain in the head and limbs, soreness of the throat, pain in the breast, a feeling of coldness all over the skin, and these followed by cough, a great discharge from the nose and eyes, and slight nausea. It was much less noticeable among the townspeople than among the troops and sailors[1]. It occurred chiefly among soldiers or sailors also at Dover and Chatham. At Bath it was marked by chills, headache, swelling of the throat, difficult swallowing, quick pulse, hot, dry skin (but not pungent as in malignant fever), ending in a sweat; no delirium, but broken sleep or vigil; the eyes scarcely affected, cough in some, but not vehement; in some, sublingual swellings which suppurated[2]. At Manchester it looked as if it had been brought in by travellers who had acquired it in London[3].

At Portsmouth a singular thing happened two or three months after the epidemic had passed. The frigate 'Rose' arrived on 4 November from Newfoundland; within a short time all the dogs on board were seized with cough and catarrh, and soon after the whole ship's company were affected in the same way[4]. Simmons says of the epidemic of 1788 in general: "During the progress of the influenza, a complaint which was evidently an inflammatory affection of the mucous membrane of the fauces, etc. was frequently observed among horses and other cattle, and was generally as violent among them as it was mild among their rational neighbours"—many dying after four or six days.

The very slight and partial influenza of July and August, 1788, happened at a time when there was much fever of a more serious kind in the country. The history of the latter belongs to another chapter; but there was in Cornwall, in the same season as the influenza, an epidemic fever which might in former times have been described as a part, and the most fatal part, of the "new disease," and may be taken in this context

---

[1] Vaughan May, surgeon to H. M. Ordnance, "Observations on the Influenza as it appeared at Plymouth, in the summer and autumn of the year 1788." Duncan's *Med. Commentaries*, Decade 2, vol. iv. p. 363.

[2] Falconer, "Influenzae Descriptio, uti nuper comparebat in urbe Bathoniae, mensibus Julio, Augusto et Septembri A.D. 1788." *Mem. Med. Soc.* III. 25.

[3] George Bew, M.D., physician at Manchester, "Of the Epidemic Catarrh of the year 1788." *Lond. Med. Journ.* IX. (1788), p. 354. "The influenza has been *very* prevalent," writes Withering, of Birmingham, to Lettsom, 19 Aug. 1788. *Mem. of Lettsom*, III. 133.

[4] Related to Dr Simmons (l. c. p. 346), by Mr Boys, surgeon, of Sandwich, who was told it by his son, a lieutenant on board the 'Rose.'

rather than in the chapter on typhus. The same physician, Dr William May, of Truro, gave an account of the influenza first[1] and of the other fever afterwards[2].

The latter began at Truro in the end of April, 1788, and was also at St Ives and other small towns in various parts of the county. A malignant fever had for near two years before been exceedingly rife among the poor (owing to distress from loss of pilchard fishing), and had carried off a great number of them; but this was something new. Yet it was "truly a fever of the typhus type," one of its symptoms being constant wakefulness. It passed through whole families, affecting all ages and constitutions. It ended on the 17th day, whereas the influenza (says May in his other paper) ended with a sweat on the fourth or fifth day. In one small neighbourhood this epidemic fever affected chiefly the aged, who were blooded owing to dyspnoea: out of ten or eleven so affected, not one recovered, an experience that reminded May of what Willis said of the village elders being swept off by the "new fever" of 1658. Surgeons at St Austel, East Looe and Falmouth are cited as having seen much of the same fever. In like manner the Manchester chronicler of the influenza of 1788 says: "Fevers of different kinds, but chiefly of the type now distinguished by the appellation of typhus, were exceedingly prevalent after the epidemic catarrh had in great measure ceased to be general; but from which, by tracing the symptoms, the fever might usually be found to have originated[3]."

For a good many years after the period last dealt with, nothing is heard in Britain either of epidemic agues or of influenza[4]. Writing in 1800, Willan said that intermittents had not, to his knowledge, been epidemic in London at any time within twenty years. He explains this by "the practice of draining, and the improved modes of cultivating land in Essex, Kent, and some other adjoining counties, from which either agues were formerly imported, or the effluvia causing them were conveyed by particular winds"—the latter being the doctrine of Lancisi for the country round Rome. But he forgets that their appearance nearly twenty years before was a strange phenomenon to the practitioners of that generation, and that Sydenham, whom he cites to prove agues in London in former times, had also remarked their absence, except in occasional cases, for as long a period as thirteen years. Of such occasional agues

---

[1] In a note to Simmons' paper, u. s., p. 342.

[2] "An Account of an Epidemic Fever that prevailed in Cornwall in the year 1788." *Lond. Med. Journal.* x. p. 117 (dated Truro, Jan. 26, 1789).

[3] Bew, u. s., p. 365. Carmichael Smyth has a similar remark on the influenza of 1782: "This epidemic distemper very soon declined. But it seemed to leave behind it an epidemical constitution which prevailed during the rest of the summer; and the fevers, even in the end of August and beginning of September, assumed a type resembling, in many respects, the fever accompanying the influenza."

[4] A solitary reference occurs to an influenza in 1792, which I have not succeeded in verifying:—B. Hutchinson, "An Account of the Epidemic Disease commonly called the Influenza, which appeared in Nottinghamshire and most other parts of the kingdom in the months of November and December, 1792." *New. Lond. Med. Journ.*, Lond. 1793, II. 174. Cited in the Washington Medical Catalogue.

acquired in London, Willan and Bateman had each one or two examples in the autumn of 1794, and the spring of 1805.

As in the case of epidemic agues, so also in the case of influenzas, there was immunity in Britain for a good many years after 1788; and, as the slight epidemic catarrh of 1788 was something less than universal, the clear interval may almost be reckoned from the summer of 1782, a space of over twenty years. Willan's monthly reports of the weather and diseases in London from March, 1796, to December, 1800, twice mention epidemic catarrhs,—in February and March, 1797, and in February, 1800, the latter chiefly among children. But to neither of them will he concede the name of "influenza," as the complaint was merely epidemical from a particular state of the atmosphere, and not propagated by contagion, nor quite general.

The symptoms, however, were headache, sometimes attended with vertigo, a thin acrid discharge from the nostrils, slight inflammation of the throat, a sense of constriction in the chest, with a frequent dry cough, pains in the limbs, a white tongue, a quick and small pulse, with a sensation of languor and general debility. These symptoms, fairly complete for influenza of the correct type, lasted about eight days and ended in a gentle sweat or in a diarrhœa. Coughs had been remarkably severe and obstinate; they were frequently attended with painful stitches and spitting of blood[1].

The Influenza of 1803.

The number of the *Medical and Physical Journal* for March, 1803, announced that "a cold attended by symptoms of a very alarming nature has been general in the city of Paris for some time"; but it said nothing of the alarming disorder being in London. It is in the next number, under the date of Soho Square, March 11th, that a correspondent identifies the Paris epidemic with "the complaint now general in this metropolis, and called by some the Influenza." In a report upon the diseases " in an Eastern District of London from February 20 to March 20, 1803," the "catarrhal fever" is thus described :

"This disease has been so general as to claim the title of the reigning epidemic, and is very similar to one which prevailed a few years ago, and was denominated Influenza. It has generally been introduced by chilliness and shivering, which have been succeeded by violent pains in the head, with some discharge from the eyes and nostrils, as in a common catarrh, together with hoarseness and cough. The pains in the head have in some cases been the first symptoms and have been succeeded by giddiness, sickness and vomiting" &c. There were also rheumatic pains in the limbs, intercostals &c.

[1] Robert Willan, M.D., *Reports on the Diseases in London, particularly during the years* 1796, '97, '98, '99 *and* 1800. London, 1801, pp. 76, 253.

Meanwhile the information from various sources showed that the old influenza was once more really in this country. Two collective inquiries were made on the influenza of 1803: one by Dr Beddoes of Bristol, who issued a circular of five queries, and received answers to them (with other information) from one hundred and twenty-four correspondents[1]; the other by the Medical Society of London[2]. The *Medical and Physical Journal* and Duncan's *Annals* each received a few independent papers on it; and several pamphlets were issued, mostly devoted to treatment—two in London[3], one at Edinburgh[4], one at Bath[5], and one at Bristol[6].

In these abundant data there is little novelty and not much variety.

The attack began with chills and severe pain in the head, along with slight running of the eyes and nose, as typhus fever might have begun. After the slightly catarrhal onset the malady was mostly a fever, with dry cough, dry and hot skin, pain in the forehead and about the eyeballs, pains in the limbs, "spontaneous" weariness and extreme prostration—a group of symptoms which led Hooper to find a rheumatic character in the malady. Among other symptoms were vertigo, nausea, vomiting and diarrhoea. Much sweating is not reported; but there was often a gentle sweat in recovering after about a week, less or more. There was the usual range from mildness to severity. Pneumonia and pleurisy were not rare, and were commonly the cause of fatalities.

The deaths were for the most part among the phthisical, the asthmatic and the aged; but these were not many, certainly not so many as in 1729, 1733 and 1743, and probably in about the same proportion as in 1762, 1775 and 1782. In the London bills the weekly deaths rose in March, to an average of 537 from an average of 429 in February, and of 375 in January, falling to an average of 417 in April. In Ireland the epidemic is said to have been seen among the troops in garrisons as early as December, 1802; it became universal in spring and summer. In Edinburgh the rise in the burials at Greyfriars churchyard was in the weeks ending 5th and 12th April, making them about a half more than usual for the brief period. When the wave of influenza was

---

[1] Published in the *Med. and Phys. Journal* from August to December, 1803.
[2] *Memoirs of the Medical Society*, vol. VI.
[3] R. Hooper, M.D., *Obs. on the Epidemic Disease now prevalent in London.* London, 1803. R. Pearson, M.D., *Obs. on the Epid. Catarrhal Fever or Influenza of* 1803. Lond. 1803.
[4] J. Herdman, *The prevailing Epid. Disease termed Influenza.* Edin. 1803.
[5] W. Falconer, M.D., *The Epidemic Catarrhal Fever commonly called tne Influenza, as it appeared at Bath &c.* Bath, 1803.
[6] John Nott, M.D., *Influenza as it prevailed in Bristol in Feb.-April,* 1803. Bristol, 1803.

past, the public health in nearly all places became unusually good, as had happened immediately after the influenza of 1782.

The question most to the front in the influenza of 1803 was its manner of spreading. Beddoes, who believed in personal contagion, had this in view in his five queries:

1. When did the influenza appear and disappear with you?
2. Was its date different in remote places within your reach?
3. After being general, did it occur for some time in single instances?
4. Did it ever seem to pass from person to person?
5. If so, is it likely that clothes or fomites conveyed it in any case?

The dates of commencement were earlier or later according to no rule of direction or of distance from London. In some large towns of Yorkshire it appeared to be unusually late, in Chester unusually early; Edinburgh, certainly, was as long behind London as London was behind Paris. Haygarth, who took the most narrow view of contagion, made out the incidence thus: London first, then the towns which have the greatest intercourse with London, such as Bath and Chester, then smaller towns, and last of all the villages around each of the more populous centres. Several towns had the brunt of the epidemic in the same weeks (of March) as London; in very few was it later than the first weeks of April. In some towns it attracted little notice. In North Devon, it was said to have been at Hartland and Clovelly a fortnight before it was seen in Bideford; the first of it seen by one of the doctors of that town was in a solitary potter's house four miles to the eastward, on a peninsula made by the confluence of a small stream with the Torridge, all the inmates of the house being attacked; in the town itself from first to last he saw but few cases, whereas there were many in the adjacent country[1].

The general rule seems to have been that the more sparse populations had it later, the nearer they were to the extremities of the kingdom, as in Cornwall, the north of Scotland, and in Ireland. Opinion was divided as to the part played by persons in carrying contagion from place to place, some holding that the facts of diffusion could be explained on no other hypothesis, while most held that the influenza was in the air. Beddoes got as many answers favouring the doctrine of personal contagion as made a respectable show for it; but when these had all been set forth to the best advantage, a practitioner wrote to say that, after all, nine-tenths of professional opinion was against the con-

[1] *Med. and Phys. Journ.* x. 104.

tagiousness of influenza.   The practical question for Haygarth, Beddoes, and other contagionists was whether influenza was not a disease, like smallpox or scarlet fever, which could be kept from spreading by means of isolation, disinfection (with the fumes of mineral acids) and other precautions.

Some curious facts came out, showing the effect of influenza upon other epidemic diseases, or the effect of other epidemic diseases upon influenza.   One writer applied to influenza what used to be said of the plague or pestilential fever, that these Leviathan constitutions swallowed up all other reigning epidemics. Holywell, a town in Flintshire, with a large cotton-weaving industry, had not been free from a bad kind of typhus for two years.   "On the appearance of the influenza the typhus entirely ceased, and only one case of fever has occurred since.   I have not for many years known this country so healthy as since the influenza disappeared[1]."   The influenza was said also to have superseded typhus fever at Navan, in Meath[2].   At St Neots typhus was peculiarly prevalent for three months before the influenza, but ceased thereafter[3].   Another relation to typhus was seen at Clifton : "In the low, confined, and ill-ventilated houses in the Hot Well road, where typhus often abounds, the influenza was very unfrequent ; while in the exposed high-lying buildings on Clifton Hill it was almost universal[4]."   As to ague, which had often before stood in a remarkable relation to epidemics of catarrhal fever, there is one possibly relevant fact related from the Lincolnshire fens.   A Wisbech physician writes :

"The influenza which ceased here about the middle of April made its appearance again in May; the leading symptoms were the same as in the first attack.   About the same time also a most malignant fever, having some symptoms in common with the influenza, began to rage in that part of Lincolnshire contiguous to us, which has proved fatal to hundreds[5]."

From 1803 to 1831, nothing is heard in England of a universal influenza, although there was one such in the end of 1805 and beginning of 1806 in Russia, Germany, France and

---

[1] Dr Currie of Chester, *Med. and Phys. Journ.* X. 213.

[2] *Ib.* X. 527, quoted by Beddoes from memory, the letter from Navan having been lost.

[3] Alvey, *Mem. Med. Soc.* VI. 462.

[4] Dr Carrick, of Bristol, in Duncan's *Annals of Med.* III.   Compare the report for Fraserburgh in 1775, supra, p. 360.

[5] Frazer, *Med. and Phys. Journ.* X. 206, dated 12 June, 1803.

Italy; and there were four great influenzas in the Western Hemisphere (1807, 1815–16, 1824–25, and 1826). Catarrhs were perhaps commoner than usual in England and Scotland in the winter of 1807–8, but they cannot be reckoned an epidemic of influenza[1]. The summer following (1808) was unusually hot and agues became more epidemic in the fens than at any time since the great aguish period of 1780 and following years[2]. Agues were again unusually rife in England in 1826, 1827 and 1828, at the same time as the remarkable epidemics of them, from inundations and subsequent drought, in Holland and along the German coast of the North Sea. Dr John Elliotson, of London, met with cases of agues in his practice in those years in the following scale:

Year	Cases		Year	Cases
1823	8		1827	53
1824	14		1828	27
1825	15		1829	8
1826	44			

They had increased, he says, throughout the country as well as in London, owing, as he thought, in agreement with Macmichael, to the higher mean temperature of the respective years; and he would apply the same law of increase to the epidemic periods of ague in Britain in former times[3]. Christison saw his first case of ague at Edinburgh in the autumn of 1827, in a labourer who had caught it working at the harvest in the fen-country of Lincolnshire.

---

[1] Hirsch cites authorities for influenza in Edinburgh, London, Nottingham and Newcastle in the winter of 1807–8. In Roberton's monthly reports from Edinburgh (*Med. and Phys. Journ.* XXI.), and Bateman's quarterly reports from London, I find only common colds recorded. Clarke for Nottingham (*Ed. Med. Surg. Journ.* IV. 429) says catarrh was so general "as to have acquired the name of influenza; but there was no reason to suppose it contagious."

[2] W. Royston, "On a Medical Topography," *Med. and Phys. J.* XXI. 1809, (Dec. 1808), p. 92: "After the unusual heat of the last summer, the frequency of intermittents in the autumn was increased in the fens of Cambridgeshire to an almost unprecedented degree; and even quadrupeds were not exempt, for distinctly marked cases of *tertian* were observed in horses. In the year 1780 a similar prevalence of this disease occurred in the same part; and though in an interval of 28 years many and frequent sporadic cases have arisen, yet its universality during that period was suspended. We have to regret that a correct record of the constitution of the year 1780, as applying to this particular district, has not been preserved in such a manner as to admit of a direct comparison with that of 1808. If it were possible, from authentic documents to compare the history of these two seasons, much light might be thrown on the obscure cause of intermittents." Clarke, of Nottingham, (l. c.) says there were some cases of irregular ague among a few privates of the regiment there, who had all come from a marshy quarter, some of them with the fever on them. The paroxysms came at unusually long intervals. Bark increased the fever.

[3] Lecture on Agues, in the *Lond. Med. Gaz.* IX. 923–4, 24 March, 1832.

The Influenza of 1831.

The next influenza in Britain fell in the early summer of 1831. It was a mild epidemic of the catarrhal type, which attracted hardly any notice in England. In one of the London medical journals there is no other notice of it but this, dated 2 July, 1831[1]: "In consequence of the sudden variations of temperature which have prevailed since the last fortnight of May an epidemic bronchitis has shown itself in Paris." Another London journal[2], on the very same day, wrote: "Influenza in a severe form is at present prevailing in London and some of the provincial towns. It commences like a common cold, but is soon discovered to be more serious, &c." The physician to the public dispensary in Chancery Lane found that more than half of the seventy applicants on 23 June came with the symptoms of influenza—severe, harsh, dry cough, in paroxysms, pain behind the sternum, a fixed pain in one side, congested state of the throat, nose and eyes, heaviness of the head, languor, debility, hot skin, foul tongue, impaired sense of taste. The symptoms went off after three or four days with a sweat in the night and a discharge from the nostrils[3].

This epidemic hardly affected the London bills of mortality, according to the following figures:

Four weeks, 25 May to 21 June, 1579 births, 1430 deaths.
Five weeks, 22 June to 26 July, 2153 births, 2010 deaths.
Four weeks, 27 July to 23 Aug., 1997 births, 1652 deaths.

The rise in the last four weeks was due to summer diarrhoea, or choleraic diarrhoea, which was unusually common in 1831. This slight influenza was also reported from Plymouth by a surgeon who had seen the disease, and suffered from it, at Manilla in September, 1830[4], and by a Plymouth practitioner, who wrote, on 14 July, that it had been extensively prevalent there and in the neighbouring towns and villages[5]. It is recorded also from the Isle of Man, Glasgow[6], and Ayr[7], and it is supposed to have been in Aberdeen[8]. But, while there are many

---

[1] *Lancet,* s. d., p. 438.   [2] *Lond. Med. Gazette,* 2 July, 1831.
[3] John Burne, M.D., *Ibid.* VIII. (1831), p. 430.
[4] G. Bennett, *Lond. Med. Gaz.* 23 July, 1831.   [5] Bellamy, *Ibid.*
[6] "Report of Diseases among the Poor of Glasgow," *Glas. Med. Journ.* IV. 444.
[7] McDerment, *ibid.* v. 230: "In June and July to an extent unequalled" etc.
[8] During the last general election before the passing of the Reform Bill, which was held in the month of June, 1831, a number of the Aberdeen radicals went out on a

accounts of this epidemic in Germany in May and June, and undoubted evidence of it in France and Italy, as well as in Sweden, and in Poland and Russia earlier in the year, the accounts of it in Britain are so meagre and casual as to make one doubt whether it really was an influenza worth reckoning.

The Influenza of 1833.

The next year, 1832, which was the first great season of Asiatic cholera in Britain, is absolutely free from records of influenza in all Europe. It was in the spring of the year following, 1833, that the really serious influenza came. The continental literature of the epidemic of 1833 is immense, the English literature of it is all but non-existent: and yet it was a very severe influenza with us, just as with other European peoples. There was no collective inquiry in Britain on this occasion, such as had been made first by Fothergill in 1775, by the College of Physicians and another Society in 1782, by Simmons in 1788, and by Beddoes and the Medical Society of London in 1803, or such as was made in the next influenza, that of 1837, by a committee of the Provincial Medical Association. But enough is known of it to place it among the severer influenzas. In London the bills of mortality, which relate only to a part of London, showed the characteristic sudden rise and fall:

		Baptisms	Burials
Four weeks,	20 Feb. to 16 March	2310	2352
Five „	17 March to 23 April	1955	2105
Four „	24 April to 21 May	2016	3350
Four „	22 May to 18 June	2070	1685

For a whole month the burials in London were nearly doubled, and for the two worst weeks they were nearly quadrupled. This mortality, by all accounts, fell most on the richer classes, to whom it was a much more serious calamity than the Asiatic cholera of the year before. The president of the Medical Society said, on the 22nd April, that he had "heard of nine lords or ladies who had been carried off by it or by its indirect agency, in the course of last week[1]." Its type in the

hot and dusty day to meet the candidate of their party who was posting from the south. It was remarked that all those who had been of this company "caught cold," unaccountably but as if from some common cause. The date would correspond to the prevalence of influenza elsewhere.

[1] Mr Kingdon, reported in the *Lancet*, s. d.

month of May was worse than in April[1]. When it was first
seen it was a somewhat short catarrhal attack, ending in a
sweat after two, three or four days, with the usual head-pains,
soreness of the ribs and limbs, languor and prostration. Later,
it became a more "adynamic" illness, beginning indeed with
slight catarrhal symptoms, but soon passing into subacute
nervous fever which might last for three weeks, involving much
risk to life[2]. Hence arose the warnings, just as in 1890–92, that
the influenza was a much more serious thing than it had been
thought when the epidemic began, and hence the delay, as it
were, in the bills of mortality to show the effects of the
epidemic until it had been two or three weeks prevalent. It is
to the month of April, before the highest death-rate was reached
in London, that the following, in the *Gentleman's Magazine,*
applies[3]:

"During the month a severe form of catarrhal epidemic, generally termed
influenza, has been extremely prevalent in London. It has laid up at once
all the members of many large households, and has attacked great numbers
in several public offices, particularly the Bank of England and some divisions
of the new police. The performers at the theatres have much suffered, and
their houses have been closed for several nights. It commences suddenly
with headache and feeling of general discomfort, attended or soon followed
by cough, hoarseness, or loss of voice; oppression, and sometimes severe
pain in the chest, tenderness about the ribs, and sense of having been
bruised about the limbs or muscles...The disease is generally attributed to
the constant north-east winds; but by some of the learned is regarded as the
epidemic influenza which has lately prevailed in the eastern parts of Europe,
and that is travelling, like many of its predecessors, to the west."

It would have been in this earlier stage of the epidemic,
when it was laying up whole households, thinning workshops
and closing theatres, that a practitioner was heard to say (as
reported by the *Lancet*): "Best thing I ever had! Quite a god-
send! Everybody ill, nobody dying!" The seriousness of the
disease was, however, at length recognized, so that the members
of the Medical Society debated the subject at three successive
meetings. One of the questions was, whether the malady called
for blooding—a question that had divided opinion as long ago
as 1658[4]. On 13 May, the following passed at the Medical
Society:

[1] Venables, *Lancet,* 11 May, 1833.
[2] Hingeston, *Lond. Med. Gaz.* XII. 199.
[3] *Gent. Magaz.,* April, 1833, p. 362.
[4] Whitmore, *Febris anomala, or the New Disease, etc.,* London, 1659, p. 109:—
"And for a plethora or fulness of blood, if that appears (though this may seem a
paradox yet 'tis certain) that it is so far in this disease from indicating bleeding that it

Mr Williams remembered the similar influenza of 1803, and said that depletion was then regarded as an injurious plan of treatment.

Mr Proctor :— Yes, but the Brunonian doctrines were then in full fling, and practitioners had not learned the full use of the lancet.

Graves states very fairly the reasons that induced them to take blood in the influenza of 1833, as well as the results of the practice[1] :

"The sudden manner in which the disease came on, the great heat of skin, acceleration of pulse, and the intolerable violence of the headache, —together with the oppression of the chest, cough, and wheezing—all encouraged us to the employment of the most active modes of depletion ; and yet the result was but little answerable to our expectations ; for these means were found to induce an awful prostration of strength, with little or no alleviation of the symptoms."

The prostration, be it said, was probably as great and as frequent in the epidemics of 1890–93, when bleeding had gone out altogether ; still it was not understood that all these signs of sthenic action in the attack were really paradoxical, as Whitmore, in the passage cited in the note, saw clearly two centuries before.

The epidemic became rapidly prevalent all over England, Scotland and Ireland in April and May, following no very definite order of progression. The Liverpool newspapers asserted that ten thousand were down with it in that town in one week. A doctor at Lincoln wrote, on 13 May, that few families there had escaped it[2]. Other towns in which it is said to have been "more or less" prevalent were Portsmouth, Sheffield, Birmingham, Leeds, York, Halifax, Glasgow, Edinburgh[3], Dublin and Armagh ; so that we may fairly assume, although we are without the detailed evidence available for earlier epidemics, that it was ubiquitous in town and country.

At Birmingham[4], among the outpatients of the Infirmary, the cases of influenza were as follows, the 25th and 26th April being the days when cases came first in rapid succession, while the middle of May was practically the limit :

stands absolutely as a contradiction to it and vehemently prohibits it. And whereas they think the heat, by bleeding, may be abated and so the feaver took off, they are mistook, for by that means the fermentation through the motion of the blood is highly increased, so as sad experience hath manifested in a great many : upon the bleeding they have within a day or two fallen delirious and had their tongues as black as soot, with an intolerable thirst and drought upon them....Petrus a Castro, who rants high for letting blood, at last as if he had been humbled with the sad success, saith etc."

[1] *A System of Clinical Medicine*, Dublin, 1843, pp. 500–501. Lecture delivered in the session 1834–35.

[2] Rawlins, *Lond. Med. Gaz.* s. d.

[3] *Ed. Med. Surg. Journ.* XLIII. 1835, p. 26.

[4] Parsons, "Report of Outcases, Birmingham Infirmary, 1 Jan. to 31 Dec. 1833." *Trans. Provin. Med. Surg. Assoc.* II. 474.

	Cases of Influenza	Males	Females
April	151	52	99
May	464	159	305
June	28	9	19
	643	220	423

The great excess of females is remarkable, but was probably due to some local circumstances. Of the 643 cases, 122 were under ten years of age. Of the females, 9 died, of the males 3. But the deaths in Birmingham caused by the epidemic directly or indirectly were many; the burial registers of four churches and chapels showed a marked increase of burials above those of the corresponding months of 1832 :

	1832	1833
April	205	245
May	211	434
June	193	230
	609	909

Medical opinion in 1833 was decidedly adverse to the contagiousness of influenza. The common remark was that it was just as little contagious as the cholera of the year before had proved to be. As in 1837 and 1847, when the doctrine of contagiousness was equally out of favour, the disease was observed to spread rapidly, in no very definite line, affecting most parts of the country in the same two or three weeks, affecting the population within a considerable radius almost at once, and the inmates of houses all together. These, it was said, are not the marks of a disease that persons hand on one to another, *quasi cursores*.

The Influenza of 1837.

Between the influenza of April–May, 1833, and that of January–February, 1837, it seems probable that there were minor catarrhal outbreaks, distinguishable from ordinary colds. One writer on the influenza of 1837 refers to those " who had it in 1834 or in the intervening period between the two epidemics." The table of diseases of the outpatients at the Birmingham Infirmary for the year 1836 contains a large total of catarrhs, and, in another line, 24 cases of " epidemic catarrh " in the summer months. The *Gentleman's Magazine* begins its notice

of the epidemic of 1837 by calling it "an influenza of a peculiar character," which shows that influenza of the ordinary kind was a familiar thing. Probably the name was a good deal misapplied in the years following every great epidemic from 1782 onwards: thus in 'St Ronan's Well,' which was written in 1823, or twenty years from the last general influenza, a tradesman's widow in easy circumstances and given to good living comes to the Spa on account of a supposed malady which she calls the *influenzy*. But our recent experiences of four great influenza seasons in succession from 1889–90 to 1893, although it is without precedent in the history, will incline us the more to credit what is recorded of influenza cases in the intervals between the years of great historical epidemics[1]. However that may be for the years following 1833, the influenza of January, 1837, was sudden, simultaneous, universal.

The first cases, which Watson compares to the first drops of a thunder-shower, were seen earlier in some places than in others; but from all parts of England it was reported that the influenza was at its height from the middle of January to the end of the first week of February. Possibly it was a few days earlier in London than in most other towns, inasmuch as the great increase of the deaths that is shown in the following table, in the second and third weeks of January, would imply a prevalence of the epidemic for at least a fortnight before.

Weekly Mortalities in London (by the old Bills).

1837

Week ending	Influenza	All causes
Jan. 10	0	284
17	13	477
24	106	871
31	99	860
Feb. 7	63	589
14	35	558
21	20	350
28	8	321
March 7	4	262

This sudden rise in the deaths from all causes is a characteristic influenza bill, comparable with those already given from

[1] In the report upon the influenza of 1837 by a Committee of the Provincial Medical Association, the preceding epidemic is uniformly referred to the year 1834. Graves, in a clinical lecture upon that of 1837, speaks two or three times of the last as that of 1834, and, in another place, he calls it the epidemic of 1833–34. But these, I think, are mere laxities of dating, of which there are many other instances where the date is recent and not yet historical.

1580 onwards. But the bill is far from showing the whole of the mortality in London in 1837. The London bills of mortality compiled by the Parish Clerks' Company had fallen into the last stage of inadequacy, and were on the eve of being superseded by the general system of registration for all England and Wales[1].

The London bills, so long as they existed, never took in the great parishes of St Pancras, Marylebone, Kensington and Chelsea. The area "within the bills of mortality" was that of London about the middle of the 18th century. But, instead of becoming more and more crowded as time went on, it had actually become much less populous, especially in the old City and Liberties, owing to the erection of warehouses, workshops, counting-houses and other non-residential buildings where dwelling houses used to be; so that the decrease of mortality "within the bills" in the 19th century is in part due to the decrease of population within the same area. This has to be kept in mind when the above table is compared with one of those for former influenzas, such as that of 1737, exactly a hundred years before.

It was thought that the 1837 influenza in London was worse than that of 1833, but the figures show the contrary as regards the number of deaths from all causes[2]. Both of them, however, were in the first rank of severity, finding their nearest parallels in the three great influenzas of the 18th century, in 1733, 1737 and 1743, when the deaths from all causes during the influenza rose, indeed, to a much larger total within the bills, but rose from a much higher mean level.

In Dublin the great increase of burials from the influenza of

[1] As early as 1612 a proposal had been made to James I. for "a grant of the general registrarship of all christenings, marriages and burials within this realm." *State Papers*, Rolls House, Ja. I. vol. LXIX. No. 54. It was a device for raising money.

[2] The account in the *Gentleman's Magazine* for February, 1837, p. 199, is almost identical with the paragraph in the number for April, 1833: "An influenza of a peculiar character has been raging throughout the country, and particularly in the Metropolis. It has been attended by inflammation of the throat and lungs, with violent spasms, sickness and headache. So general have been its effects that business in numerous instances has been entirely suspended. The greater number of clerks at the War Office, Admiralty, Navy Pay Office, Stamp Office, Treasury, Post-Office and other Government Offices have been prevented from attending to their daily avocations....Of the police force there were upwards of 800 incapable of doing duty. On Sunday the 13th the churches which have generally a full congregation presented a mournful scene &c....the number of burials on the same day in the different cemeteries was nearly as numerous as during the raging of the cholera in 1832 and 1833. In the workhouses the number of poor who have died far exceed any return that has been made for the last thirty years."

1837 fell at the same time as in London, according to the following comparison with the year before for Glasnevin Cemetery[1]:

1835–36		1836–37	
Dec. 1835	355	Dec. 1836	413
Jan. 1836	392	Jan. 1837	821
Feb. „	362	Feb. „	537
Mar. „	392	Mar. „	477
	1501		2248

At Glasgow the deaths from influenza were as follows[2]:

1837

	Males	Females	Total
January	111	118	229
February	37	62	99
March	9	20	29
	157	200	357

But the heading of "influenza" did not nearly show the full effects of the epidemic upon the mortality, which was enormous in Glasgow in January, as compared with the same month of 1836:

	All causes	Catarrh	Aged	Asthma	Fever	Decline
Jan. 1836	790	4	73	31	45	124
Jan. 1837	1972	229	274	185	201	247

There was also a great increase in the deaths of infants by bowel complaint. The only period of life which did not show a great rise of mortality was from five to twenty; the greatest rise was between the ages of forty and seventy, corresponding to the London experience in the epidemic of 1847.

At Bolton, Lancashire, the great rise in the deaths, as compared with the average of five years before, was in February:

	Average of five years 1831–36	1837
January	111·2	115
February	79·0	205
March	97·8	100
	288·0	420

At Exeter, the burials in the two chief graveyards were 227

[1] Graves, u. s., p. 545.
[2] Robert Cowan, M.D., *Journ. Stat. Soc.* III. 257.

in January and February, 1837, as compared with 125 in the same months of 1836. These mortalities, although large, were but a small ratio of the attacks. In 2347 cases enumerated in the collective inquiry, there were 54 deaths, a ratio of two deaths in a hundred cases being considered a full average. The attacks were mostly in middle life, and the deaths nearly all among the asthmatic, the consumptive and the aged. The ages of one hundred persons attacked at Birmingham were as follows[1]:

Ages	1—	5—	10—	20—	30—	40—	50—	60—	70—	80—90
Cases	3	2	12	23	21	19	12	7	0	1

At Evesham only five out of 93 were under five years. At Leamington, in a list of 170 cases, there were 26 under fourteen years, 119 from fourteen to sixty-five years, and 25 above the age of sixty-five[2]. In some places males seemed to be most attacked, just as at Birmingham in 1833 there was a great excess of female cases; but the collective inquiry showed that the sexes shared about equally all over. The type of the malady was on the whole catarrhal, as in 1833. Nearly all the cases had symptoms of sneezing, coughing, and defluxions; many cases had nothing more than the symptoms of a severe feverish cold; the more dangerous cases had dyspnoea, pneumonia and the like; while all had the languor, weariness, and soreness in the bones which mark every influenza, whether it incline more to the moist type of catarrhal fever or to the dry type of the old " hot ague."

The influenza of 1837 having been remarkably simultaneous, sudden and brief, the doctrine of personal contagiousness found little favour, just as in 1833. The 12th query sent out by the committee of the Provincial Medical Association was: " Are you in possession of any proof of its having been communicated from one person to another?" The answers are said to have been nearly all negative; namely, that there was " no proof of the existence of any contagious principles by which it was propagated from one individual to another." Shapter, a learned physician at Exeter, inclined to a certain modified doctrine of

[1] Peyton Blakiston, *A Treatise on the Influenza of* 1837, *containing an analysis of one hundred cases observed at Birmingham between* 1 *Jan. and* 15 *Feb.* Lond. 1837.
[2] These and some former particulars are from the " Report upon the Influenza or Epidemic Catarrh of the winter of 1836–37," compiled by Robt. J. N. Streeten, M.D. for the Committee of the Provincial Medical Association. *Trans. Prov. Med. Assoc.* VI. 501.

contagion by persons. Blakiston, of Birmingham, an exact mathematician, declared that the question as ordinarily stated did not admit of an answer.

At Liverpool there was an interesting observation made, exactly parallel with those made at Gravesend in 1782 and Portsmouth in 1788. The influenza of 1837 was practically over by the first or second week of March; but "that the atmosphere of Liverpool was still contaminated by the epidemic influence up to the middle and latter end of April was apparent from the fact that many of the officers and men of the American ships, and generally the most robust, were violently attacked shortly after their arrival in port,"—the same being the case also with black sailors on ships arriving from the Brazils and the West Coast of Africa[1]. At the naval stations of Sheerness, Portsmouth, Plymouth and Falmouth, every one of the ships of war had been attacked in January, the ships cruising on the south coast of Spain, or lying at Barcelona, in February, the ships at Gibraltar in April, and those at Malta in May. The 'Thunderer,' on the passage from Malta to Plymouth, had the first cases of influenza at sea on the 3rd of January, four days before reaching Plymouth[2], as if she had sailed into an atmosphere of it somewhere near the coast of Brittany.

For fully ten years, from March or April 1837 to November 1847, there was no great and universal influenza in England. But there were several undoubted minor, and perhaps localized, outbreaks of an epidemic malady which was in each case judged to be truly the influenza, and not a common cold. The earliest of these was in the spring of 1841. It was recognized by the Registrar-General to have been in London from 20 February to 24 April, the mortality having been little affected by it. It was also recognized in Dublin in March, and remarked upon by two physicians to the Cork Street Fever Hospital; it was characterized by the usual languor, weariness, and pains in the head, by defluxions of the eyes, nose and throat, but not by any affection of the lungs, and was in all respects mild[3]. Exactly a year after, in March, 1842, influenza was described as epidemic

[1] Streeten's Report, u. s., p. 505.
[2] *Statist. Report on Health of Navy*, 1837–43.
[3] Jackson, *Dubl. Med. Press*, VIII. 69; Brady, *Dubl. Journ. Med. Sc.* XX. (1842), 76.

at York[1]: it was noted also in London in March[2], and is mentioned as having been again in Ireland in 1842[3]. The next undoubted influenza is reported from a rural part of Cheshire (Holme Chapel) in January, 1844, in the wake of an epidemic of scarlatina; it continued in all kinds of weather until June, and had a remarkable intercurrent episode, for some weeks from the middle of March, in the form of an epidemic of pneumonia among young children, which passed into mild bronchitis in the cases last attacked[4]. Coincidently with the influenza in Cheshire, there is a report of a series of catarrhal cases in Dublin about the beginning of January, 1844, in which the sense of constriction and suffocation under the sternum and the paroxysmal character of the attacks seemed to point to influenza[5]. Two years after, a Dublin physician in extensive practice among the rich wrote, at the request of a medical editor, an account of an epidemic of influenza in January and February, 1847; he had sixty cases among children under fourteen in his private practice, usually several children in one house, and sometimes the adults in the house[6]. This was in the midst of the great epidemic of relapsing fever in Dublin and all over Ireland, due to the potato famine. The same prevalence of influenza to a slight extent is recorded also for London at the end of 1846 and beginning of 1847[7]. It is easy to object that these "influenzas" between 1837 and 1847 were but the ordinary catarrhal maladies of the seasons. But the physicians who took the trouble to record them—probably more might have done so—were, of course, aware of the distinction that had to be made between many common feverish colds concurring in the ordinary way, and a truly epidemic influenza, however slight.

The Influenza of 1847–48.

The great influenza of 1847 began in London about the 16th or 18th of November, was at its height from the 22nd to the

---

[1] Laycock, *Dubl. Med. Press*, VII. 234. Several cases of sudden and great enlargement of the liver and of suppression of urine were judged to be part of the epidemic.

[2] Ross, *Lancet*, 1845, I. p. 2.

[3] Report of Holywood Dispensary for 1842, *Dublin Med. Press*, IX. 204.

[4] Hall, *Prov. Med. Journ.* 1844, p. 315.

[5] M'Coy, *Med. Press*, XI. 133.

[6] Fleetwood Churchill, *Dubl. Quart. Journ.*, May, 1847, p. 373.

[7] Farr, in *Rep. Reg.-Gen.*

30th, had "ceased to be very prevalent" by the 6th or 8th of December, but affected the bills of mortality for some time longer, as in the following table :

Weekly Mortalities in London.

1847

Week ending	All causes	Influenza	Pneumonia	Bronchitis	Asthma	Typhus
Nov. 20	1086	4	95	61	12	86
27	1677	36	170	196	77	87
Dec. 4	2454	198	306	343	86	132
11	2416	374	294	299	78	136
18	1946	270	189	234	52	131
25	1247	142	131	107	14	83
Jan. 1	1599	127	148	138	26	74

In the thirteen weeks of the first quarter of 1848 the influenza deaths declined as follows : 102, 102, 89, 56, 59, 47, 27, 33, 18, 11, 10, 16, 8.

This was the first great epidemic of influenza under the new system of registration. According to the Superintendent of Statistics, it caused an excess of 5000 deaths during the six weeks that it lasted, of which about a fourth part only were set down to influenza, and the rest to pneumonia, bronchitis, asthma, etc. During the three worst weeks it raised the deaths in the age of childhood 83 per cent., in the age of manhood 104 per cent., in old age 247 per cent., whereas the deaths between fifteen years and twenty-five were but little raised by it, and those between ten and fifteen hardly at all. It raised the deaths during six weeks in St George's-in-the East to a rate per annum of 73 per 1000 living : in some other parishes it increased the death-rate very little. But it had the usual effect of lengthening enormously the obituary columns of the newspapers, which shows that it fell, as usual, to a large extent upon the richer classes. It went all over England in a short time, the month of December being the time of excessive mortality in the towns, according to the following sample totals of deaths from all causes :

1847

	Manchester (Ancoats)	Sheffield (West)	York (Walmgate)	Places in Scotland
October	169	27	61	521
November	135	27	52	728
December	270	85	99	1001

In some parts of England, as in Kendal, a district of Anglesea and in the Isle of Wight, the mortality of the last

quarter of 1847 was actually lower than that of the year before. From St Albans the sub-registrar reported that there had been "no epidemic." In most parts of the country, including the medium-sized towns, the mortality directly or indirectly due to influenza was lower than in London. The principal returns did not come in from the country until after the new year, the effects of the epidemic having been, as usual, later in rural districts. Hence, while London had 1253 deaths put down to "influenza" in 1847 (nearly all in December), and 659 in 1848 (nearly all in the first quarter), the rest of England had 4881 influenza deaths before the New Year, and 7963 after it[1]. This influenza in the mid-winter of 1847–8 made a great impression everywhere[2]. As regards its range and its fatality, it was like those of 1833 and 1837 ; and it had once more so much of the catarrhal type, that the name of influenza became still more firmly joined to the idea of a feverish cold or defluxion.

By the year 1847, agues had almost ceased to be written of in England, although they still occurred in the Fens. But Peacock begins his account of the influenza of that winter with an enumeration of prevailing diseases, which reads somewhat like an old "constitution" by Sydenham or Huxham. The summers and autumns of 1846 and 1847, he says, were both highly choleraic, and dysentery (as well as enteric fever) was unusually common in the former year. Fatal cases of "ague and remittent fever" were also more numerous than usual. Then came much enteric fever, "not unfrequently complicated with catarrhal symptoms." Throughout the spring and early summer of the influenza year, 1847, "intermittent fevers were common, and in March, April and May, purpura was frequently met with, either as a primary or secondary disease. Scurvy also, owing to the deficiency of fresh vegetables, and from the general failure of the

[1] Farr, in the *Report of the Registrar-General for* 1848. He cites (p. xxxi) Stark for Scotland, that it "suddenly attacked great masses of the population twice during November"—on the 18th, and again on the 28th.

[2] A curious trace of the temporary interest excited by influenza in 1847–8 remains in a great book of the time, Carlyle's *Letters and Speeches of Cromwell*, the third edition of which, with new letters, was then under hand. One of the new letters related to the death of Colonel Pickering from the camp-sickness among the troops of Fairfax at Ottery St Mary in December, 1645. Carlyle's comment is: "has caught the epidemic 'new disease' as they call it, some ancient *influenza* very prevalent and fatal during those wet winter operations." "New disease" was the name given by Greaves to the war-typhus in Oxfordshire and Berkshire in 1643, but neither that nor the sickness at Ottery (which is not called "new disease" in the documents) had anything of the nature of influenza.

potato crop in the previous year was occasionally seen." Then follows much concerning a fever called remittent, which reads more like relapsing fever than anything else[1]. "The remittent form of fever was frequent in the course of the epidemic [of influenza], though seldom registered as the cause of death." Peacock says truly that the rather unusual concurrence of so many sicknesses was "not peculiar to the recent influenza alone;" and he can "scarcely refrain from acknowledging that these several affections are not merely coetaneous but correlative, and types and modifications of one disease, with which they have a common origin. Assuming this inference to be admitted, we may advance to the solution of the further question of what is the essential nature or proximate cause of the disease." But the inquiry led him to no result: the precise cause he leaves "involved in the obscurity that veils the origin of epidemics generally"—which are surely not all equally obscure[2].

Influenza having continued epidemic for a few weeks in the beginning of 1848, ceased thereafter to attract popular notice in Britain during a period of more than forty years. But a certain number of "influenza" deaths continued to appear steadily year after year in the registration tables. In 1851 this number was nearly doubled, in 1855 it was more than trebled; and those two years were undoubtedly seasons (about January and February) of real influenza epidemics in Europe, recorded by several but not by English writers. A slight epidemic was described for Scotland in 1857, and one for Norfolk in 1878, neither of which seems to have influenced the registration returns in an obvious degree. After the undoubted influenza of 1855, the annual total of deaths in England set down to that cause steadily declined from four figures, to three figures, and then to two figures, standing at 55 in the bill of mortality for 1889. It is improbable that those small annual totals of deaths in all England and Wales were caused by the real influenza; the name at that

---

[1] But Dr Rose Cormack, who had known relapsing fever well in Edinburgh, wrote from Putney, near London, in October, 1849: "For some months past the majority of cases of all diseases in this neighbourhood have...presented a well-marked tendency to assume the remittent and intermittent types." "Infantile Remittent Fever," *Lond. Journ. of Med.*, Oct. 1849, reprinted in his *Clinical Studies*, 2 vols., 1876.

[2] T. B. Peacock, M.D., *On the Influenza, or Epidemic Catarrhal Fever of 1847-8.* London, 1848.

time was synonymous with a feverish cold, and would have been given here or there to fatalities from some such ordinary cause. An epidemic ague was reported from Somerset in 1858[1].

The Influenzas of 1889–94.

More than a generation had passed with little or no word of epidemic influenza in this country, when in the early winter of 1889 the newspapers began to publish long telegrams on the influenza in Moscow, St Petersburg, Berlin, Paris, Madrid and other foreign capitals. This epidemic wave, like those immediately preceding it in the Eastern hemisphere, in 1833, 1837 and 1847, and like one or more, but by no means all, of the earlier influenzas, had an obvious course from Asiatic and European Russia towards Western Europe[2]. In due time it reached London, and produced a decided effect upon the bills of mortality for the first and second weeks of January, 1890, but a moderate effect compared with that of 1847, which was the first to be recorded under the same system of registration. It spread all over England, Scotland and Ireland in the months of January and February, 1890, proving itself everywhere a short and sharp influenza of the old kind, but with catarrhal symptoms on the whole a less constant feature than in the epidemics of most recent memory. At the end of February it looked as if Great Britain and Ireland had got off lightly from the visitation which had caused high mortalities in many countries of Continental Europe. But this epidemic in the beginning of 1890 was only the first of four, and less severe than the second and third. It returned in the spring and early summer of 1891, in the first weeks of 1892, and in the winter of 1893–94. To understand this influenza prevalence as a whole, its four great seasons should be compared. The following tables show its incidence upon London on each occasion:

[1] Haviland, *Journ. Pub. Health*, IV. 288, (94 cases in June—Aug. in a village).
[2] See F. Clemow, M.D., of St Petersburg, "The Recent Pandemic of Influenza: its place of origin and mode of spread." *Lancet*, 20 Jan. and 10 Feb. 1894. These papers bring together and discuss the Russian opinions, official and other. The Army Medical Report favoured the view that the birthplace of this pandemic in the autumn of 1889 was an extensive region occupied by nomadic tribes in the northern part of the Kirghiz Steppe. There is evidence of its rapid progress westwards over Tobolsk to the borders of European Russia. Influenza is said to be constantly present in many parts of the Russian Empire; but the circumstances that have, on four or five occasions in the 19th century, set the infection rolling in a great wave westwards from the assumed source are wholly unknown.

Four epidemics of Influenza in London, 1890–94.

1890

Week ending	Annual death-rate per 1000 living	Deaths from all causes	Influenza	Bronchitis	Pneumonia
Jan. 4	28·0	2371	4	530	215
11	32·4	2747	67	715	253
18	32·1	2720	127	630	281
25	26·3	2227	105	468	193
Feb. 1	21·8	1849	75	339	145
8	20·6	1749	38	369	117

1891

Week ending	Annual death-rate per 1000 living	Deaths from all causes	Influenza	Bronchitis	Pneumonia
April 25	21·0	1809	10	240	179
May 2	23·3	2006	37	280	241
9	25·6	2069	148	302	230
16	27·7	2245	266	352	207
23	27·6	2235	319	337	219
30	28·9	2337	310	353	189
June 6	27·0	2189	303	320	176
13	23·3	1886	249	255	166
20	23·0	1865	182	248	159
27	19·0	1538	117	151	113
July 4	16·8	1363	56	108	103

1891–92

Week ending	Annual death-rate per 1000 living	Deaths from all causes	Influenza	Bronchitis	Pneumonia
Dec. 26	21·9	1771	19	355	131
Jan. 2	42·0	3399	37	927	256
9	32·8	2679	95	740	246
16	40·0	3271	271	867	285
23	46·0	3761	506	1035	317
30	41·0	3355	436	844	255
Feb. 6	30·6	2500	314	492	215
13	24·6	2010	183	368	140
20	20·7	1693	79	259	137

1893–94

Week ending	Annual death-rate per 1000 living	Deaths from all causes	Influenza	Bronchitis	Pneumonia
Nov. 4	20·2	1695	8	191	125
11	21·4	1679	20	220	137
18	24·4	2016	22	318	228
25	26·5	2190	36	384	215
Dec. 2	27·1	2235	74	426	248
9	31·0	2556	127	491	266
16	29·1	2401	164	421	232
23	26·3	2170	147	387	203
30	23·3	1920	108	306	157
Jan. 6	24·5	2040	87	342	169
13	29·5	2462	75	490	211
20	23·7	1975	69	320	172
27	19·8	1655	41	232	152

It will be seen that the third epidemic, that of Jan.–Feb. 1892, had the highest maximum weekly mortality from influenza (506) as well as the highest maxima from bronchitis and pneumonia not specially associated in the certificates with influenza; that the second epidemic, of 1891, had the next highest maxima, and that the first and last of the four outbreaks were both milder than the two intermediate ones. All but the second, which fell in early summer, are strictly comparable as regards season (mid-winter). But although the second, in 1891, had the advantage of falling in some of the healthiest weeks of the year, it was more protracted than the original outbreak, much more fatal than it in the article influenza, more fatal also in the article pneumonia, and less fatal only in the article bronchitis. The third outbreak was not only more protracted than the first, in the same season of the year, but much more fatal in all the associated articles. As to the deaths referred to influenza (whether as primary or secondary cause), the numbers are not strictly comparable in all the outbreaks; they are probably too few in the first table, more nearly exact in the second, third, and fourth, the diagnosis having at length become familiar and the fashion of nomenclature established. It is undoubted that many of the deaths from bronchitis and pneumonia in January, 1890, were due to the epidemic; for, "while the ordinary rise of mortality in cold seasons is mainly among the very aged, the increased mortality in this fatal month was mainly among persons between 20 and 60 years" (Ogle).

While the first epidemic of the series was universal and of short duration all over the kingdom, the second and third were more partial in their incidence and more desultory or prolonged. The second, which began in Hull (and at the same time on the borders of Wales), produced the following highest weekly death-rates per annum from all causes among 1000 persons living:

Highest Weekly Death-rates in the Second Influenza.

1891

	Week ending	Annual death-rate from all causes per 1000 living		Week ending	Annual death-rate from all causes per 1000 living
Hull	Apr. 11	42·5	Huddersfield	May 16	54·5
Sheffield	May 2	70·5	Leicester	,, 16	44·6
Halifax	,, 2	42·1	Oldham	,, 23	50·4
Leeds	,, 9	48·5	London	,, 30	28·9
Manchester	,, 9	43·6	Salford	,, 30	45·9
Bradford	,, 16	56·7	Blackburn	June 6	48·5

The third was heard of first in the west of Cornwall and in the east of Scotland, in the last quarter of 1891. It was in the following English towns that it produced the maximum weekly death-rates per annum from all causes:

Highest Weekly Death-rates in the Third Influenza.

1892

Town	Week ending	Annual death-rate from all causes per 1000 living
Portsmouth	Jan. 16	57·0
London	,, 23	46·0
Norwich	,, 23	44·7
Brighton	,, 23	60·9
Croydon	,, 30	47·2

These highest death-rates in the third successive season of influenza were all in the southern or eastern counties; in the latter, Colchester also had a maximum death-rate during one week of about 80 per 1000 per annum. Liverpool, among the northern great towns, appears to have had most of the third influenza. The fourth outbreak, in the end of 1893, was noticed first in the Midlands (Birmingham especially), and was afterwards heard of in the mining and manufacturing districts of Stafford-shire, South Wales, Lancashire, Yorkshire and Durham, as well as in Scotland and Ireland, London, as in the table, having a share of it. The tables given of the London mortality in each of the four outbreaks, from influenza and the chest-complaints which were its most usual secondary effects, are a fair index both of the period and of the severity of the disease all over the kingdom in each of its successive appearances[1]. Everywhere the first and the fourth were the mildest, the second and third the most fatal. Deaths from "influenza" were reported from all the counties of England and Wales in the first and second epidemics, the highest rates of mortality per 1000 inhabitants in the corresponding calendar years having been in the following counties, while in all the counties the greater fatality of the second epidemic is equally marked:

[1] The collective inquiry on the epidemics was made by the medical department of the Local Government Board, the result being given in two reports: *Report on the Influenza Epidemic of* 1889-90, *Parl. Papers,* 1891, and *Further Report and Papers on Epidemic Influenza,* 1889-92, *Parl. Papers,* Sept. 1893. By H. Franklin Parsons, M.D. Statistical tables comparing the epidemics in London with those in some other capitals were published by F. A. Dixey, M.D., *Epidemic Influenza,* Oxford, 1892.

1890		1891	
Cumberland	·35	Rutland	1·36
North Wales	·28	Lincolnshire	1·19
Herefordshire	·28	North Wales	1·09
Salop	·28	Westmoreland	1·02
Wilts	·28	Monmouth	1·00
Somerset	·26	E. Riding Yorks	·98
Dorset	·25	Herefordshire	·98
Bucks	·25	Northamptonshire	·95

In London the entry of influenza is in the weekly bills of mortality throughout the whole period, with the exception of a few weeks; but the deaths were often reduced to unity, and there was perhaps only one occasion, besides the four great outbursts, namely the months of March and April, 1893, when cases were so numerous or so close together in households or neighbourhoods as to constitute a minor epidemic.

The type of the influenza of 1890–93 was not quite the same as on the last historical occasions. When it was announced as approaching from the Continent, everyone looked for "influenza colds"; but the catarrhal symptoms, although not wanting, were soon found to be unimportant beside the nameless misery, prostration and ensuing weakness. Some, indeed, contended that the disease was not influenza but dengue, so pronounced were the symptoms of break-bone fever[1]. Many cases had a decided aguish or intermittent character. The name of ague itself was once more heard in newspaper paragraphs, and more freely used in private talk; but, as we have long ceased to write of epidemic agues, equally as of marsh intermittents, in this country, it is not probable that there will remain any record of agues in Britain accompanying the influenzas of the years 1890–94. On the other hand the complications and after-effects of our latest influenza, more especially as affecting the nervous system, have been very fully studied[2].

That which chiefly distinguishes the influenza of the end of the 19th century from all other invasions of the disease is the

[1] The notable difference between the type of this epidemic and that of the epidemics of 1833, 1837 and 1847, from which the conventional notion of "influenza cold" was derived, is perhaps the explanation of the following apt and erudite remark by Buchanan, on "influenza proper," in his introduction to the first departmental report, 1891: "It would be no small gain to get more authentic methods of identifying influenza proper from among the various grippes, catarrhs, colds and the like—in man, horse, and other animals—that take to themselves the same popular title" (p. xi).

[2] The volume by Julius Althaus, M.D., *Influenza: its Pathology, Complications and Sequelae*, 2nd ed., Lond. 1892, includes a summary and bibliography of recent observations.

revival of the epidemic in three successive seasons, the first recurrence having been more fatal than the original outbreak, and the second recurrence more fatal (in London at least) than the first. The closest scrutiny of the old records, including the series of weekly bills of mortality issued by the Parish Clerks of London for nearly two hundred years, discovers no such recurrences of influenza on the great scale in successive seasons. It is true that several of the old influenzas came in the midst of sickly periods of two or more years' duration, such as the years 1557–58, 1580–82, 1657–59, 1678–80, 1727–29 and 1780–85. But in those periods the bulk of the sickness was aguish, the somewhat definite episodes of catarrhal fever having been distinguished from the epidemic agues by Willis in 1658, by Sydenham in 1679, by several in 1729, and by Baker, among others, in 1782. It is probable, indeed, that there were two strictly catarrhal epidemics in successive years in the periods 1657–59 and 1727–29, just as we know that, in New England, there was a catarrhal epidemic in the autumn of 1789 and an equally severe influenza, less catarrhal in type, in the spring of 1790[1]. But history does not appear to supply a parallel case to the four successive influenzas in the period 1889–94, unless we count the seasonal epidemic agues of former "constitutions" as equivalent to influenzas for the purpose of making out a series.

The Theory of Influenza.

Influenza is not an infection which lends itself to a simple theory of its nature or a neat formula of its cause. All that one can do is to indicate the direction in which the truth lies. Something broad, comprehensive, steady from age to age, telluric if not cosmic, must be sought for. Some have thought that the legendary or representative universal sickness at the siege of Troy was influenza, because it began upon the horses and dogs, as so many historical influenzas have done. But it will be sufficient to show that influenza was the same in the Middle Ages as now; for what circumstances make a broader contrast than medieval and modern? The first writer in England to mention influenza—of course not under that name—was a dean of St Paul's in the reign of Henry II., Radulphus de

---

[1] Noah Webster, *Brief History of Epidemick Diseases*, I. 288; Warren, of Boston, to Lettsom, 30 May, 1790, *Lettsom's Memoirs*, III. 238: "whether this [the second] is a variety of influenza, or a new disease with us, I am at a loss to determine."

Diceto[1]. He is narrating the journey to Rome of the arch-bishop-elect of Canterbury: his election in England was in June, 1173, he had got as far as Placentia by Christmas, whence he turned aside to Genoa, and at length reached Rome, to have his election confirmed by the pope in the nones of April, 1174. It is in the midst of this account of the archbishop's journey, that reference is made to an influenza, otherwise known, from German and Italian chronicles, to have happened in December, 1173: "In those days the whole world was infected by a nebulous corruption of the air, causing catarrh of the stomach and a general cough, to the detriment of all and the death of many"—*universus orbis infectus ex aeris nebulosa corruptione.* What kind of infection can that be which has befallen men on both sides of the Alps within the same short time in the 12th century as in the 19th? And what kind of infection is it which has outlived so many changes in the great pestilences of mankind, has seen the extinction of plague and the rise of cholera, and all other variations, most of them for the better, in the reigning types of epidemic sickness? To have lasted unchanged through so many mutations of things, from medieval to modern, and from modern to ultra-modern, and to have become more in-veterate or protracted at the end of the 19th century than it had ever been, is unique in this history. Influenza appears to correspond with something broadly the same in human life at all times. Or is it rather a thing telluric, of the crust of the earth or the bowels of the earth? Or is it perhaps cosmic, affecting men as the vintage is affected by a comet, or as if it came from the upper spheres? My belief is that we need not transcend the globe to look for its source, and that, upon the earth, we need not go deeper than the surface, nor beyond the inhabited spots. I shall come back to this from giving the history of English opinion upon it.

The best known influenzas of the 16th century all came in summer, as some of the later ones have done, so that no one thought of them as exaggerated common colds. But it hap-pened that the influenzas observed by Willis in 1658, and by Sydenham in 1675 and 1679, came in spring or winter and in such weather as to suggest to each of those physicians that the catarrhal symptoms corresponded to the season. Robert Boyle, their great philosophical contemporary, was also a witness of

---

[1] In Twysden's *Decem Scriptores*, col. 579.

one or more of these influenzas, and it appeared to him that there was more than season and weather in them.

"I have known a great cold," he says, "in a day or two invade multitudes in the same city with violent, and as to many persons, fatal symptoms; when I could not judge (as others also did not), that the bare coldness of the air could so suddenly produce a disease so epidemical and hurtful; and it appeared the more probable that the cause came from under ground, by reason that it began with a very troublesome fog[1]."

I am unable to say whether Boyle was the first to apply the doctrine of telluric or subterranean emanations to influenza; he was certainly not the first to apply it to pestilences in general, for it is found in Seneca among the ancients[2], and it is clearly stated in Ambroise Paré's essay "Sur les Venins," having been probably a familiar notion of the sixteenth century, although a mystical and undefined one. Sydenham also, who must have discussed these questions with Boyle, referred all the more obscure or "stationary" epidemic constitutions to effluvia discharged into the air from "the bowels of the earth": those hypothetical miasmata were for him the τὸ θεῖον of Hippocrates, the mysterious something which had to be assumed so as to explain plague, pestilential fever, intermittent and remittent fevers, the "new fever" of 1685–6, and all other epidemic constitutions which were not caused by obvious changes of season and weather. But it does not appear, and it is not probable, that he ascribed to that mysterious cause the two transient waves of influenza which fell within his own experience, those of November, 1675, and of November, 1679. On the other hand, Boyle certainly did so; he included influenza in his hypothesis explicitly; and if one examines its general terms, it will appear as if it had been made specially for influenza.

Boyle's general expression, for both endemial and epidemic maladies, is that they are due to subterranean effluvia sent up into the air. As a chemist, and as dealing with the new knowledge then most in vogue, he assumed the sources of these miasmata to be for the most part mineral deposits in the crust of the globe, especially "orpimental and other mischievous fossiles"; but later in his writing he says:

---

[1] Boyle's *Works*, 6 vols., London, 1772, v. 52.
[2] Seneca, *Nat. Quaest.* § 27, cited by Webster. After earthquakes, "subitae continuaeque mortes, et monstrosa genera morborum ut ex novis orta causis." The passage cited from Baglivi (p. 530) looks like a repetition of this: "imo nova et inaudita morborum genera...post terraemotus."

"To speak candidly I do not think that these minerals are the causes of even all those pestilences whose efficients may come from under ground"; there were many mischievous fossils of which physicians and even chymists had no knowledge, and "the various associations of these, which nature may, by fire and menstruums, make under ground and perhaps in the air itself, may very much increase the number and variety of hurtful matters."

He makes provision, also, for the hurtful matters multiplying in their underground seats, according to a principle which we know now to be true for organic, instead of mineral matters, and to be true for them above ground, or in the air, as well as under ground :

"I think it possible that divers subterraneal bodies that emit effluvia may have in them a kind of propagative or self-multiplying power. I will not here examine whether this proceeds from some seminal principle, which many chymists and others ascribe to metals and even to stones; or (which is perhaps more likely) to something analogous to a ferment, such as, in vegetables, enables a little sour dough to extend itself through the whole mass, or such as, when an apple or pear is bruised in one part, makes the putrefied part by degrees to transmute the sound into its own likeness ; or else some maturative power...as ananas in the Indies, and medlars...after they are gathered, acquire (as it were spontaneously) in process of time a consistence and sweetness and sometimes colour and odour, and, in short, such a state as by one word we call maturity or ripeness."

Other of Boyle's fruitful principles (I am separating them out from amidst much other matter not specially related to influenza) are these :

"It is possible that these effluvia may be, in their own nature, either innocent enough, or at least not considerably hurtful, and yet may become very noxious if they chance to find the air already imbued with certain corpuscles fit to associate with them."
Again, the effluvia sent up into the air may pass by certain places without causing an epidemic, because these "are not inhabited enough to make their ill qualities taken note of; but, more frequently, because by being diffused through a greater tract of air, they are more and more dispersed in their passage, and thereby so diluted (if I may so speak) and weakened as not to be able to do any notorious mischief."
Again, the effluvia may not produce epidemic disease at the part of the globe where they had emerged from under ground; an illustration of which may be intended in the case of the Black Death, which, as he says, came from China, yet plague is little heard of in that country, a Jesuit, Alexander de Rhodes, who spent thirty years in those parts, testifying that the plague is not so much as spoken of there. Again, why are some epidemics of so short duration at a given place? Either, he answers, because the morbific expiration from under ground had ascended almost at once, and been easily spent; or the subterraneal commotion which sends up the miasmata "may pass from one place to another and so cease to afford the air incumbent on the first place the supplies necessary to keep it impregnated with noxious exhalation ; and it agrees well with this conjecture that sometimes we may observe certain epidemical diseases to have, as it were, a progressive motion, and leaving one town free, pass on to another" —as notably in the case of sweating sickness and influenza.

Lastly there are ever new forms of epidemic disease appearing, not to count every variation of an autumnal ague "which the vulgar call a New Disease." Of the really new types Boyle offers the following explanation : "Some among the emergent variety of exotick and hurtful steams may be found capable to disaffect human bodies after a very uncommon way, and thereby to produce new diseases, whose duration may be greater or smaller according to the lastingness of those subterraneal causes that produce them. On which account it need be no wonder that some new diseases have but a short duration, and vanish not long after their appearing, the sources or fumes being soon destroyed or spent; whereas some others may continue longer upon the stage, as having under ground more settled and durable causes to maintain them."

As a chemist, Boyle sought for the source of the pestilential emanations in underground minerals, in the new combinations of these under the action of "fire and menstruums," in their self-multiplying power as if by subterraneous fermentation ("which many chymists and others ascribe to metals and even to stones"), and in their meeting with suitable "corpuscles" in the air of an inhabited spot wherewith to combine for their morbific effects. He assumed, also, their discharge into the air at particular spots of the globe (where they might not be directly morbific in their effects), or in a series of localities from the wave-like progress of the underground commotion ; in which assumption he seems to be applying the very old idea of classical times that earthquakes and volcanic eruptions were a cause or antecedent of epidemics. Sometimes his mineral fossils were deep in the crust of the globe, touched only by the greater cataclysms ; and then we might expect novelties in the forms of epidemic disease. But he does not exclude emanations from the earth's surface proceeding more gently or insensibly.

It would be a mistake to set aside Boyle's hypothesis of epidemical miasmata as made altogether void by his choosing strange minerals to be the source of them, and by his assuming a kind of fermentation in these inorganic matters so as to explain the continuance and spreading of the infections. Substitute organic matters in the soil for minerals in the crust of the earth, and read a modern meaning into the doctrine of underground or aërial fermentation or leavening, and we shall find Boyle's hypothesis, especially as applied to influenza, far from obsolete. Some such adaptation of the doctrine of miasmata was made two generations later by Dr John Arbuthnot in his 'Essay concerning the Effects of Air upon Human Bodies,' the immediate occasion of which was the London influenza of 1733. There is nothing to note between Boyle and Arbuthnot ; for

Willis and Sydenham, using the Hippocratic language of "constitutions," explained, as we have seen, the epidemic catarrhs of the spring or winter as the reigning febrile constitution modified to suit the season and weather.

Arbuthnot's essay makes more modern reading than Boyle's. He assumes emanations from the ground, but they are no longer from the bowels of the earth, or from deposits of strange minerals requiring earthquakes to set them free, or "fire and menstruums" to give potency to them. Of all the things that pass into the atmosphere, he makes most of the various steams and other volatile decomposing matters of men and animals; and when he brings in the earth, it is as the storehouse or receptacle of such matters, in a surface stratum no deeper than the effects of drought and rainfall could reach. While he accepts the Hippocratic doctrine of epidemic constitutions, and recognizes the air with its various organic contents as the τὸ θεῖον, the *quid divinum* or mysterious something of epidemical causation, he does not forget that the earth is inhabited by creatures, human and other, who befoul the atmosphere by "their own steams"; again, he lays stress upon alternations of drought and moisture in the soil and subsoil as a cause of morbific emanations, not, indeed, stating the matters of fact in the very terms of Pettenkofer's law, but assuming the presence of special organic matters in the soil as much as that does. Although Arbuthnot was hardly a serious epidemiologist, any more than Boyle, yet in the growth of opinion on the subject of morbific matters in the air, he may be said to have shifted the interest from inorganic or mineral substances and gases, to organic matters chiefly of human or animal origin, and from the deeper regions of the globe, such as only earthquakes reach, to the surface stratum of soil and subsoil which is affected by every rise and fall of the ground-water. I shall now give a few extracts, to bear out the above summary, from Abuthnot's essay.

"Air," he says, "is the τὸ θεῖον in diseases, which Hippocrates takes notice of. Air is what he means by the powers of the universe, which, he says, human nature cannot overcome; and he lays it down as a maxim 'that whoever intends to be master of the art of physick must observe the constitution of the year; that the powers and influence of the seasons (what are seldom uniform) produce great changes in human bodies.'" He then pays a compliment to Sydenham as ."endowed with the genius of Hippocrates," and passes on to his own analytic method. "Many great effects must follow, and many sudden changes may happen in human bodies by absorbing outward air with all its qualities and contents.

Nothing accounts more clearly for epidemical diseases seizing human creatures inhabiting the same tract of earth, who have nothing in common that affects them except air: such as that epidemical catarrhous fever of 1728 and of this present year [1733]...It seems to be occasioned by effluvia, uncommon either in quantity or quality, infecting the air...It is likewise evident that these effluvia were not of any particular or mineral nature, because they were of a substance that was common to every part of the surface of the earth: and therefore one may conclude that they were watery exhalations, or, at least, such mixed with other exhalable substances that are common to every spot of ground."

In his account of the qualities and contents of the air, he enumerates them, not so much as detected in the air on analysis, but as having of necessity passed into it, and in some instances been deposited again from it, as in strange dews. One class of substances that pass into the air are the oils, salts, seeds and insensible abrasions of vegetables. Also all excrements and all the carcases of animals vanish into air. Another ingredient of the air is the perspirable matters of animals, the amount of which for human beings he works out by a curious calculation of a column of their own steams raised so many feet high in so many days. Perhaps there are insects in the air invisible to human eyes: one may observe, in that part of a room which is illuminated with the rays of the sun, flies sometimes darting like hawks as if it were upon a prey. Some have imagined the plague to proceed from invisible insects: this system agrees with many of the appearances in the progress or manner of propagation of that disease, but is altogether inconsistent with others. Air replete with the steams of animals, especially such as are rotting, has often produced pestilential fevers in that place: of which there are many instances.

But why should certain years or seasons have a pestilential atmosphere, for example the season of the catarrhous fever of 1733? There had been, he says, an unusual drought for these two years past, the best estimate of the dryness of the surface of the earth being taken from the falling of the springs, "the consequence of which has been unusual diseases amongst several animals, and a great mortality amongst mankind. It is true, this did not happen during the dry weather...The previous great drought must have been particularly hurtful to mankind. Great droughts exert their effects after the surface of the earth is again opened by moisture, and the perspiration of the ground, which was long suppressed, is suddenly restored. It is probable that the earth then emits several new effluvia hurtful to human bodies: this appeared to be the case by the thick and stinking fogs which succeeded the rain that had fallen before."

Arbuthnot knew the progress of the influenza of 1732–33. Its worst week in London was from the 23rd to the 30th January, 1733; but he tells us that it had been at a height in Saxony from the 15th to the 29th November, 1732, had been earlier in Holland than in England, earlier in Edinburgh than in London, in New England before Great Britain. Again, it appeared in Paris in February, somewhat later than in London, and in Naples in March. This progress, he says, was often against the wind. Nor does he assume a progressive infection of regions of atmosphere. The effluvia, he says, were of a substance that was common to every part of the surface of the earth; they were exhalable substances that were common to every spot of

ground ; the excessive drought of two years, followed by heavy rains in the end of 1732, is also assumed to have been common, for, in Germany and France, especially in November, 1732, the air was filled with frequent fogs. It is clear that Arbuthnot traced the universality of influenza, the uniform symptoms of which he recognized, to certain conditions of soil and atmosphere common to all the countries visited by the epidemic.

Throughout the rest of the 18th century there were numerous and varied experiences of influenza, in summer and winter, spring and autumn, coming up from the south as if from Africa, or from the east as if from Central Asia, or appearing in America sooner than in Europe—experiences which made a theory of the disease difficult. Some inclined to Arbuthnot's view of unusual seasons and weather producing the same effects everywhere ; others favoured the hypothesis of contagion from a remote source, which might be China or might be some other territory. Geach, a surgeon at Plymouth who was a Fellow of the Royal Society, actually went back to the astrological cause, pointing out that Jupiter and Saturn were in a certain conjunction during the influenza of 1775. The only elaborate theory of the strange disease that calls for notice, besides those of Boyle and Arbuthnot, is that of Noah Webster, the famous lexicographer of Hartford, Connecticut.

While Webster was a journalist in New York about the years 1794–6, the subject of yellow fever, which was then of great practical moment, set him reading and speculating about pestilences in general. Writing to Priestley, he said that in the course of his inquiries he found the American libraries ill supplied with books[1]; but he certainly made diligent and skilful use of his literary materials, and produced in his ' Brief History of Epidemic and Pestilential Diseases,' a work which was better than any before it in the chronological part, and remains to the present time unique in its philosophical part for the boldness of its generalities[2]. He saw that influenza was the crux of epidemiology, and paid special attention to it.

In looking for the antecedents of influenza, he kept in view the greater telluric changes and convulsions, such as earthquakes and volcanic eruptions. He did not regard these as the cause of

[1] Cited by Horace E. Scudder, in *Noah Webster*. New York and London, 1881, p. 105.
[2] *Brief History of Epidemic and Pestilential Diseases.* 2 vols., Hartford, 1799.

influenza, but as the index of some hidden cause to which both they and the universal catarrh were due.

"It is probable to me," he says, "that neither seasons, earthquakes, nor volcanic eruptions are the causes of the principal derangements we behold in animal and vegetable life, but are themselves the *effects* of those motions and invisible operations which affect mankind. Hence catarrh and other epidemics often appear *before* the visible phenomena of eruptions and earthquakes[1]." As to influenza, he found "reason to conclude the disease to be the effect of some access of stimulant powers to the atmosphere by means of the electrical principle. No other principle in creation, which has yet come under the cognizance of the human mind, seems adequate to the same effects."

And again: "It is more probable that it is to be ascribed to an insensible action of atmospheric fire, which is more general and violent about the time of eruptions, and which fire is probably agitated in all parts of the globe, although it produces visible effects in explosions in some particular places only." It is due to Webster to give his reason for preferring a physical force to an organic poison: "If a deleterious vapour were the cause, I should suppose its effects would be speedy, and its force soon expended, the atmosphere being speedily purified by the winds. But if stimulus is the cause, it may exist for a long time in the atmosphere, and the human body not yield to its force in many weeks or months. This would better accord with facts. For, although diseases appear soon after an earthquake, yet the worst effects are often many months or years after[2]."

Dr Blagden also saw a difficulty in "the prodigious quantity of matter required in the air to infect the space not only of the Chinese land, but to a hundred leagues of the coast, or, as in this instance [1782] all Europe and the circumjacent sea," and was accordingly driven to Arbuthnot's view of an origin in the unusual weather of each locality.

Webster drew up a chronological table of influenzas in either Hemisphere, with the volcanic eruptions, earthquakes, comets, etc., to suit[3]. A few instances from near the beginning may serve as samples:

1647. First catarrh mentioned in American annals, in the same year with violent earthquakes in South America, and a comet.

1655. Influenza in America, in the same year with violent earthquakes in South America and an eruption of Vesuvius. It began about the end of June.

1658. Influenza in Europe after a severe winter: the summer cool.

---

[1] *Brief History of Epidemic and Pestilential Diseases*, II. 15.

[2] *Id.* II. 34, 84. Dr Robert Williams, in his work on *Morbid Poisons* (II. 670) argues for Webster's electrical theory of influenza without knowing, or at least without saying, that it was Webster's. The much-advertised writings of Mr John Parkin on *The Volcanic Theory of Epidemics* (or other title) follow Webster very closely both in the main idea and in its ramifications, but without acknowledgment to the American *philosophe*. Milton's rule was that one might take from an old author if one improved upon him; but neither Williams nor Parkin has improved upon Webster.

[3] *Ibid.* II. 30.

1675. Influenza in Europe while Etna was still in a state of explosion: the winter mild.

1679–80. Influenza in Europe during or just after the eruption of Etna: the season wet: a comet.

1688. Influenza in Europe in the same year with an eruption of Vesuvius, after a severe winter, and earthquakes: it began in a hot summer.

1693. Influenza in Europe in the same year with an eruption in Iceland and great earthquakes: the season cool.

1697–98. Influenza in America after a great earthquake in Peru: a comet the same year: the winter severe.

In most instances the region of the earthquake is not specified in the table; but it is sometimes named in the text of the annals under the respective years. Volcanoes are on the whole made more of than earthquakes, Webster's object being to find evidence of "electrical stimulus," and not of material miasmata discharged into the air. Etna and Hecla are much in request. Any earthquake suits, as if "earthquake" and "volcano" were like algebraic symbols, always *a* and *b*, and never anything but *a* and *b*, "influenza" being always *x*. One begins to realize the difficulties of the volcano or earthquake theory of influenza on turning to Mallet's Catalogue of Earthquakes[1]. Here, indeed, is an embarrassing choice between China and Peru, Asia Minor and North Africa, Portugal and Sicily or Calabria, Iceland and Jamaica, the Azores and the Philippines, Caracas or Acapulco and Valparaiso, Hungary and Savoy, Kamtschatka and Amboina; between earthquakes great and small; between earthquakes and volcanoes. Any influenza year might be suited with one or more earthquakes, perhaps in either Hemisphere; but there are some long clear intervals between the greater influenzas in Europe, for example the interval from 1803 to 1831, which seem to occupy as many pages of the catalogue of earthquakes as the years wherein influenzas came thickest, for example from 1729 to 1743, or from 1831 to 1847.

None the less, Webster, like Boyle, obeyed a true impulse when he looked for the cause of influenzas in something telluric, occasional, phenomenal. A wave of influenza comes up unexpectedly from a particular point of the compass, passes quickly over many degrees of latitude and longitude, lasting a few weeks at any given place, disappears in the distance, and does not return again perhaps for a whole generation. Influenza has the qualities of suddenness, swiftness, transitoriness; it has a certain

[1] "Catalogue of Recorded Earthquakes from 1606 B.C. to A.D. 1850." *British Assocn. Reports,* 1852–54.

sameness in its symptoms; it can be identified as certainly in the brief phrases of medieval chronicles as in elaborate modern descriptions; it has had no season for its own, as plague and cholera have had the summer and autumn, but has reached a height in Europe sometimes in midsummer, sometimes in mid-winter. No other epidemic malady can compare with it in these respects; all the rest seem to have been provoked more or less by the turns and changes in human affairs, some being of a medieval colour, others of a modern, each in its own way admitting of explanation from unwholesome living, or from famine, or from over-population, or from something more re-condite but still within the sphere of things insanitary in an intelligible sense. Other plagues besides influenza were, it is true, once reckoned mysterious, or associated in the popular mind with earthquakes and comets. But several such plagues have disappeared from among us, while their alleged causes, the earthquakes or comets, continue as before. Influenza alone returns at intervals as of old, untouched by civilization, by sani-tation, by the immense differences between medieval and modern, making the same impression upon England in the year 1890 as it did in 1173, or 1427, or 1580, or, if changed at all, then changed for the worse inasmuch as the epidemic came back more severely in 1891, and still more severely in 1892. It is not surprising that for such a disease something telluric or even cosmic should have been assigned as the cause, something as occasional as itself, phenomenal, if not cataclysmic. It may be proper, therefore, that we should try over again the philosophic generalities of Boyle, Arbuthnot and Webster, peradventure a combination of them may yield a true theory. From Boyle we may take the great principle of a progressive infection through regions of air (or leagues of ground), which was expressed once for all by Lucretius in the sixth book of the 'De Rerum Natura':

> ...atque aer inimicus serpere coepit;
> Ut nebula ac nubes paulatim repit, et omne
> Qua graditur, conturbat et immutare coactat;
> Fit quoque ut in nostrum quum venit denique coelum
> Corrumpat reddatque sui simile atque alienum.

From Arbuthnot we may take the organic source and nature of the influenzal miasmata, and the association with changes in the level of the water in the soil. From Webster we may take the idea that the historic influenzas, having been sudden,

occasional or phenomenal, must have had phenomenal causes somewhere in either Hemisphere. Instead of sketching a theory in the abstract, and safeguarding it by following all its ramifications, I shall proceed by the way of instances, choosing them so as to bring out particular points in order.

The only generality which may be indicated at starting is one that has presented itself time after time in the foregoing history, namely that there is something more than accident in the association between epidemics of influenza and epidemics of ague. So close was this association in former times that both the influenza and the widely prevalent ague were included together under such names as "the new ague," "the new fever," "the new distemper." As late as 1679, Morley did not distinguish the epidemic of influenza from the epidemic agues in the midst of which it was set, although the distinction was real, and was actually made by Sydenham on that occasion, as it had been made by Willis and in a manner by Whitmore on the occasion immediately preceding, and as it was made by everyone on the last great occasion when an influenza made an interlude among epidemic agues in the year 1782. It has often been suspected that influenza was related to some other infection: at one time it was taken for a volatile emanation of plague, in our own time it has been regarded as a volatile emanation of Asiatic cholera. In a wider historical view the question may arise, whether the real relation is not rather to those remarkable agues which have been epidemic in company with influenza when there was no plague and no cholera.

I come now to certain influenzas, as illustrating particular points of theory, in order.

I.

It is probable that Webster's theory of influenza as related to earthquakes and volcanoes, first published in 1799, was suggested to him by a communication to the Royal Society on the volcanic waves seen at Barbados on the 31st of March, 1761, and on the epidemic of influenza thereafter ensuing all over the island. At Bridgetown, in the afternoon of the 31st of March, 1761, the water in the bay and harbour ebbed and flowed to the extent of eighteen inches or two feet at intervals of eight minutes, and continued to do so for the space of three hours, the oscillation regularly decreasing till night when it was no more

observable. These tidal waves were due to volcanic upheavals somewhere; and it was found that the centre of disturbance had been in the Atlantic near the coast of Portugal, and the time some hours earlier than the waves were felt at Bridgetown. The Barbados chronicler procèeds :

"It is very remarkable that since that time the island has been in a very deplorable condition, having suffered under the severest colds that have been ever known. The distress has been so general that I may venture to assert (with confidence) that nineteen twentieths of the inhabitants of the island have felt the effects of the contagion; and to some it has been repeated several times. It has puzzled all the adepts in pharmacy to find out the cause and cure of it. One favourable circumstance has attended it, viz. few have died with it. The Leeward Islands have not escaped, it having raged there more violently and more fatal. His Majesty's ships have severely felt the effects of it, some of them not being capable of keeping the seas for want of men fit for service. This happening at a season of the year remarkably the healthiest, makes it the more surprising[1]."

This is as good an instance as we shall find, of explaining something sudden, swift, and phenomenal, by something else sudden, swift, and phenomenal, in a purely empirical way and without pausing to ask whether the latter could have been a *vera causa* of the former. That the influenza came to Barbados in the wake, as it were, of the volcanic waves, had been a common subject of talk among the residents; and that common opinion of the colony had found expression in the paper sent to the Royal Society. The influenza was not only in Barbados, in the Leeward Islands, and in the ships on the West Indian Station, but also in New England and "over the whole country" of the North American Colonies. Dr Tufts, of Weymouth, New England, wrote to Webster that "it began in April, and in May ran into a malignant fever which proved fatal to aged persons. It spread over the whole country and the West India Islands[2]." It was not until some nine months after that influenza appeared in Europe, at first in the east of that continent,—Hungary, Vienna, Breslau, Copenhagen—in February and March, 1762, in central Germany and Scotland in April, in London about the first of May and all over England and Ireland thereafter, but not in France until June and July. Precisely the same order was followed by the influenza twenty years after : it began in North America in March, 1781, and, says Webster, spread over that continent; it appeared in

[1] Abraham Mason, *Phil. Trans.* LII. Part 2, p. 477.
[2] Webster, I. 150.

the East Indies in October and November, 1781, and on the eastern confines of Europe in January, 1782, having been traced from Tobolsk, made a slow progress westwards, and was at its height in London about the end of May or beginning of June. Assuming, says Webster, that the American influenza of 1781 had been continuous with the European of 1782, it must have "passed the Pacific in high northern latitudes," traversed Siberia and Tartary, and so reached Russia in Europe. In like manner, if the European influenza of 1762 were continuous with the American of 1761, it must have made the circuit of the globe in the same order, as if it were following the first impulse of the volcanic waves across the Atlantic from the coast of Portugal westwards, and so round the earth until it came back to Europe on its eastern frontier. So much may be fairly advanced on the ground of a particular set of facts. But then there were many other facts, both in 1761–62, and in 1781–82. Meanwhile let us take another instance of volcanic waves felt at Barbados six years before, on the same afternoon as the great earthquake of Lisbon.

II.

At Bridgetown, on the 1st November, 1755, Dr Hillary saw the peculiar flux and reflux of the water in the harbour from 2.20 p.m. to 9 p.m. and pronounced that there must have been an earthquake somewhere. The waves came at first at intervals of five minutes, and at last at intervals of twenty minutes. The day was calm, and the ships in the bay were not touched; but small craft lying in the channel over the bar were driven to and fro with great violence. There was no motion of the earth, and no noise. The distance from Lisbon was 3400 miles, the vibrations having taken seven and a half hours to reach Barbados. The one notable effect in the harbour of Bridgetown was that the water flowed in and out with such a force that it tore up the black mud in the bottom of the channel, so that a great stench was sent forth and the fishes caused to float on the surface, many of them being driven a considerable distance on to the dry land where they were taken up by the negroes[1].

It so happened that there was an epidemic catarrh prevalent at that very time all over the island of Barbados, chiefly among

[1] Hillary, *Changes of the Air, etc.*, p. 82.

children, few or none of whom, white or black, escaped it. It had begun in October, says Hillary[1] (who chronicled the epidemiology very exactly), and continued into November, so that it both preceded and followed the great convulsion in the bed of the Atlantic, which destroyed Lisbon and tore up the mud in the harbour of Bridgetown, disengaging a great stench therefrom and poisoning the fish. Webster's theory of a relation between earthquakes and influenzas provides for such discrepancies in the dates of each: it is probable, he says, that seasons, earthquakes and volcanic eruptions are themselves the effects of those motions and invisible operations which affect mankind, so that catarrh and other epidemics often appear *before* the visible phenomena of eruptions and earthquakes. In like manner, the chronicler of the earthquake of Lisbon in the *Philosophical Transactions* drew attention to the fact that there had been a remarkable drought for several years before, and that some of the springs near Lisbon were actually dried up at the time. That droughts precede earthquakes is perhaps the most instructive generality that has yet been reached as to the cause of the latter.

Let us see, then, whether any such remote antecedents, in a possible relation to the influenza epidemics, hold good for the island of Barbados. Hillary's chronicle is sufficiently full to let us answer the question.

Following the seasons and prevalent maladies backwards from the influenza of children in October–November, 1755, we find a catarrhal fever all over Barbados in February of the same year, which "few escaped having more or less of." The immediate precursor of that influenza had been a very definite constitution, eighteen months long, of a "slow nervous fever," from February, 1753 to September, 1754, which corresponds in every respect to the "remittent" fever of nearly the same period in England and Ireland, described by Fothergill, Rutty, Huxham and Johnstone, and to the famous Rouen fever described by Le Cat. Hillary is clear that the "slow nervous fever" was not seen again so long as he remained in the colony (1758). Just before it began, there had been an influenza so general in December, 1752, and January, 1753, "that few people, either white or black, escaped having it," and that, in turn, was preceded by a season of agues, which, says Hillary, "are never seen in Barbados now [1758], unless brought hither from some place of the Leeward Islands."

So many influenzas in Barbados, and so many things possibly relevant to them among their antecedents. So also in New England, the influenza which seemed to follow the earthquake

[1] Hillary, *Changes of the Air, etc.*, p. 80.

along the coast of Portugal on the 31st of March, 1761, had the
same remittent and intermittent fevers among its antecedents.

In the winter and spring of 1760–61 there had been much fever in New
England, which was believed to be malarious. Webster, however, says:
" There is no necessity of resorting to marsh exhalations for the source of
this malady. The same species of fever [as at Bethlem] prevailed in that
winter and the spring following in many other parts of Connecticut where no
marsh existed. In Hartford it carried off a number of robust men, in two or
three days from the attack...In North Haven it attacked few persons, but
everyone of them died. In East Haven died about forty-five men in the
prime of life, mostly heads of families. The same disease prevailed in New
Haven among the inhabitants and students in college." In Bethlem the
sickness began in November, 1760, and carried off about forty of the
inhabitants in the winter following. This was the fever, generally reckoned
malarious, which preceded the influenza of April and May, 1761 [1].

III.

The next great influenza, twenty years after, which was in
America in the spring of 1781 and in Europe in the winter and
spring following, will repay the same kind of scrutiny. There had
been influenza here or there in Europe since the beginning of
1780, but no great epidemic of it ; and in England, as elsewhere,
there had been epidemic agues and dysenteries since that year,
or the autumn before. The epidemic agues became worse in
England in 1783, 1784, and 1785, appearing in places which had
never been thought malarious. The whole period from 1780
to 1784 was remarkable for hot and dry summers and great
earthquakes. Italy and Sicily were troubled by earthquakes to
an unusual extent in 1780, 1781, 1782, and 1783 ; they were so
frequent in 1781 that the pope ordered public prayers. The
great earthquake of the period was in Calabria at half an hour
after noon of the 5th of February, 1783, about six months after
the great influenza of the period was over. Sir William
Hamilton, the British ambassador at Naples, visited the
numerous scenes of the earthquake in Calabria and Sicily
in the first fortnight of May, 1783, and sent to the Royal
Society an account of what he saw. At several places he found
fever epidemic, part of it from the overcrowding and filth of
the temporary barracks in which the people were living, part of
it malarious from the damming of water by changes in the river
beds. At Palmi the spilt oil mixed with the corn of the overthrown
granaries, and the corrupted bodies, had a sensible effect on the

[1] Webster, I. 250.

air, which threatened an epidemic; at the village of Torre del Pezzolo an epidemical disorder had already manifested itself[1].

But the most striking effect of the earthquake was that a dry fog began in Calabria in February, and overspread until autumn the greater part of Europe, extending even to the Azores. This fog, though not consisting apparently of moisture, was so dense that the sky was quite obscured, appearing a light grey colour instead of blue, while the sun became a blood-red disc. In Calabria the darkness was so great that lights were needed in the houses, and ships came into collision at sea. There was a most disagreeable odour[2]. The fog spreading over all Europe from Calabria was not at all mythical, as we are apt to suppose that similar recorded phenomena of the wonder-loving Middle Ages may have been. The phenomenon was independently re-produced in Iceland the same year, from the 1st to the 11th of June, causing the same darkness at sea, the same atmospheric effects at a distance, but not to so great a distance, and some amount of sickness, but seemingly not aguish or febrile, among the population[3].

Those two great convulsions of the year 1783, each of them the cause of a widely spreading dry fog, may have been con-ceivably the cause of pestiferous miasmata in the air, such as the corresponding hypothesis of influenza requires; but how little comparable or equivalent were the miasmata—in the one case from the ancient and well-peopled soil of Southern Italy, in the other from the inhospitable Danish colony just without the Arctic Circle! In any case, the earthquakes of 1783 were both too late for the great influenza of the period. The antecedent common alike to the influenza and the earthquakes was the extraordinary droughts, which caused famine and famine-fever in Iceland, and, according to old experience, was probably related to the epidemic prevalence of agues in Britain and on the continent of Europe.

---

[1] Hamilton, *Phil. Trans.* LXXIII. 176.   [2] Mallet's Catalogue, u. s.
[3] Holm, *Vom Erdbrande auf Island im Jahre* 1783, Kopenhagen, 1784, says: "Since the outbreak began, the atmosphere of the whole country has been full of vapour, smoke and dust, so much so that the sun looked brownish-red, and the fishermen could not find the banks....Old people, especially those with weak chests, suffered much from the smell of sulphur and the volcanic vapours, being afflicted with dyspnoea. Various persons in good health fell ill, and more would have suffered had not the air been cooled and refreshed from time to time by rains," pp. 57, 60. The real sickness of Iceland in those years had been before the volcanic eruptions, in 1781 and 1782, when some parts of the island were almost depopulated by the famine and pestilential fevers that followed the unusual seasons.

IV.

What kind or kinds of epidemic sickness earthquakes may produce as an effect immediate and at the place, will appear from other instances. One of the most remarkable of earthquakes was that which destroyed Port Royal and nearly all the planters' houses and sugar-works throughout the island of Jamaica on the 7th of June, 1692. Jamaica had been an English colony for little more than thirty years, during which time it had passed from its state of lethargy under the Spaniards into an emporium of commerce with a rapidly growing population of slaves and whites. The business capital was at Port Royal, wholly built since the British occupation. The site of it was a sandy key or shoal which was said to have risen perceptibly within the memory of original settlers ; a writer in September, 1667, said of it: "wherever you dig five or six feet, water will appear which ebbs and flows as the tide. It is not salt, but brackish[1]." A quay had been built along this spit of land, at which vessels of 700 tons could lie afloat. . It was here that the havoc of the earthquake was most complete.

Sloane, who had visited Jamaica a few years before, said that the inhabitants expect an earthquake every year, and that some of them were of opinion that they follow their great rains[2]. The year 1692 began in Jamaica with very dry and hot weather which continued until May: then came gales and heavy rains until the end of the month, and from that time until the day of the earthquake, the 7th of June, the weather was excessively hot, calm and dry. The shakes began at 11.40 a.m., and at the third shake, the ground of nearly all Port Royal fell in suddenly, so that in the course of a minute or two most of the houses were under water and the whole wharf was covered by the sea to the depth of several fathoms. The loss of life was, of course, greatest where population was densest ; but in the interior of the island the effects on the soil were greater than at the shore: in the north a thousand acres of land sank and thirteen people with it ; mountains on either side of a narrow gorge came together and blocked the way ; wide chasms appeared in the

---

[1] *Phil. Trans.* II. (1667), p. 499.
[2] *Ibid.* March–Apr. 1694, p. 81. Sloane had himself felt several shocks at Port Royal on the 20th October, 1687, between four and six o'clock in the morning, which were due to the same earthquake that destroyed Lima in Peru.

ground, and on one mountain side there were some dozen
openings from which brackish water spouted forth. The first
effect in the streets of Port Royal was that men and women
seemed all at once to be floundering up to the neck in the wet
shifting sand, and were speedily drowned or floated away by
the inrushing water. The shakes ceased for days at a time, and
then began again, five or six perhaps in twenty-four hours; so
that those who had escaped to ships in the bay remained on
board for two months, being afraid to come ashore. The
weather was hotter after the earthquake than before, and mos-
quitoes swarmed in unheard of numbers.

During the upheavals or subsidences in Port Royal, and
the rushing of water into or from the gapings in the ground, "ill
stenches and offensive smells" arose, so that "by means of the
openings and the vapours at that time belcht forth from the
earth into the air, the sky, which before was clear and blue, was
in a minute's time become dull and reddish looking (as I have
heard it compared often) like a red-hot oven." A very great
mortality followed among those who had escaped the earthquake. Some of them settled at Leguanea, others at the place
on the bay which became the Kingston of later history, enduring many hardships in their hastily built shelters, from the
heavy rains that followed the earthquake, and from want of
clothes, food and comforts.

One writes: "Our people settled a town at Leguanea side; and there is
about five hundred graves already [20th September, 1692], and people every
day is dying still. I went about once to see it, and I had like to have tipt
off." Another says: "Almost half the people that escaped upon Port
Royal are since dead of a malignant fever": and another, referring to the
hasty settlement on the bay at Kingston, says "they died miserably in
heaps." But the most interesting information is his next sentence : "Indeed
there was a general sickness (supposed to proceed from the hurtful vapours
belched from the many openings of the earth) all over the island, so general
that few escaped being sick: and 'tis thought it swept away in all parts of
the island three thousand souls, the greatest part from Kingstown, only yet
an unhealthy place[1]."

That great mortality from a malignant fever after the earthquake of 7th June, 1692, is usually counted an epidemic of the
yellow fever which became established at Kingston and Port
Royal from that time for at least a century and a half. I have
not found any contemporary medical account of it, but all the

[1] *Phil. Trans.* XVIII. p. 83 (March–April, 1794). Series of reports from Jamaica
collected by Sloane.

later writers on yellow fever at Kingston and Port Royal have accepted the tradition that it was yellow fever. But there was one peculiarity, which marks it off from all subsequent epidemics of yellow fever—the sickness was all over the island, so general that few escaped being sick, and was supposed to proceed from the hurtful vapours belched from the many openings of the ground in and near Port Royal. In all subsequent experience yellow fever has been almost confined to the shore or to the ships in the bay[1]. Certainly it has never been all over the island as in 1692, "so general that few escaped being sick": that is rather in the manner of influenza, although there is nothing to show that the sickness of the interior was so different from that of the shore as to be counted an influenza, or that the mortality of the sick was other than that of a "malignant fever."

The earthquake at Port Royal in 1692 produced "ill stenches and offensive smells." The tidal waves, or the subterranean vibrations which caused them, in tearing up the mud at the bottom of the channel at Bridgetown, Barbados, in 1755, had in like manner sent forth a great stench which poisoned the fish. Such offensive vapours were supposed in former times to come, as in a figure, from "the bowels of the earth"; and undoubtedly the sulphurous fumes which have overhung the region of Sicilian earthquakes must have had a source as deep as the strange minerals or "fossils" of Boyle's hypothesis. But, while the commotion of an earthquake is deep, it is also superficial; whatever miasmata issue from the ground in the ordinary alternations of wet and drought, would be discharged into the atmosphere in unusual quantity and with unusual force in such disturbances of soil as sunk Port Royal in 1692 or were felt at Barbados across the whole width of the Atlantic in 1755. Nor is that effect upon miasmata instantaneous or quickly past; in Jamaica the rumblings and shakes lasted for nearly two months, during which time the pressure upon the gases in the subsoil must have been such as to make them pass into the atmosphere in stronger ascending currents than the mere alternations of moisture and drought would have done. And just as the ordinary seasonal changes in the level of the ground-water are

---

[1] A few cases have been exceptionally seen at Spanish Town, six miles from the head of the bay, the infection of which was supposed to have been brought from the shore by sailors, and it has also prevailed in the barracks on the high ground of Newcastle not far from the shore.

of little or no account for miasmatic-infective disease unless the soil in which they occur be full of organic impurities from human occupancy, so one may reason that the great cataclysmic changes of the earth's crust are, in this hypothesis of influenza, of most account as touching the stratum of soil wherein lie organic impurities, and as touching those areas of the surface,— the sites of cities, the populous plains, the shores of bays, the bottoms of harbours or any other definite spots—in which the products of organic decomposition are present in largest amount and, perhaps, of somewhat special kind. Such impurities of the soil are indeed a *vera causa* of infective disease, known to be capable of the effect which has to be accounted for; and, as discharged into the air in great volume and with great force by some upheaval, they would make a local beginning of that "aer inimicus" which the Roman poet figures as creeping like a mist from one region of the heavens to another so that it corrupts each successive tract of air with its own baleful qualities, "reddatque sui simile atque alienum."

But, as soon as we begin to apply this formula to particular historic cases, difficulties and ambiguities arise[1]. To come back to the instance of Jamaica in 1692, did the general sickness of the island, manifestly miasmatic as it was, and due to disturbances of soil, become an influenza for other regions of the globe? About fifteen months after there was, indeed, a universal catarrh in Britain and Ireland, of no great fatality, which is said by Molyneux, of Dublin, to have prevailed also in the northern parts of France, Flanders, and Holland, but is not reported in the usual way from Europe generally nor from America. Let us suppose a miasmatic cloud formed over the

[1] Without seeking to argue for the connexion between particular earthquakes and influenzas, but merely to illustrate the possibilities, I append here an instance that ought not to be overlooked. On the 1st of November, 1835, there was a great earthquake in the Moluccas, which so completely changed the soil of the island of Amboina, that it became notably subject to deadly miasmatic or malarious fevers from that time forth. For three weeks before the earthquake the atmosphere had been full of a heavy sulphurous fog, so that miasmata were rising from the soil by some unwonted pressure before the actual cataclysm. There is no doubt at all that Amboina became "malarious" in a most marked degree from the date of the earthquake; it is a classical instance of the sudden effect of great changes in the earth's crust upon the frequency and malignity of remittent and intermittent fevers, according to the testimony of physicians in the Dutch East Indian service. The influenza nearest to the earthquake was about a year after, at Sydney, Cape Town, and in the East Indies, during October and November, 1836. The epidemic appeared about the same time in the north-east of Europe, spread all over the continent, and reached London in January, 1837. There was again influenza in Australia and New Zealand in November, 1838, two years after the last outbreak in that region.

island of Jamaica in June, July, August and September, a cloud of infective particles which might produce influenza at a distance from its place of origin, whatever disease the miasmata after the earthquake may have produced in Jamaica itself. Let this invisible cloud, or emanation, get into the warm atmosphere over the great oceanic current that sets out from the Gulf of Mexico. The vehicle lies ready to hand,—to receive the miasmata not far from their place of origin, to carry them far into the Atlantic, and to bring them, perhaps, to the shores of Britain. This may seem a sufficiently plausible source of the influenza of October and November, 1693, which appears to have been felt only in the British Isles and on the opposite shores of the North Sea. But Webster's own choice is the volcanic eruption in Iceland in the same year as the influenza; and if we prefer, in this hypothesis, an earthquake to an active volcano, there is a rival source for the British influenza of 1693, nearer both in place and time than that of Jamaica in 1692, and not less important in respect of miasmatic disease in its own locality. This was the disastrous series of earthquakes in Calabria and Sicily, culminating on the 9th of January, 1693. The following extracts from the account sent to the Royal Society will show how great was the commotion of soil, of underground water, and of atmosphere, and how close the connexion of these with the sickness ensuing[1]:

"In the plain of Catania, an open place, it is reported that from one of the clefts in the ground, narrow but very long and about four miles off the sea, the water was thrown forth altogether as salt as that of the sea, [as in Jamaica the year before]. In Syracuse and other places near the sea, the waters in many wells, which at first were salt, are become fresh again... The fountain Arethusa for the space of some months was so brackish that the Syracusans could make no use of it, and now that it is grown sweeter the spring is increased to near double. In the city of Termini all the running waters are dried up...It was contrary with the hot-baths, which were augmented by a third part.

Darkness and obscurity of the air has always been over us, but still inferior to that on the 10th and 11th of January; and often these clouds have been thin and light, and of a great extent, such as the authors call *rarae nubeculae.* The sun often and the moon always obscured at the rising and setting, and the horizon all day long dusky...

The effects it has had on humane bodies (although I do not believe they have all immediately been caused by the earthquake) have (yet) been various : such as foolishness (but not to any great degree), madness, dulness, sottishness, and stolidity everywhere : hypochondriack, melancholick and cholerick distempers. Every-day fevers have been common, with many continual and tertian : malignant, mortal and dangerous ones in a great

[1] *Phil. Trans.* for the year 1694, p. 5.

27—2

number, with deliria and lethargies. Where there has been any infection caused by the natural malignity of the air, infinite mortality has followed. The smallpox has made great destruction among children."

Thus we find in Sicily a great disturbance of soil followed, as in Jamaica, by a great increase of local sickness, and by an atmosphere visibly charged with products of the earthquake for months after. This is a nearer source than the Jamaican for the British influenza of Oct.-Nov. 1693,—nearer in time, if that be any advantage for the theory, nearer also in place. There are, however, no intermediate stages to connect the influenza on the northern edge of the European continent with the disturbance of soil and the miasmata arising therefrom in Sicily and Calabria. If there had been any such dry fog as spread all over Europe from the Calabrian earthquake of January, 1783, it would have been a help at least to the imagination in bridging over a gulf of space and time.

As to the interval of time, it should at all events be kept in mind that the same difficulty has to be reckoned with in any hypothesis of influenza and in every great historic instance. In the instance still before us, the infection began in England, according to Molyneux, in October, 1693, and was in Dublin a month later. But we must assume it to have been in the air for some time before it became effective upon mankind. Influenza has been observed, with curious uniformity, to attack the horses, say of London, of Plymouth, of Edinburgh, or of Dublin (as on the occasion before this, 1688) two months or more in advance of the inhabitants of the respective places; and if it had waited, so to speak, for two months before it showed its effects upon men, it may have waited equally long, or longer, before it showed its effects upon horses. That would give at least four months; and then we know, from such an influenza as that of 1743, that there may be weeks, perhaps months, between its prevalence in Naples, Rome or Milan, and its prevalence in London or Edinburgh, and, from the influenza of 1693 itself, that it was a month later in Dublin than in London. An earthquake in Sicily on the 9th of January, 1693, with effects there for months after upon the water, the air, and the prevalent diseases, is not excluded by lapse of time from being a *vera causa* of an influenza in England in October of the same year, and in Ireland in November. The sort of proof which most men desire, a proof such as we rarely get, and one

that is suspiciously neat when we do get it, would be to find an influenza in Sicily and Calabria following the earthquake, and to trace the same step by step over Europe. But the miasmatic sickness in the countries of the earthquakes was not influenza, so far as is known; and there was no epidemic catarrh, so far as is known, in any other part of Europe but the British Isles and the neighbouring shores of the North Sea.

V.

Molyneux, who recorded with a good deal of circumstance the influenza of 1693, is the principal authority, along with Dr Walter Harris, of London, for another influenza in 1688, seemingly peculiar to the British Isles. Its effects can be discovered with the utmost certainty in the London bills of mortality for two or three weeks at the end of May and beginning of June, and it is mentioned as "the new distemper" in letters of the time. Is it possible to find an earthquake for it? Webster's note is: "in the same year with an eruption of Vesuvius, after a severe winter and earthquakes"—which is somewhat general. Turning to Evelyn's diary, where these matters are often recorded, we find, in the very weeks when the influenza was at a height in London, this entry: "News arrived of the most prodigious earthquake that was almost ever heard of, subverting the city of Lima and country in Peru, with a dreadfull inundation following it"—as if the influenza and the news of the earthquake had reached London at the same time. This was the earthquake of 20th October, 1687, which destroyed Lima, Callao and an immense district along the coast of Peru. The rocking of the earth was most violent, the sea retreated like a sudden immense ebb and filled again like a sudden immense flood, the effect of the commotion being felt on board ships a hundred and fifty leagues out in the Pacific. It was remarked that wheat and barley would not thrive in Peru after that earthquake[1]. Here was undoubtedly a great disturbance of soil and of subsoil, almost certainly attended with the discharge of effluvia or miasmata into the air, as in other great earthquakes. But the universal slight fever of the British Isles in the months of June and July, 1688, is remote from the earth-

[1] Mallet, "First Report on the Facts of Earthquake Phenomena." *Trans. Brit. Assoc. for* 1850, Lond. 1851. Cited from von Hoff.

quake of Lima in place ; and, if it be a question of earthquakes at all, there are others nearer to it both in place and time, such as that in the Basilicata province of Naples in January, 1688, and the Jamaica earthquake, felt through all the island, on the 1st of March, 1688. The greatest of them all, that of Smyrna, on the 10th of July, was a few weeks too late for the hypothesis.

VI.

A continent so subject to earthquakes as South America might be expected, in this hypothesis, to have had some corresponding influenzas. It has indeed had influenzas, some of them peculiar to itself. The Western Hemisphere as a whole has, on several great occasions, had influenzas which were not felt in the Old World. Again, there are one or two instances in which the infection, while it spread widely over the table-lands of Bolivia and Peru, does not appear by existing testimony to have been carried north of the Isthmus. One of these was the influenza of 1720, as special to a region of South America as that of 1688 was to the British Isles. The account of it was given in an essay by Botoni 'On the Circulation of the Blood,' published at Lima in 1723[1]. He calls it *catarro maligno*; it was popularly known as *fierro chuto* or "iron cap." It appeared at Cuzco in the end of March, or beginning of April, 1720, and was over about November. Four thousand are said to have died of it in the diocese of Cuzco, and it is said to have made so great a scarcity of hands that the first harvest after it was imperfectly gathered. It had all the marks of an influenza, with the addition of bleeding from the nose and lungs. It had also the grand characteristic common to influenza and epidemic ague: "the symptoms were so diverse and even contradictory that no correct diagnosis, or curative plan, could be fixed." The Lima writer of 1723 says that it followed an eclipse of the sun on the 15th of August, 1719, having begun on the eastern side of the Andes, in the basin of La Plata, about that time, and travelled northwards and westwards, as the South American influenza of 1759 did.

This is a localized influenza in a country of earthquakes. But the two great earthquakes in 1719 are not South American.

---

[1] Archibald Smith, M.D., "Notices of the Epidemics of 1719–20 and 1759 in Peru," etc. *Trans. Epid. Soc.* II. pt. 1, p. 134. From the *Medical Gazette of Lima*, 15 March, 1862.

They both happened in July: one along the coast of Fez and Morocco, which ruined many villages and a part of the city of Morocco (there is also a later disturbance in the Azores in December, followed by the upheaval of a new island), the other in North China. Here we have the choice of following the "aer inimicus" of Lucretius either from China or from the African coast; and if it be the case that the influenza began in the latter part of the year 1719 in the basin of the La Plata, to cross the Andes next year, it may seem, in this hypothesis, that a course from east to west, bringing the infection across the Atlantic from Africa, is to be preferred to a course from west to east, bringing it across the Pacific from North China. In either case there need be no difficulty in finding local clouds of miasmata. Some traces of the corresponding great earthquake in China were found in November of the following year, by Bell, an English traveller who crossed from Moscow to Peking:

"Jumy," he says, "suffered greatly by the earthquakes that happened in the month of July the preceding year [1719], above one half of it being thereby laid in ruins. Indeed more than one half of the towns and villages through which we travelled this day had suffered much on the same occasion, and vast numbers of people had been buried in the ruins. I must confess it was a dismal scene to see everywhere such heaps of rubbish[1]."

The atmospheric effects of Chinese earthquakes have been pictured since medieval times, in obviously superstitious colours; and there are reasons why a great disturbance of soil in that country should produce remarkable miasmata. The surface soil of China is peculiar in having the bodies of the dead dispersed at large in it, insomuch that excavations for the foundations of houses, or for roads and railway cuttings, can hardly be made without the constant risk of exposing graves[2].

If the soil of China is peculiar in one way, that of the West Coast of Africa is peculiar in another. Without entering on the large question of "malaria" in each of them, I shall take an old illustration of the miasmata of the West Coast of Africa as a

---

[1] Bell's Travels, in Pinkerton, VII. 377.
[2] See an article "Railways—their Future in China," by W. B. Dunlop, in *Blackwood's Magazine*, March, 1889, pp. 395–6. A letter in the *Pall Mall Gazette*, dated 23 May, 1891, and signed "Shanghai," recalled the outbreak of Hongkong fever, "the symptoms of which bore a curious resemblance to the influenza epidemic," at the time when much building was going on upon the slope of Victoria Peak : "It was said at the time—I do not know with what truth—that in this turning-up of the soil, several old Chinese burying-places were included."

cause of dengue-fever, a disease curiously like influenza in its symptoms, and like it also in its occasional wave-like dispersion over wide regions. The authority is Dr Aubrey, who resided many years on the coast of Guinea, saw much of the slave-trade, and wrote a very sensible book in 1729, called 'The Sea Surgeon, or the Guinea Man's Vade Mecum.' He describes quite clearly the fever which was long after described by West Indian physicians as dengue, or three-days' fever, or break-bone fever, including in his description the characteristic exanthems of it and the penetrating odour of the sweat. He gives also, in clinical form, a series of cases on board the galley 'Peterborough' in December, 1717, which are exquisite examples of break-bone fever. This disease, he says, " many times runs over the whole ship, as well negroes as white men, for they infect one the other, and the ship is then in a very deplorable condition unless they have an able man to take care of them." But the original source of infection, he believed, was the fogs that hung at nightfall over the estuaries of the rivers; and he gives an experimental proof, remarkable but not quite incredible, of the poisonous nature of the miasmata:

"But to let you see the evil, malevolent, contagious, destructive quality of those fogs that fall there in the night, and how far they are inimical to human nature, I will tell you of an experiment of my own. I made a lump of paste with oat-meal somewhat hard, and about the bigness of a hen's egg, which was exposed to the fog from twilight to twilight, i.e. from the dusk of the evening till daybreak in the morning; after which I crumbled it, and gave it to fowls, which we had on board, and soon after they had eaten it, they turned round and in a kind of vertigo dropt down and expired."

A great mortality in Guinea in 1754 or 1755 was ascribed by Lind, the least credulous in such matters, to "a noxious stinking fog[1]."

What the alternations of heat and chill, of moisture and drought, produce ordinarily in the way of miasmata, the same, we may suppose, is produced on the great scale, as a phenomenon at some particular time and place, by one of those cataclysms which break the surface of the earth or the bed of the sea, lower or raise the level of wells and springs, and fill the air with particles of dust or vapour which may overhang the locality for months and visibly disperse themselves to a great distance. Nothing relating to miasmata in the air need be hard

[1] *Essay on the Most Effective Means of preserving the Health of Seamen in the Royal Navy.* London, 1757, p. 83.

for belief after the wonderful diffusion and permanence in the atmosphere of the whole globe, for two years or more, of finely divided particles shot up by the earthquakes and eruptions of Krakatoa in the Straits of Sunda on the 27th and 28th of August, 1883[1].

A theory of influenza constructed from such generalities as those of Boyle, Arbuthnot and Webster will have attractions for many over the theory that influenza is always present in some remote country and becomes dispersed now and then over the world by contagion from person to person : it will have superior attractions, for the reason that influenza is a phenomenal thing which needs a phenomenal cause to account for it. But if anyone were to attempt to fit each historic wave of influenza with its particular earthquake, or to find the precise locality where clouds of infective matter had arisen, or the particular circumstances in which they arose, he would certainly find his fragile structure of probabilities pulled to pieces by the professed discouragers and depravers. I make no such attempt ; but I am not the less persuaded of the direction in which the true theory of influenza lies.

Influenza at Sea.

There is no point more essential to a correct theory of influenza than to find out in what circumstances it has occurred among the crews of ships on the high seas. If it be true that a ship may sail into an atmosphere of influenza, just as she may sail into a fog, or an oceanic current, or the track of a cyclone, then the possible hypotheses touching the nature, source, and mode of diffusion of influenza become narrowed down within definite limits.

One of the first observations was made in the case of a Scotch vessel in the influenza of 1732–33[2]. The epidemic was earlier in Scotland than in England; it began suddenly in Edinburgh on 17 December, 1732, the horses having been attacked with running of the nose towards the end of October. About the time when the disease began among mankind, in December, a vessel, the 'Anne and Agnes' sailed from Leith for Holland. One sailor was sick on this voyage. She sailed on the return voyage to Leith, with the other ten of her crew in perfect health. Just as she made the English coast at Flamborough Head on the 15th of January, 1733, six of the sailors fell ill together, two more the next day, and one more on the day after

[1] See *The Eruption of Krakatoa and subsequent phenomena.* Report of the Krakatoa Committee of the Royal Society....Edited by G. J. Symons, London, 1888.
[2] *Edin. Med. Essays and Obs.* II. 32.

that, so that when the vessel anchored in Leith Roads there was only one man well, and he fell ill on the day following the arrival. The symptoms were the common ones of the reigning epidemic. The dates are not given more precisely or fully than as above. Influenza was prevalent in Germany and Holland somewhat earlier than in Scotland or England; the men may, of course, have imbibed the infection when they were in the Dutch port, just as it is almost certain that the crews of Drake's fleet in 1587 had received during a ten days' stay upon the island of St Jago, of the Cape de Verde group, the miasmatic infection of which they suddenly fell sick in large numbers together in mid-Atlantic some six days after sailing to the westward.

This early case of the 'Anne and Agnes' in 1733 may pass as an ambiguous one. The next occasion when influenza on board ship attracted much notice was the epidemic of 1782.

On the 6th of May, Admiral Kempenfelt sailed from Spithead with seven ships of the line and a frigate, on a cruize to the westward; on the 18th May, he came into Torbay, and sailed again soon after; on the 30th May he came again into Torbay with eight sail of the line and three frigates, and on 1 June sailed again to the westward. Sometime before his squadron put into Torbay for the second time, influenza had appeared among them at sea, it is said in the 'Goliath' on the 29th of May[1]. A letter from Plymouth, of the 2nd June, after referring to the violence of influenza in that town, at the Dock, and on board the men-of-war lying there, says that the 'Fortitude' of 74 guns, and 'Latona' frigate came in that afternoon with 250 sick men from the fleet under Admiral Kempenfelt, mostly with fevers. Another Plymouth letter two days later (4 June) says: "Kempenfelt is returning to Torbay: he could keep the sea no longer, on account of the sickness that rages on board his fleet. More than 400 men have been brought to the hospital this morning. Our men drop down with it by scores at a time. The 'Latona' frigate, that sailed the other day is returned, the officers being the only hands that could work the ship[2]."

This outbreak on board ships in the Channel was fully as early as the great development of influenza in 1782 on shore, whether in London or Plymouth; but there were almost certainly cases of it at the latter port before the 'Latona' sailed to join Kempenfelt's squadron. Robertson, however, who was surgeon on the 'Romney' in the Channel service at that time, says that "hundreds in different ships, towns, and counties, which had *no* communication with one another, were seized nearly as suddenly and so nigh the same instant as if they had been electrified.... The companies of many of the ships were very well at bed-time, and in the morning there were hardly enough able to do the common business of the ship[3]." This is confirmed by McNair, surgeon of the 'Fortitude,' who told Trotter that two hundred

[1] *Trans. Col. Phys.* III. 62. [2] *Gent. Magaz.* 1782, p. 306.
[3] R. Robertson, M.D., *Observations on Jail, Hospital or Ship Fever from the 4th April, 1776, to the 30th April,* 1789. Lond. 1789, New ed., p. 411.

of her men, as she lay in Torbay, were seized in one night and were unable to come on deck in the morning[1].

There was another English fleet in the North Sea at the same time, under Lord Howe, watching the Dutch fleet or seeking to intercept the Dutch East Indiamen.

Howe sailed from St Helen's on the 9th May, with twelve ships of the line. Towards the end of that month he had his fleet in the Texel; the men were in excellent health, "when a cutter arrived from the Admiralty, and the signal was given for an officer from each ship [to come on board the admiral]. An officer was accordingly sent with a boat's crew from every vessel, and returned with orders, carrying with them also, however, the influenza"—which soon prostrated the crews to the same extraordinary extent as in the ships under Kempenfelt at the other end of the Channel. This was the oral account given to Professor Gregory of Edinburgh, by a lieutenant on board a sixty-four gun ship[2]. Another account says that the disorder first appeared in Howe's fleet on the Dutch coast about the end of May, on board the 'Ripon,' and in two days after in the 'Princess Amelia'; other ships of the same fleet were affected with it at different periods, some indeed, not until their return to Portsmouth about the second week of June. "This fleet, also, had no communication with the shore until their return to the Downs, on their way back to Portsmouth, towards the 3d and 4th of June[3]."

But, apart from the story of the Admiralty despatch-boat carrying the influenza to Howe's squadron, it appears that both Kempenfelt and Howe were joined from time to time by additional ships, which might have carried an atmosphere of influenza with them[4]. Still, it was an influenza atmosphere that they had carried, and not merely so many sick persons. The doctrine of contagion from person to person would have to be so widened as to become meaningless, if all those experiences of the fleet in 1782 were to be brought within it. In the history both of sweating sickness and of influenza, there are instances of the disease breaking out suddenly in a place after someone's arrival; but the new arrival may not have had the disease, it was enough that he came from a place where the disease was[5]. That was, perhaps, the reason why Beddoes, in his inquiry of 1803, framed one of his questions so as to elicit information about the dispersal of influenza by *fomites.*

[1] Trotter, *Medicina Nautica*, I. 1797. p. 367.
[2] Notes of a lecture on Influenza, by Gregory, taken by Christison about the year 1817, in the *Life of Sir Robert Christison*, I. 82.
[3] College of Physicians' Report, *Trans. Col. Phys.* III. 63.
[4] This is inferred from the varying number of ships in the two fleets in the several notices of their movements in the *Gentleman's Magazine*, for May and June, 1782.
[5] Brian Tuke to Peter Vannes, 14 July, 1528: "For when a whole man comes from London and talks of the sweat, the same night all the town is full of it, and thus it spreads as the fame runs." *Cal. State Papers, Henry VIII.* IV. 1971.

It is not easy to prove that a ship may meet with an atmosphere of influenza on the high seas; but many have believed that ships have done so. Webster says: "The disease invades seamen on the ocean in the same [western] hemisphere, when a hundred leagues from land, at the same time that it invades people on shore. Of this I have certain evidence from the testimony of American captains of vessels, who have been on their passage from the continent to the West India Islands during the prevalence of this disease[1]." There are several instances of this, authenticated with times, places, and other data of credibility.

The best known of these is the voyage of the East Indiaman 'Asia' in September, 1780, through the China Sea from Malacca to Canton: "When the ship left Malacca, there was no epidemic disease in the place; when it arrived at Canton it was found that at the very time when they had the *Influenza* on board the Atlas (*sic*) in the China seas, it had raged at Canton with as much violence as it did in London in June, 1782, and with the very same symptoms[2]."

In the present century, the cases nearly all come from the medical reports of the navies of Great Britain, France, Germany and the Netherlands, and they relate to ships on foreign service —in the East Indies, the Pacific, Africa, or other foreign stations. In some of the instances influenza went through a ship's company in port or in a roadstead, others are examples of outbreaks at sea:

1837: "The ship's company of the ' Raleigh,' were attacked by epidemic catarrh—influenza—first in March, while at sea between Singapore and Manilla, and again, although less severely, in June and July while on the coast of China...Influenza also made its appearance amongst the crew of the ' Zebra ' in April while she lay at Penang; it was supposed to have been contracted by infection from the people on shore, as they were then suffering from it. No death occurred under this head[3]."

1838: In the ' Rattlesnake,' at Diamond Harbour, in the Hooghly River, a large proportion of the men were suffering from epidemic catarrh. Intermittent fever made its appearance; "the change from the catarrhal to the febrile form was sudden and complete, the one entirely superseding the other[4]."

1842: In the ' Agincourt ' on a voyage from the Cape of Good Hope to Hongkong in August and September, the greater part of 102 cases of catarrh occurred; many of these were accompanied with inflammation of tonsils and fauces, and in some there was deafness with discharge from the ear. This is not claimed as an instance of epidemic influenza, but as an aggregate of common colds, due to cold weather in the Southern Ocean and to wet decks[5].

[1] Webster, II. 63.
[2] College of Physicians' Report. *Trans. Col. Phys.* III. (1785), p. 60–61. "Information has been received" of the incident.
[3] *Statist. Report of Health of Navy*, 1837–43. Parl. papers, 1 June, 1853, p. 8.
[4] *Ibid.* p. 14.   [5] *Ibid.* s. d.

1857: "Influenza broke out in the 'Monarch' while at sea, on the passage from Payta [extreme north of Peru] to Valparaiso. She left the former place on the 23d August, and arrived at the latter on the last day of September. About the 12th of the month [twenty days out], the wind suddenly changed to the south-west, when nearly every person in the ship began to complain of cold, although the thermometer did not show any marked change in the temperature. On the 12th and 13th seven patients were placed on the sick list with catarrhal symptoms; and during the following ten days, upwards of eighty more were added, but by the end of the month the attacks ceased. [She carried 690 men, and had 191 cases of "influenza and catarrh," in the year 1857.] Some of the cases were severe, ending either in slight bronchitis or pneumonia, accompanied with great prostration of the vital powers. On the arrival of the ship at Valparaiso, the surgeon observes: 'We found the place healthy, but in the course of a few days some cases of influenza made their appearance, and very soon afterwards the disease extended over the whole town. It was generally believed that we imported it, and the authorities took the trouble to send on board a medical officer to investigate the matter.' He further observes that the whole coast, from Vancouver's Island southward to Valparaiso was visited by the epidemic." It made its appearance on board the 'Satellite' at Vancouver's Island in September, and among the residents ashore, both on the island and mainland, at the same time [1].

1857: Catarrh "assumed the form of influenza in the 'Arachne' [149 men, 114 cases] while the vessel was cruizing off the coast of Cuba, "with which, however, she had no communication. There was nothing in the state of the atmosphere to attract special attention. A question therefore arises whether it might not have been caused by infection wafted from the shore." It was prevalent at the time at Havana [2].

1857: "Australian Station :—An eruption of epidemic catarrh occurred in the 'Juno' [200 men, 131 cases], but long after she left the station [3]."

Whilst the influenza was on the American Pacific coast in September, 1857, it was on the coast of China three months earlier—on board the 'Inflexible' at Hongkong on the 18th of May, and in the 'Amethyst' and 'Niger' in a creek near Hongkong early in June [4]. But it had been on the Pacific coast of South America the year before, according to the following:

"1856: Epidemic catarrh broke out in the 'President' when lying off the island of San Lorenzo in the bay of Callao, first on the 20th October, and the last cases were placed on the sick list on 1st November,—the usual period which influenza takes to pass through a frigate ship's company. About sixty required to be placed on the sick list." It had occurred on board English ships of war at Rio de Janeiro, on the other side of the continent, some two months before, in August, 1856 [5].

1863: The following, in the experience of the French navy, has been elaborately recorded [6]: The frigate 'Duguay-Trouin' left Gorée, Senegambia, for Brest, in February. There were no cases of influenza in Gorée when she left; but four days out, an epidemic of influenza began on board, the weather being fine and the temperature genial at the time. Another French frigate, which had left Gorée, on the same voyage to Brest, two days earlier, did not have a single case.

The following instance, here published for the first time, belongs to the most recent pandemics of influenza, 1890–93. It

---

[1] *Report on Health of Navy*, 1857, p. 69.   [2] *Ibid.* p. 41.
[3] *Ibid.* p. 131.   [4] *Ibid.* p. 112.   [5] *Report for* 1856, p. 100.
[6] Chaumezière, *Fievre catarrhals épidemique, observée à bord du vaisseau 'Le Duguay-Trouin' aux mois de Fevr. et Mars*, 1863. Paris, 1865. Cited by Hirsch.

relates to only a single case of influenza, in the captain of a merchantship ; it would have been a more satisfactory piece of evidence, if there had been several cases in the ship ; but among the comparatively small crew of a merchantman, the same groups of cases are not to be looked for that we find on board crowded men of war ; and in this particular case the only other occupants of the quarter-deck were the first mate and the steward.

The ship 'Wellington,' sailed from the Thames, for Lyttelton, New Zealand, on the 19th December, 1891. The epidemic of influenza in London in that year had been in May, June and July ; the mate of the 'Wellington' had had an attack of it ashore, on that occasion, but not the captain nor the steward. On the 2nd of March, 1892, when seventy-four days out and in latitude 42° S., longitude 63 E., near Kerguelen's Land, the captain began to have lumbago and bilious headaches, for which he took several doses of mercurial purgative followed by saline draughts. The treatment at length brought on continual purging, which, together with three days' starving from the 22nd to the 24th of March, caused him a loss of weight of eight pounds. The navigation had meanwhile been somewhat difficult and anxious, owing to a long spell of easterly head winds. Quite suddenly, on the 26th March, when the ship was in latitude 44 S., longitude 145 E., or about two hundred miles to the south of Tasmania, he had an aguish shake followed by prolonged febrile heat, which sent him to his berth. The symptoms were acute from the 26th to the 30th March,—intense pain through and through the head, as if it were being screwed tight in an iron casing, pain behind the eyeballs, a perception of yellow colour in the eyes when shut, a feeling of soreness all over the body, which he set down at the time to his uneasy berth while the ship was ploughing through the seas at about twelve knots, and a pulse of 110. The head pains were by far the worst symptom, and were so unbearable as to make the patient desperate. This acute state lasted for four days, and suddenly disappeared leaving great prostration behind. The captain, who had long experience with crews and passengers, and a considerable amateur knowledge of medicine, summed up his illness as a bilious attack, passing into "ague" with "neuralgia of the head." While the acute attack lasted the ship had covered the distance from Tasmania to the southern end of New Zealand, and on the 31st of March the captain by an effort came on deck to navigate the vessel in stormy weather up the coast to Lyttelton, which was reached on the 2nd of April. The pilot coming on board found the captain ill in his berth, and on being told the symptoms, at once said, "It is the influenza : I have just had it myself." The doctor who was sent for found the captain "talking foolishly," as he afterwards told him, and had him removed to the convalescent home at Christchurch, where he remained a fortnight slowly regaining strength. The doctor[1] could find no other name for the illness but influenza, although he had not supposed such a thing possible in mid-ocean. They had just passed through an epidemic of it in New Zealand, and it is reported about the same time in New South Wales, afterwards in the Tonga group, and still later in the summer in Peru. The symptoms of this case are sufficiently distinctive: the intense constricting pain of the head is exactly the "*fierro chuto*" or "iron cap" of South American epidemics ; the pain in the eyeballs, the soreness of the limbs and body, and the unparalleled depression and despair, are the marks of influenza without catarrh. The

---

[1] Dr Guthrie, of Lyttelton.

patient was of abstemious habits, and had made the same voyage year after year for a long period without any illness that he could recall. He had reduced himself by purging and starving, on account of a bilious attack during a fortnight of foul winds from the eastward, and had doubtless become peculiarly susceptible of the influenza miasm before the ship came into the longitude of Tasmania on the 26th March.

The Influenzas of Remote Islands.

The full and correct theory of influenza will not be reached by the great pandemics only. On the other hand some very localized epidemics may prove to be signal instances for the pathology, although they do not bear upon the source of the great historic waves of influenza. The instances in view are the influenzas started among a remote community on the arrival of strangers in their ordinary health. This phenomenon has been known at the island of St Kilda, in the Outer Hebrides of Scotland, since the year 1716, when it was recorded in the second edition of an essay upon the island by Martin. Some thought these "strangers' colds" mythical, so much so that Aulay Macaulay, in preparing a work upon St Kilda, was advised to leave them out; he declined to do so, and Dr Johnson commended him for his magnanimity in recording this marvel of nature. There is now no doubt about the fact. H.M.S. 'Porcupine' visited the island in 1860; a day or two after she sailed again, the entire population, some 200 souls, were afflicted with "the trouble," and another visitor, who landed ten days after the 'Porcupine's' visit, saw the epidemic of influenza in progress. The same thing happened in 1876, on the occasion of the factor landing, and again in 1877 on the occasion of a crew coming ashore from a wrecked Austrian ship. A medical account of this epidemic catarrh was given in 1886: The patient complains of a feeling of tightness, oppression and soreness of the chest, lassitude in some cases, pains in the back and limbs, with general discomfort and lowness of spirits. In severe cases there is marked fever, and great prostration. A cough ensues, at first dry, then attended with expectoration, which may go on for weeks[1].

In the remote island of Tristan d'Acunha, in the South Atlantic midway between the River Plate and the Cape of Good Hope, the same thing happens "invariably" on the arrival

[1] Macdonald, _Brit. Med. Journ._, 14 July, 1886.

of a vessel from St Helena[1]. It is reported also as a common phenomenon of the island of Wharekauri, of the Chatham Group, about 480 miles to the eastward of New Zealand. Residents, both white and coloured, suddenly fall into an illness, one symptom of which is that they feel "intensely miserable." It lasts acutely for about four days, and gradually declines. It resembles influenza in all respects, and is known by the name of *murri-murri*, which is curiously like the old English name of *mure* or *murre*. "The mere appearance of murri-murri is proof to the inhabitants, even at distant parts of the island, which is thirty miles long, that a ship is in port, insomuch that, on no other evidence, people have actually ridden off to Waitangi to fetch their letters[2]."

About equally distant in the Pacific from Brisbane, as Wharekauri from Christchurch, lies Norfolk Island, originally colonized by the mutineers of the 'Bounty.' A writer in a newspaper says:

"During a seven years' residence in Norfolk Island, I had opportunities of verifying the popular local tradition that the arrival of a vessel was almost invariably accompanied by an epidemic of influenza among the inhabitants of the island. In spite of the apparent remoteness of cause and effect, the connexion had so strongly impressed itself on the mind of the Norfolk Islanders that they were in the habit of distinguishing the successive outbreaks by the name of the vessel during whose visit it had occurred[3]."

Something similar has long been known in connexion with the Danish trade to Iceland, the first spring arrivals from the mother country bringing with them an influenza which the crews did not suffer from during the voyage, nor, in most cases, during the progress of the epidemic in Reikjavik. The experience at Thorshaven, in the Faröe Islands, has been the same[4].

These are important indications for the pathology of influenza in general. They point to its inclusion in that strange class of infections which fall most upon a population, or upon those orders of a population, who are the least likely to breed disease by anything that they do or leave undone. Veterinary as well

---

[1] *Cruise of H.M.S. 'Galatea' in* 1867-8.
[2] R. A. Chudleigh, in *Brit. Med. Journal*, 4 Sept. 1886. The experiences are not altogether recent, for they were noted for "the Chatham Islands and parts of New Zealand" by Dieffenbach, in his German translation of Darwin's *Naturalist's Voyage round the World*. See English ed. 1876, p. 435 *note*.
[3] *Pall Mall Gazette*, 11 Dec. 1889.
[4] Hirsch, *Geograph. and Histor. Pathol.* I. 29. Engl. Transl.

as human pathology presents instances of the kind[1]. In seeking for the source of such an infectious principle, we are not to look for previous cases of the identical disease, but for something else of which it had been an emanation or derivative or equivalent, something which may have amounted to no more than a disparity of physical condition or a difference of race. And as the countries of the globe present now as formerly contrasts of civilized and barbarous, nomade and settled, rude and refined, antiquated and modern, with the aboriginal varieties of race, it may be said, in this theory of infection, that mere juxtaposition has its risks. But, in the theory of influenza, the first requisite is an explanation of its phenomenal uprisings and wave-like propagation, at longer or shorter intervals, during a period of many centuries.

[1] See the chapter on Sweating Sickness in the first volume of this History, p. 269, and the author's other writings there cited.

CHAPTER IV.

SMALLPOX.

THE history of smallpox in Britain is that of a disease coming gradually into prominence and hardly attaining a leading place until the reign of James I. In this respect it is unlike plague and sweating sickness, both of which burst upon the country in their full strength, just as both made their last show in epidemics which were as severe as any in their history. In the former volume of this work I have shown that smallpox in the first Tudor reigns was usually coupled with measles, that in the Elizabethan period the Latin name *variolae* was rendered by measles, and that smallpox, where distinguished from measles, was not reputed a very serious malady[1]. From the beginning of the Stuart period, smallpox is mentioned in letters, especially from London, in such a way as to give the impression of something which, if not new, was much more formidable than before; and that impression is deepened by all that is known of the disease later in the 17th century, including the rising figures in the London bills of mortality.

An early notice of a particular outbreak of smallpox is found in the Kirk Session records of Aberdeen in 1610, under the date of 12 August: "There was at this time a great visitation of the young children with the plague of the pocks[2]."

---

[1] See the first volume, pp. 456–461. I shall add here a reference to smallpox among young people in Henry VIII.'s palace at Greenwich in 1528. Fox, newly arrived from a mission to France, writes to Gardiner, 11 May, 1528 (Harl. MS. 419, fol. 103): The king "commanded me to goe unto Maystress Annes chamber, who at that tyme, for that my Lady prynces and dyvers other the quenes maydenes were sicke of the small pocks, lay in the gallerey in the tilt yarde."

[2] *Selections from the Records of the Kirk Session, Presbytery and Synod of Aberdeen.* Edited by John Stuart, for the Spalding Club, Aberd. 1846, I. 427.

In 1612 there are various references to deaths from smallpox in
London in rich houses. In 1613, the Lord Harrington, who
is said in a letter of Dr Donne's to be suffering from "the pox
and measles mingled," died of smallpox (probably haemorrhagic)
on the Sunday before 3 March, at which date also the Lady
Burghley and two of her daughters were sick of the same
disease. Those two years were probably an epidemic period.
Another epidemic is known from a letter of December, 1621:
"The smallpox brake out again in divers places, for all the last
hard winter and cool summer, and hitherto we have had no
sultry summer nor warm winter that might invite them. The
Lord Dudley's eldest son is lately dead of them, and the young
Lady Mordaunt is now sick." On 28 January, 1623, "the
speech that the smallpox be very rife there [Newmarket] will
not hinder his [James I.'s] journey." The years 1623 and 1624
were far more disastrous by the spotted fever all over England;
but smallpox attended the typhus epidemic, as it often did in
later experience, the two together having "taken away many of
good sort as well as mean people."

The first epidemic of smallpox in London, from which some
figures of the weekly mortalities have come down, was in 1628:
this was the year before the Parish Clerks began to print their
annual bills, but they had kept the returns regularly since 1604,
and appear to have made known in one way or another the
weekly mortality and the chief diseases contributing thereto.
The smallpox deaths in London in the week ending 24 May,
1628, were forty-one, in the following week thirty-eight, and in
the third week of June fifty-eight[1]. Such weekly mortalities
in a population of about 300,000 belong to an epidemic of the
first degree; and it is clear from letters of the time that the
London smallpox of 1628 made a great impression. Lord
Dorchester, in a letter of 30 August, calls it "the popular
disease[2]." Several letters relating to a fatal case of smallpox in
June in the house of Sir John Coke in the city (Garlick Hill)
bear witness to the dread of contagion through all that circle of
society[3]. One of the letters may be cited:

[1] Mead to Stutteville, in *Court and Times of Charles I.*, I. 359. Joan, Lady Coke
to Sir J. Coke, 26 June, 1628. *Cal. Coke MSS.*
[2] Lord Dorchester to the Earl of Carlisle, 30 Aug. 1628, in *C. and T. Charles I.*:
"Your dear lady hath suffered by the popular disease, but without danger, as I
understand from her doctor, either of death or deformity."
[3] Gilbert Thacker to Sir J. Coke at Portsmouth, 9 June, 1628; Thomas Alured to
the same, 21 June; Richard Poole to the same, 23 June. *Cal. Coke MSS.*, I.

"It pleased God to visit Mrs Ellweys [Coke's stepdaughter] with such a disease that neither she nor any other of her nearest and dearest friends durst come near her, unless they would hazard their own health. The children and almost all our family were sent to Tottenham before she fell sick, and blessed be God are all in health. Mrs Ellweys was sick with us of the smallpox twelve days or thereabouts." Before she was out of the smallpox, she was taken in labour on 15 June, and died the next morning at five o'clock, being buried the same night at ten, with only Sir Robert Lee and his lady of her kindred at the funeral. The letter proceeds: "God knows we have been sequestered from many of our friends' company, who came not near us for fear of infection, and indeed we were very circumspect, careful, and unwilling that any should come to us to impair their health." Lady Coke was fearful to go to Tottenham because of the children who had been removed thither.

All the indications, whether from letters of the time, from poems and plays, or from statistics, point to the two first Stuart reigns as the period when smallpox became an alarming disease in London among adults and in the upper class. The reference to smallpox at Aberdeen in 1610 is to the disease among children; and so also is an unique entry, opposite the year 1636, on the margin of the register of Trinity parish, Chester: "For this two or three years, divers children died of smallpox in Chester[1]." In London, the disease had not yet settled down to that steady prevalence from year to year which characterized it after the Restoration. On the other hand, the periodic epidemics were very severe while they lasted. The epidemic of 1628 was followed by three years of very slight smallpox mortality in London; then came a moderate epidemic in 1632 and a severe one in 1634, with again two or more years of comparative immunity, as in the following table from the earliest annual printed bills:

Smallpox deaths in London, 1629–36[2].

Year	Smallpox deaths	Deaths from all causes
1629	72	8771
1630	40	10554
1631	58	8532
1632	531	9535
1633	72	8393
1634	1354	10400
1635	293	10651
1636	127	23359

Thomas Alured's house "hath been visited in the same kind, once with the measles and twice with the smallpox, though I thank God we are now free; and I know not how many households have run the same hazard."

[1] Harl. MS., No. 2177.

[2] The original heading in the Bills of Mortality was "flox and smallpox." "Flox" meant flux, or confluent smallpox, which was so distinguished, as if in kind, from the ordinary discrete form, seldom fatal. Huxham, in 1725, *Phil. Trans.* XXXIII. 379,

For the next ten years, 1637–46, the London figures are lost[1], excepting the plague-deaths and the totals of deaths from all causes, but it is known from letters that there was a great epidemic of smallpox in one of them, the year 1641: the deaths were 118 in the week ending 26 August, and 101 in the week ending 9 September[2], totals seldom reached a century later, when the population had nearly doubled. In those weeks of 1641, it was second only to the plague as a cause of dread, and was, along with the latter, the reason that "both Houses grow thin," for all the political excitement of the time. The next London epidemic was in 1649, when the annual bill gives 1190 deaths from smallpox. Willis says that the epidemic was also at Oxford that year, not so very extensive, "yet most died of it" owing to the severe type of the disease[3]. Five years after, in 1654, "at Oxford, about autumn, the smallpox spread abundantly, yet very many escaped with them." The London deaths from smallpox for a series of years were as follows:

Year	Smallpox deaths	Year	Smallpox deaths
1647	139	1655	1294
1648	401	1656	823
1649	1190	1657	835
1650	184	1658	409
1651	525	1659	1523
1652	1279	1660	354
1653	139	1661	1246
1654	832		

Smallpox after the Restoration.

The period which must now concern us particularly, from the Restoration onwards, opens with two deaths from smallpox in the royal family within a few months of the return of the

still used these terms: "When the pustules broke out in less than twenty-four hours from the seizure, they were always of the flux kind, as is commonly observed . . . Pocks which at first were distinct would flux together during suppuration." Dover, *Physician's Legacy*, 1732, p. 101, has "the flux smallpox, or variolae confluentes," as one of the varieties: and again, pustules "fluxing in some parts, in others distinct."

[1] Having been omitted by Graunt in his table. *Op. cit.* 1662.

[2] *Cal. State Papers*, under the dates. The epidemic seems to have revived in 1642. An affidavit among the papers of the House of Lords, excusing the attendance of a witness, states that Thomas Tallcott has recently lost his wife and one child by smallpox, and that he himself, six of his children and three of his servants are now visited with the same disease. 13 July, 1642, *Hist. MSS. Com.* v. 38. The Mercurius Rusticus, 1643, says that Bath was much infected both with the plague and the smallpox. Cited in Hutchins, *Dorsetshire*, III. 10.

[3] *Remaining Works.* Transl. by Pordage. Lond. 1681. "Of Feavers," p. 142. In one of his cases Willis was at first uncertain as to the diagnosis, because "the smallpox had never been in that place."

Stuarts. When Charles II. left the Hague on 23 May, 1660, to assume the English crown, his two brothers, the Duke of York and the Duke of Gloucester, accompanied him in the fleet. In the first days of September, the Duke of Gloucester was seized at Whitehall with an illness of which various accounts are given in letters of the time[1]. On 4 September, "the duke hath been very sick, and 'tis thought he will have the smallpox." On the 8th "the doctors say it is a disease between the smallpox and the measles; he is now past danger of death for this bout, as the doctors say"; or, by another account, "the smallpox come out full and kindly, and 'tis thought the worst is past." On the 11th the duke is "in good condition for one that has the smallpox." But a day or two afterwards his symptoms took an unfavourable turn; the doctors left him, apparently with a good prognosis, one evening at six o'clock, but shortly after he bled at the nose three or four ounces, then fell asleep, and on awaking passed into an unconscious state, in which he died. When his body was opened, the lungs were full of blood, "besides three or four pints that lay about them, and much blood in his head, which took away his sense." Pepys says his death was put down to the great negligence of the doctors; and if we can trust a news-letter of the time, their negligence was such as would have been now approved, for "the physicians never gave him anything from first to last, so well was he in appearance to everyone[2]." Three days after his funeral, the king and the Duke of York went to Margate to meet their sister, the princess Mary of Orange, on her arrival from the Hague. Her visit to the Court extended into the winter, and about the middle of December she also took smallpox, of which she died on the 21st. Pepys, dining with Lady Sandwich, heard that "much fault was laid upon Dr Frazer and the rest of the doctors for the death of the princess." Her sister, the princess Henrietta, who had come on a visit to Whitehall with the Queen-mother in October, was removed to St James's on 21st December, "for fear of the smallpox"; but she must have been already sickening, for on the 16th January it is reported that she "is recovered of the measles."

These deaths at Whitehall of a brother and sister of Charles II. happened in the autumn and winter of 1660; but

[1] *Histor. MSS. Commis.* v. 156–184. Sutherland Letters.
[2] Sutherland Letters, *u. s.* Andrew Newport to Sir R. Leveson at Trentham.

it was not until next year that the smallpox rose to epidemic
height in London, the deaths from it having been only 354
in 1660, rising to 1246 in 1661, and 768 in 1662. In 1661 it
appears to have been epidemic in other parts of England:
Willis, who was then at Oxford, says that smallpox began to
rage severely before the summer solstice (adding that it was
"a distemper rarely epidemical"), and there are letters from
a squire's wife in Rutlandshire to her husband in London, which
speak of the disease raging in their village in May and June[1].

There was much fever of a fatal type in London in 1661,
which is more noticed than smallpox itself in the diary of
Pepys. The town was in a very unhealthy state; and it would
have been in accordance with all later experience if the
"pestilential constitution" of fevers, which continued more or
less until the plague burst forth in 1665, had been accompanied
by much fatal smallpox. The occasion was used by two
medical writers to remark upon the fatality of smallpox as
something new. The second of the two essays (1663), was
anonymous, and bore the significant title of *Hactenus Inaudita*,
the hitherto unheard of thing being that smallpox should prove
so fatal as it had been lately. The author adopts the dictum of
Mercurialis, with which, he says, most men agree: "Smallpox
and measles are wont for the most part to terminate favourably";
and he makes it clear in the following passage that the blame of
recent fatalities was laid, justly or unjustly, at the door of the
doctors, as, indeed, we know that it was from the gossip of
Pepys:

"And I know not by what fate physicians of late have more lost their
credit in these diseases than ever: witness the severe judgment of the world
in the cases of the Duke of Gloucester and the Princess Royal: so that now
they stick not to say, with your Agrippa, that at least in these a physician is
more dangerous than the malady[2]."

The other essay was by one of the king's physicians,
Dr Tobias Whitaker, who had attended the Court in its exile at

[1] Mary Barker to Abel Barker, 26 May and 2 June, 1661. *Hist. MSS. Com.*
v. 398: "There is many dy out in this town, and many abroad that we heare of";
the squire's mother is living "within a yard of the smallpox, which is also in the
house of my nearest neighbour"; her own children had whooping cough, but do not
appear to have taken smallpox.
[2] *Hactenus Inaudita, or Animadversions upon the new found way of curing the
Smallpox.* London, 1663. Dated 10 July, 1662. The burden of his own complaint
is of a prominent personage in the smallpox who was killed, as he maintains, by
enormous doses of diacodium, an opiate with oil of vitriol, much in request among the
partisans of the cooling regimen.

St Germain and the Hague. He was by no means an empiric, as some were whom Charles II. delighted to honour; and, although he protests warmly against the modish injudicious treatment of smallpox by blooding and cooling, he has little of the recriminating manner of the time, which Sydenham used from the one side and Morton from the other. He is, indeed, all for moderation : "upon this hinge of moderation turneth the safety of every person affected with this disease." His moderation is somewhat like that of Sir Thomas Browne (whose colleague he may have been for a few years at Norwich), and is apt to run into paradox. In 1634 he wrote in praise of water, including the waters of spas and of the sea, and in 1638 he wrote with even greater enthusiasm in praise of wine[1]. He says of his "most learned predecessor" at Court, Harvey, that his demonstration of the circular motion of the blood was a farther extension of what none were ignorant of "though not expert in dissection of living bodies." On his return to London in 1660, he seemed to find as great a change in smallpox as in the disposition of the people towards the monarchy. His statement as to the change for the worse that had come over smallpox within his memory would be of the highest historical importance if we could be sure it was not illusory; it is difficult to reconcile with the London experiences of smallpox in 1628 and 1641, but, such as it is, we must take note of it :

"It is not as yet a complete year since my landing with his Majesty in England, and in this short time have observed as strange a difference in this subject of my present discourse as in the variety of opinions and dispositions of this nation, with whom I have discoursed." This disease of smallpox, he proceeds, "was antiently and generally in the common place of *petit* and *puerile*, and the cure of no moment....But from what present constitution of the ayre this childish disease hath received such pestilential tinctures I know not; yet I am sure that this disease, which for hundreds of yeares and before the practice of medicine was so exquisite, hath been as commonly cured as it hapned, therefore in this age not incurable, as upon my own practice I can testifie....Riverius will not have one of one thousand of humane principles to escape it, yet in my conjecture there is not one of one thousand in the universe that hath any knowledge or sense of it, from their first ingress into the world to their last egress out of this world ; which could

[1] His first book was Περὶ ὑδροποσίας, or *A Discourse of Waters, their Qualities and Effects, Diaeteticall, Pathologicall and Pharmacuiticall.* By Tobias Whitaker, Doctor in Physicke of Norwich. Lond. 1834. In 1638, being then Doctor in Physick of London, he published *The Tree of Humane Life, or the Bloud of the Grape. Proving the Possibilitie of maintaining humane life from infancy to extreame old age without any sicknesse by the use of wine.* An enlarged edition in Latin was published at Frankfurt in 1655, and reprinted at the Hague in 1660, and again in 1663. The passages cited in the text occur in his *Opinions on the Smallpox.* London, 1661.

not be, if it were so inherent or concomitant with maternal bloud and seed," referring to the old Arabian doctrine, which Willis adhered to, that every child was tainted in the womb with the retained impure menstrual blood of the mother, and that smallpox (or measles) was the natural and regular purification therefrom. "But smallpox," he continues, "is dedicated to infants more particularly which are moist, and some more than others abounding with vitious humours drawn from maternal extravagancy and corrupt dyet in the time of their gestation; and by this aptitude are well disposed to receive infection of the ayre upon the least infection[1]."

When Whitaker calls smallpox a "childish disease," a disease that was "antientiy and generally in the common place of *petit* and *puerile*, and the cure of no moment," he says no more than Willis and others say of smallpox as it affected infants and children. Says Willis: "there is less danger if it should happen in the age of childhood or infancy"; and again: "the sooner that anyone hath this disease, the more secure they are, wherefore children most often escape"; and again: "the measles are so much akin to the smallpox that with most authors they have not deserved to be handled apart from them," although he recognizes that measles is sooner ended and with less danger. Nor was Willis singular among seventeenth-century physicians in his view—"the sooner that anyone hath this disease the more secure they are." Morton in two passages remarks upon the greater mildness of smallpox in "infants": "For that they are less anxious about the result, infants feel its destructive force more rarely than others"; and again: "Hence doubtless infants, being of course ἀπαθεῖς, are afflicted more rarely than adults with the severe kinds of confluent and malignant smallpox[2]."

In the very first treatise written by an English physician specially on the Acute Diseases of Infants, the work by Dr Walter Harris, there is a statement concerning the mildness of "smallpox and measles in infants" (who are defined as under four years of age), which goes even farther than Morton's:

"The smallpox and measles of infants, being for the most part a mild and tranquil effervescence of the blood, are wont to have often no bad character, where neither the helping hands of physicians are called in nor the abounding skill of complacent nurses is put in requisition[3]."

[1] His only reference to the deaths in the royal family, which were currently set down to professional mismanagement, comes in where he opposes the prescription of Riverius to bathe the hands and feet in cold water: "this hath proved fatall," he says, "in such as have rare and tender skins, as is proved by the bathing of the illustrious Princess Royal. Therefore I shall rather ordain aperient fomentations in their bed, to assist their eruption and move sweat."

[2] *Pyretologia*, II. 94, 112.

[3] Walter Harris, M.D., *De morbis acutis infantum*, 1689. There were several editions, some in English.

It has to be said, however, that Morton's statement about infants is made to illustrate a favourite notion of his that apprehension as to the result, which infants were not subject to, made smallpox worse; and that Harris's assertion of the natural mildness of the "smallpox and measles" of infants comes in to illustrate the evil done by the heating regimen of physicians and nurses, who are mentioned in obviously sarcastic terms. So also Sydenham says that "many thousands" of infants had perished in the smallpox through the ill-timed endeavours of imprudent women to check the diarrhoea which was a complication of the malady, but was in Sydenham's view, although not in Morton's, at the same time a wholesome relieving incident therein. If we may take it that infants and young children had smallpox in a mild form, or more rarely confluent than in adults, we may also conclude that many of them died, whether from the alexipharmac remedies which Morton advised and Sydenham (with his follower Harris) denounced, or from the attendant diarrhoea which Sydenham thought a natural relief to the disease and Morton thought a dangerous complication.

Making every allowance for motive or recrimination in the statements, from their several points of view, by Willis, Sydenham, Morton, Harris (Martin Lister might have been added), as to the naturally mild course of smallpox in infants, or when not interfered with by erroneous treatment, it cannot but appear that infantile smallpox at that time was more like measles in its severity or fatality than the infantile smallpox of later times. It is perhaps of little moment that Jurin should have repeated in 1723 the statements of Willis and others ("the hazard of dying of smallpox increases after the birth, as the child advances in age")[1], for he had little intimate knowledge of epidemics, being at that time mainly occupied with mathematics, and with smallpox from the arithmetical side only. But it is not so easy to understand why Heberden should have said the same a generation after[2]; or how much credit should attach to the remark of "an eminent physician from Ireland," who wrote to Dr Andrew, of Exeter, in 1765: "Infants usually have the natural pock of as benign a kind as the artificial[3]."

[1] Jurin, *Letter to Cotesworth.* Lond. 1723, p. 11.
[2] Speaking of malignant sore-throat, he says: "The younger the patients are, the greater is their danger, which is contrary to what happens in the measles and smallpox." *Commentaries on Diseases,* p. 25.
[3] Andrew's *Practice of Inoculation impartially considered.* Exeter, 1765, p. 60.

Whatever may have been its fatality or severity among infants and children, it was chiefly as a disease of the higher ages that smallpox in the Stuart period attracted so much notice and excited so much alarm. The cases mentioned in letters and diaries are nearly all of adults; and these were the cases, whatever proportion they may have made of the smallpox at all ages, that gave the disease its ill repute. About the middle of the 18th century we begin to have exact figures of the ages at which deaths from smallpox occurred: the deaths are then nearly all of infants, so much so that in a total of 1622, made up from exact returns, only 7 were above the age of ten, and only 92 between five and ten; while an age-incidence nearly the same continued to be the rule until after the great epidemic of 1837–39, when it began gradually to move higher[1]. But we should err in imagining that state of things the rule for the 17th century, just as we should err in carrying it forward into our own time. Not only are we told that smallpox of infants was like measles in that the cure was of no moment (which is strange), but we do know from references to smallpox in the familiar writings of the Stuart period that many of its attacks, with a high ratio of fatalities, must have happened to adults. Thus, to take the diary of John Evelyn, he himself had small-pox abroad when he was a young man, his two daughters died of it in early womanhood within a few months of each other, and a suitor for the hand of one of them died of it about the same time. Medical writings leave the same impression of

---

[1] Duvillard (*Analyse et Tableaux de l'Influence de la Petite Vérole sur la Mortalité à chaque Age.* Paris, 1806) gives the ages at which 6792 persons died of smallpox at Geneva from 1580 to 1760, according to the registers of burials:

Total at all ages.	0—1,	—2,	—3,	—4,	—5,	—6,	—7,	—8,	—9,	—10,	—15,	—20,	—25,	—30.
6792	1376	1300	1290	898	603	381	301	189	109	78	126	54	39	31

The public health of Geneva altered very much for the better in the course of two centuries from 1561 to 1760. From 1561 to 1600, in every hundred children born, 30·9 died before nine months, on an annual average, and 50 before five years. From 1601 to 1700 the ratios were 27·7 under nine months, and 46 before five years. From 1701 to 1760 the deaths under nine months had fallen to 17·2 per cent., and under five years to 33·6 per cent. (Calculated from a table in the *Bibliothèque Britannique, Sciences et Arts,* IV. 327.) Thus, with an increasing probability of life, the age-incidence of fatal smallpox may have varied a good deal within the period from 1580 to 1760. It is given by Duvillard separately for the years 1700–1783 (inclusive of measles): during which limited period a smaller ratio died under nine months, and a larger ratio above the age of five years, than in the aggregate of the whole period from 1580 to 1760. Whatever may have been the rule at Geneva, it cannot be applied to English towns; for, while some 30 per cent. of the smallpox deaths were at ages above five in the Swiss city (1700–1783), only 12 per cent. were above five in English towns such as Chester and Warrington in 1773–4.

smallpox attacking many after the age of childhood. Willis gives four cases, all of adults. Morton gives sixty-six clinical cases of smallpox, the earliest record of the kind, and one that might pass as modern: twelve of the cases are under six years of age, nine are at ages from seven to twelve, eleven from thirteen years to twenty, seven from twenty-two to forty, and all but two of the remaining twenty-four clearly indicated in the text, in one way or another, as adolescents or adults, the result being that 23 cases are under twelve and 43 cases over twelve[1].

That ratio of adults to children may have been exceptional. Morton was less likely to be called to infants than to older persons, even among the middle class; and no physician in London at that time knew what was passing among the poorer classes, except from the bills of mortality. But if Morton had practised in London two or three generations later, say in the time of Lettsom, when "most born in London have smallpox before they are seven," his casebook would not have shown a proportion of forty-three cases over twelve years to twenty-three under that age. Whatever things contributed to the growing evil repute of smallpox among epidemic maladies, there is so much concurrent testimony to the fact itself that we can hardly take it to have been wholly illusion. In some parts the mildness of smallpox was still asserted as if due to local advantages. Thus Dr Plot, who succeeded Willis in his chair of physics at Oxford, wrote in 1677: "Generally here they are so favourable and kind that, be the nurse but tolerably good, the patient seldom miscarries[2]."

The reason commonly assigned for the large number of fatalities in smallpox after the Restoration was erroneous treatment. That is the charge made, not only in the gossip of the town, as Pepys reported it, but in Sydenham's animadversions on the heating regimen, in Morton's on the cooling regimen, and in the sarcasms of both physicians upon the practice of "mulierculae" or nurses. One may easily make too much of this view of the matter; it is certain that the incidence of smallpox, its fatality and its frequency in general, were determined in the Stuart period, as at other times, by many things besides. Still, the treatment of smallpox has always had the first place in its epidemiological history. The fashion of it that concerns us at

[1] *Pyretologia*, 2 vols. Lond. 1692–94, vol. II.
[2] *Natural History of Oxfordshire.* Oxford, 1677, p. 23.

this stage was the famous cooling regimen, commonly joined with the name of Sydenham.

Sydenham's Practice in Smallpox.

Sydenham occupied his pen largely with smallpox, and gained much of his reputation by his treatment of it. At the root of his practice lay the distinction that he made between discrete smallpox and confluent. His practice in the discrete form was to do little or nothing, leaving the disease to get well of itself. Whether the eventual eruption were to be discrete or confluent, he could not of course tell for certain until two or three days after the patient sickened; but in no case was the sick person to be confined to bed until the eruption came out. If the latter were sparse or discrete, the patient was to get up for several hours every day while the disease ran its course, the physician having small occasion to interfere with its progress: "whoever labours under the distinct kind hardly needs the aid of a physician, but gets well of himself and by the strength of nature." One may see how salutary a piece of good sense this was at the time, by taking such a case as that of John Evelyn, narrated by himself[1]. He fell ill at Geneva in 1646, and was bled, leeched and purged before the diagnosis of smallpox was made. "God knows," he says, "what this would have produced if the spots had not appeared." When the eruption did appear, it was only the discrete smallpox; the pimples, he says, were not many. But he was kept warm in bed for sixteen days, during which he was infinitely afflicted with heat and noisomeness, although the appearance of the eruption had eased him of his pains. For five whole weeks did he keep his chamber in this comparatively slight ailment. When he suggested to the physician that the letting of blood had been uncalled for, the latter excused the depletion on the ground that the blood was so burnt and vicious that the disease would have turned to plague or spotted fever had he proceeded by any other method[2].

As there were many such cases, Sydenham's radical distinction between discrete and confluent smallpox, with his

---

[1] In his *Diary*, under the year 1646, homeward journey from Rome.
[2] The physician was "a very learned old man," Dr Le Chat, who had counted among his patients at Geneva such eminent personages as Gustavus Adolphus and the duke of Buckingham.

advice to leave the former to itself, was of great value, and is justly reckoned to his credit. But in the management of confluent smallpox he advised active interference. If there were the slightest indication that the disease was to be confluent (that is to say, the eruption copious and the pocks tending to run together), he at once ordered the patient to receive a vomit and a purge, and then to be bled, with a view to check the ebullition of the blood and mitigate the violence of the disease. Even infants and young children were to have their blood drawn in such an event. This heroic treatment at the outset was according to the rule of *obsta principiis*; by means of it he thought to divert the attack into a milder course. The initial depletion once over, Sydenham had resort to what is known as the cooling regimen. He set his face against the "sixteen days warm in bed," which Evelyn had to endure even in a discrete smallpox. It was usually a mistake for the patient to take to bed continually before the sixth day from his sickening or the fourth day from the appearance of the eruption; after that stage, when all the pustules would be out, the regimen would differ in different confluent cases, and, of course, in some a continuance in bed would be inevitable as well as prudent. In like manner cardiac or cordial remedies, which were of a heating character, were indicated only by the patient's lowness. The more powerful diaphoretic treacles, such as mithridate, were always a mistake. The tenth day was a critical time, and then paregoric was almost a specific. In the stage of recovery it was not rarely prudent to prescribe cordial medicines and canary wine. Thus, on a fair review of Sydenham's ordinances for smallpox in a variety of circumstances, it will appear that he did not carry the cooling regimen to fanatical lengths and that he was sufficiently aware of the risks attending a chill in the course of the disease[1].

Apart from his rule of leaving cases of discrete smallpox to recover of themselves, Sydenham's management of the disease

[1] Dr Dover has left us an account of Sydenham's practice in the smallpox as he himself experienced it: " Whilst I lived with Dr Sydenham, I had myself the small-pox, and fell ill on the twelfth day. In the beginning I lost twenty ounces of blood. He gave me a vomit, but I find by experience purging much better. I went abroad, by his direction, till I was blind, and then took to my bed. I had no fire allowed in my room, my windows were constantly open, my bedclothes were ordered to be laid no higher than my waist. He made me take twelve bottles of small beer, acidulated with spirit of vitriol, every twenty-four hours. I had of this anomalous kind to a very · great degree, yet never lost my senses one moment." *The Ancient Physician's Legacy.* London, 1732, p. 114.

was neither approved generally at the time, nor endorsed by posterity. His phlebotomies in confluent cases, usually at the outset, but sometimes even after the eruption was out if the patient had been under the heating regimen before, were an innovation borrowed from the French Galenists. The earlier writers had, for the most part, excepted smallpox among the acute maladies in which blood was to be drawn. But the Galenic rules of treatment were made more rigorous in proportion as they were challenged by the Paracelsist or chemical physicians, and it was among the upholders of tradition that blood-letting was extended to smallpox. Whitaker says that, when he was at St Germain with the exiled Stuarts, the French king was blooded in smallpox ten or eleven times, and recovered; "and upon this example they will ground a precept for universal practice."

The ambiguity of the diagnosis at the outset, and the desire to lose no time, may have been the original grounds of this indiscriminate fashion of bleeding. Evelyn's doctor at Geneva in 1646, "afterwards acknowledged that he should not have bled me had he suspected the smallpox, which brake out a day after," but eventually he defended his practice as having made the attack milder. In like manner Sir Robert Sibbald, of Edinburgh, (1684) took four ounces of blood from a child of five, who was sickening for some malady; when it turned out to be smallpox, the mother expressed her alarm that blood should have been drawn; but Sibbald pointed to the favourable character of the eruption as justifying what he had done: "Optime enim eruperunt variolae, et ab earum eruptione febris remissit[1]."

The ill effects of blood-letting, says Whitaker, may be observed in French children, which by this frequent phlebotomizing are "withered in *juvenile* age." Therefore, he concludes, blooding in smallpox should not be a common remedy, "but in such extremity as the person must lose some part of his substance to save the whole." He calls it the rash and inconsiderate practice of modish persons; "and if the disease be conjunct [confluent], with an undeniable plethory of blood, which is the proper indication of phlebotomy, yet such bleeding ought to be by scarification [upon the arms, thighs or back] and cupping-glasses, without the cutting of any major vessel." Another English physician of the time, Dr Slatholm, of Buntingford in Hertfordshire, who wrote in 1657[2], says that he had known physicians in Paris not to abstain from venesection in children of tender age, even in sucklings. He had never approved the

---

[1] *Scotia Illustrata.* Lib. II., cap. 10.
[2] *De Febribus &c.*, Lond. 1657: cap. ix. "De Variolis et Morbillis," p. 141.

letting of blood in such cases, lest nature be so weakened as to be unable to drive the peccant matter to the skin. For the most part, he says, an ill result follows venesection in smallpox; and although it sometimes succeeds, yet that is more by chance than by good management. As to exposing the sick in smallpox to cold air, he declares that he had known many in benign smallpox carried off thereby, instancing the case of his brother-in-law, the squire of Great Hornham, near Buntingford, whose death from smallpox in November, 1656, in the flower of his age, he set down to a chill brought on "ejus inobedientia et mulierum contumacia[1]."

The cooling regimen, as well as the danger of it, was familiar long before Sydenham's time. There could be no better proof of this than a bit of dialogue in Beaumont and Fletcher's 'Fair Maid of the Inn' (Act II. scene 2), a comedy which was licensed in January, 1626:

Host. And you have been in England? But they say ladies in England take a great deal of physic....They say ladies there take physic for fashion.
Clown. Yes, sir, and many times die to keep fashion.
Host. How! Die to keep fashion?
Clown. Yes: I have known a lady sick of the smallpox, only to keep her face from pit-holes, take cold, strike them in again, kick up the heels, and vanish.

Sydenham says that the heating regimen was the practice of empirics and sciolists. Per contra his distinguished colleague Morton says that every old woman and apothecary practised the cooling regimen, and he points the moral of its evil consequences in a good many of his sixty-six clinical cases[2]. He pronounces the results of the cooling regimen to have been disastrous; he had been told that Sydenham himself relaxed the rigour of his treatment in his later years. There was so

---

[1] "First of all," he says, "let the patient be kept with all care and diligence from cold air, especially in winter, so that the pores of the skin may be opened and the pocks assisted to come out. Therefore let him be kept in a room well closed, into which cold air is in no manner to enter, and let him be sedulously covered up in bed. . . . I desire the more to admonish my friends in this matter, for that Robert Cage, esquire, my dear sister's husband," etc.

[2] Besides cases to show the ill effects of blooding, vomits, purges and cooling medicines such as spirit of vitriol, he gives examples as if to refute Sydenham's favourite notion that salivation, diarrhoea and menstrual haemorrhage were relieving or salutary. Morton's chief object was to bring out the eruption, and to get it to maturate kindly; an eruption which languished, or did not rise and fill, was for him the most untoward of events. Sydenham, on the other hand, argued that the danger was in proportion to the number of pustules and to the total quantity of matter contained in them; and he sought, accordingly, to restrain cases which threatened to be confluent by an evacuant treatment or repressive regimen.

little smallpox for some fifteen years after the date of Morton's book (1694) that the controversies on its treatment appear to have dropped. But, on the revival of epidemics in 1710 and 1714, essays were written against blooding, vomits and purges in smallpox[1].

In 1718, Dr Woodward, the Gresham professor of physic and an eminent geologist, published some remarks on "the new practice of purging" in smallpox, which were directed against Mead and Freind. In 1719 Freind addressed a Latin letter to Mead on the subject (the purging was in the secondary fever of confluent smallpox), and a lively controversy arose in which Freind referred to Woodward anonymously as a well-known empiric. On the 10th of June, 1719, about eight in the evening, Woodward was entering the quadrangle of Gresham College when he was set upon by Mead. Woodward drew his sword and rested the point of it until Mead drew his, which he was long in doing. The passes then began and the combatants advanced step by step until they were in the middle of the quadrangle. Woodward declared (in a letter to the *Weekly Journal*) that he was getting the best of it, when his foot slipped and he fell. He found Mead quickly standing over him demanding that he should beg his life. This Woodward declined to do, and the combat degenerated to a strife of tongues[2]. Next year the controversy over the treatment of smallpox assumed a triangular form. The third side was represented by Dr Dover, who had been something of a buccaneer on the Spanish main and was now in practice as a physician. An old pupil of Sydenham's, he still adhered to blood-letting in smallpox; and in the spring of 1720, when the disease was exceedingly prevalent among persons of quality in London, he claimed to have rescued from death a lady whom Mead had given over, by pulling off the latter's blisters and ordering a pint of blood to be drawn. "He hath observed the same method with like success with several persons of quality this week, and is as yet in very great vogue... He declaims against his brethren of the faculty [especially Mead and Freind], with public and

[1] Walter Lynn, M.B., *A more easy and safe Method of Cure in the Smallpox founded upon Experiments, and a Review of Dr Sydenham's Works*, Lond. 1714; *Some Reflections upon the Modern Practice of Physic in Relation to the Smallpox*, Lond. 1715. F. Bellinger, *A Treatise concerning the Smallpox*, Lond. 1721.
[2] Letter from Woodward to the *Weekly Journal*, 20 June, 1719, in Nichols, *Lit. Anecd.* VI. 641.

great vehemence, and particularly against purging and blistering in the distemper, which he affirms to be the death of thousands[1]."

Huxham, another Sydenhamian, appears to have practised not only blooding in smallpox, but also blistering, purging and salivating[2]. But in that generation the practice was exceptional; so much so that when it revived in some hands about 1752 (including Fothergill's), it was thus referred to in a letter upon the general epidemic of smallpox in that year: " I have heard that bleeding is more commonly practised by some of the best physicians nowadays than it was formerly, even after the smallpox is come out[3]." In smallpox the lancet, like other methods, has been in fashion for a time, and then out of fashion ; but the old teaching that smallpox did not call for blood-letting was ultimately restored. When Barker, in 1747, gave a discourse before the College of Physicians on the " Agreement betwixt Ancient and Modern Physicians," he did not venture to defend Sydenham's blooding in smallpox, although he would not admit that he was " a bloodthirsty man[4]."

Causes of Mild or Severe Smallpox.

Besides the errors of the heating or the cooling regimen respectively, there is another thing that may have had something to do with the greater fatality of smallpox, as remarked by many, about the middle of the 17th century. " How is it," asks Sydenham, " that so few of the common people die of this disease compared with the numbers that perish by it among the rich[5]?" Sydenham may not have known how much smallpox mortality there was in the poorer quarters of London. But the Restoration was certainly a great time of free living in the

[1] Rev. Dr Mangey to Dr Waller, 4 March, 1720, London. Nichols' *Lit. Anecd.* I. 135.
[2] Huxham, *Phil. Trans.* XXXII. (1725), 379.
[3] *Gent. Magaz.*, Sept. 1752.
[4] John Barker, M.D., *Agreement betwixt Ancient and Modern Physicians*, Lond. 1747. Also two French editions. It is on Van Helmont that Barker pours his scorn for " breaking down the two pillars of ancient medicine—bleeding and purging in acute diseases." That upsetting person forbore to bleed even in pleurisy; the only thing that he took from the ancient medicine was a thin diet in fevers ; " and yet this scheme, as wild and absurd as it seems, had its admirers for a time."
[5] Lynn (u. s. 1714-15) agrees as to the matter of fact, namely, that the mortality from smallpox was greater among the richer classes, who were too much pampered and heated in their cure, than among the poorer, who had not the means to fee physicians and pay apothecaries' bills.

upper classes of society, and it is equally certain that smallpox was apt to prove a deadly disease to a broken constitution. Willis believed that excesses even predisposed people to take the infection: "I have known some to have fallen into this disease from a surfeit or immoderate exercise, when none besides in the whole country about hath been sick of it." There were, of course, families in which smallpox was for some unknown reason peculiarly fatal. Again, the origins of constitutional weakness are lost in ancestry, the poor stamina of children being often determined by the lives of their grandfathers or great-grandfathers. In the royal family of Stuart smallpox proved more than ordinarily fatal, but it was among the grand-children and great grand-children of James I. that those fatalities happened. Of the children of Charles I., the Duke of Gloucester and the Princess of Orange died of smallpox within a few months of each other in the year of the Restoration. The disease was not less fatal a generation after in the family of the Duke of York (James II.). Dr Willis fell into disgrace with that prince because he bluntly told him that the ailment of one of his sons was "mala stamina vitae." All his sons, says Burnet, died young and unhealthy, one of them by smallpox. Of his two daughters, Queen Mary died of haemorrhagic smallpox in 1694, and the Duke of Gloucester, only child of the other, Princess Anne of Denmark (afterwards Queen Anne), died at the age of eleven, of a malady which was called smallpox by some, and malignant sorethroat by others[1].

Among the medical writers of this period, who gave reasons why smallpox should be so severe or deadly in some while it was so slight in others, Morton was the most systematic. He made three degrees of smallpox—benign, medium and malignant: these did not answer quite to the discrete, confluent and haemorrhagic of other classifiers, for his malignant class included so many confluent cases that in one place he uses *malignae* as the equivalent of *confluentes seu cohaerentes*, while his middle class was made up of some confluent cases,—perhaps such medium cases as had confluent pocks on the face but not

---

[1] He was under the tutelage of John Churchill, duke of Marlborough, who does not give a name to the malady (Coxe's *Life of Marlborough*). Dr James Johnstone, junr., of Worcester, in his *Treatise on the Malignant Angina*, 1779, p. 78, claims the death of the Duke of Gloucester as from that cause, on the evidence of Bishop Kennet's account.

elsewhere,—and a certain proportion of discrete. The medium kind were the most common (*frequentissimae sunt et maxime vulgares variolae mediae*). Still, it was the benign type that he made the *norma* or standard of smallpox, from which the disease was "deflected" towards the medium type, or still farther deflected towards the malignant. He gives a list of fourteen things that may serve to deflect an attack of smallpox from the *norma* of mildness to the degrees of mean severity or malignity:

1. If the eruption come out too soon or too late.
2. If the patient be sprung from a stock in which smallpox is wont to prove fatal, as if by hereditary right.
3. If the attack fall in the flower of life, when the spirits are keener and more inclined to febrile heats.
4. If the patient be harassed by fever, or by sorrow, love or any other passion of the mind.
5. If the patient be given to spirituous liquors, vehement exercise or anything else of the kind that tends to irritate the spirits.
6. If the attack come upon women during certain states of health peculiar to them.
7. If cathartics, emetics and blooding had been used.
8. If the heating regimen had been carried to excess, or other ill-judged treatment followed.
9. If the patient had met a chill at the outset, checking the eruption.
10. If the attack happen in summer.
11. If the attack happen during a variolous epidemic constitution of the air.
12. If the patient be pregnant or newly married.
13. If the patient be consumptive or syphilitic.
14. If the patient be apprehensive as to the result.

Morton having made the benign type the norm, made the medium type the commonest; and that was really true of the first great epidemic in London in his experience, in the years 1667–68. Sydenham says of it that the cases were more than he ever remembered to have seen, before or after: "nevertheless, as the disease was regular and of a mild type, it cut off comparatively few among the immense number of those who took it." Pepys enters this epidemic under the date of 9 Feb. 1668: "It also hardly ever was remembered for such a season for the smallpox as these last two months have been, people being seen all up and down the streets newly come out after the smallpox." Let us pause here for a moment to ask what Pepys may have meant by recognising the people all up and down the streets newly come out after the smallpox. Did he mean that they were pock-marked? We may answer the question by the testimony of Dr Fothergill for a correspondingly mild and extensive preva-

lence of smallpox in London some three generations later, which I shall take out of its order because it bears upon the question of pitting. His report for December 1751 is:[1]

"Smallpox began to make their appearance more frequently than they had done of late, and became epidemic in this month. They were in general of a benign kind, tolerably distinct, though often very numerous. Many had them so favourably as to require very little medical assistance, and perhaps a greater number have got through them safely than has of late years been known." The January (1752) report is: "A distinct benign kind of smallpox continued to be the epidemic of this month; a few confluent cases, but rarely." In February he writes: "Children and young persons, unless the constitution is very unfavourable, get through it very well; and the height to which the weekly bills are swelled ought to be considered, in the present case, as an argument of the frequency, not the fatality, of this distemper." In June the type was still favourable: "Crowds of such whom we see daily in the streets without any other vestige than the remaining redness of a distinct pock."

This was an epidemic such as Sydenham alleges that of 1667–68 to have been; and the vestiges of smallpox by which Pepys recognized those who were newly come out of the disease were probably the same that Fothergill saw in 1752.

A practitioner at Chichester does indeed say as much of those treated by himself about the same date: "when the distemper did rage so much in and about Chichester, ten or a dozen years since [written in 1685], it was a great many that fell under my care, I believe sixty at the least, and yet I lost but one person of the disease. Nor was one of my patients marked with them to be seen but half a year after[2]." As these experiences must have been somewhat exceptional I shall give a section to the general case.

Pockmarked Faces in the 17th Century.

The smallpox of 1667–68 had among its numerous victims one of the king's mistresses, the beautiful Frances Stewart, duchess of Richmond, residing in Somerset House, who caught

---

[1] In the *Gentleman's Magazine*, under the dates.

[2] *A Direct Method of ordering and curing People of that Loathsome Disease the Smallpox*, being the twenty years' practical experience of John Lamport alias Lampard, London, 1685. The writer was probably an empiric, "Practitioner in Chyrurgery and Physick," dwelling at Havant, and attending the George at Chichester on Mondays, Wednesdays and Fridays, the Half Moon at Petersfield on Saturdays. He says: "One great cause of this disease being so mortal in the country is because the infection doth make many physicians backward to visit such patients, either for fear of taking the disease themselves or transferring the infection to others." He has another fling at the regular faculty: "Do not run madding to Dr Dunce or his assistance to be let blood." Empirics, although they were commonly right about blood-letting, were under the suspicion of not speaking the truth about their cures.

the disease in March 1668 and was "mighty full of it." Pepys, who records the fact, had seen her portrait taken shortly before: "It would make a man weep," he exclaims, "to see what she was then and what she is likely to be by people's discourse now." Happily the worst fears were not realized. Pepys saw her driving in the Park in August, and remarks, without a strict regard to grammar, that she was "of a noble person as ever I did see, but her face worse than it was considerably by the smallpox." The king, unlike the Lord Castlewood of romance, suffered no loss of ardour for his mistress, having visited her over the garden wall, as Mr Pepys relates, on the evening of Sunday, the 10th of May. It is rather the idea, and especially the historical idea, of these horrors that "would make a man weep," and it has moved a great and eloquent historian of our own time to deep pathos[1]. If there be anything that can counteract the effects of agreeable rhetoric it is perhaps statistics. The following numerical estimate of the proportion of pockmarked faces in London after the Restoration is accordingly offered with all deference. It applies mainly to the criminal and lower classes, who were as likely as any to bear the marks of smallpox.

In the *London Gazette*, the first advertisement of a person "wanted" appears in December, 1667; and thereafter until June, 1774, there are a hundred such advertisements of runaway apprentices, of footmen or other servants who had robbed their masters, of horse-stealers, of highwaymen, and the like. There is always a description more or less full; and in the consecutive hundred I have included only such persons as are so particularly described in feature that pock-pits would have been mentioned if they had existed. It is not until the ninth case that "pock-holes in his face" occurs in the description, the eleventh case following close, with the same mark of identity. Then comes a long interval until the twenty-fourth and twenty-fifth cases, both with pock-holes, two of a band of highwaymen concerned in an attempt to rob the Duke of Ormond's coach near London, one of them having emerged from Frying-pan Alley in Petticoat Lane. Fifteen cases follow, all described by distinctive features, without mention of pock-marks, until

[1] Macaulay, *History of England*, IV. 532. The moving passage on the former horrors of smallpox, *à propos* of the death of Queen Mary in 1694, is familiar to most, but it may be cited once more in the context of a professional history: "That disease, over which science has since achieved a succession of glorious and beneficent victories, was then the most terrible of all the ministers of death. The havoc of the plague had been far more rapid: but plague had visited our shores only once or twice within living memory; and the smallpox was always present, filling the churchyards with corpses, tormenting with constant fears all whom it had not yet stricken, leaving on those whose lives it spared the hideous traces of its power, turning the babe into a changeling at which the mother shuddered, and making the eyes and cheeks of the betrothed maiden objects of horror to the lover." It is not given to us all to write like this; but it is possible that the loss of picturesqueness may be balanced by a gain of accuracy and correctness.

we come to the fortieth, a boy of twelve or thirteen, who "hath lately had the smallpox." The next is the forty-ninth, a Yorkshireman, long-visaged, and "hath had the smallpox," and close upon him the fiftieth "marked with smallpox." Then come four in quick succession, the 56th, 59th, 61st and 63d; next the 71st; and then a long series with no marks of smallpox, until the 95th, 97th, 99th and 100th, three of these last four having been negroes.

The result is that sixteen in the hundred are marked more or less with smallpox, four of them being black men or boys. One had "lately had the smallpox," another had "newly recovered of the smallpox." One was a cherry-cheeked boy of twelve, "somewhat disfigured with smallpox," who had run away from Bradford school. Two are described as much disfigured, some as a little disfigured, several others as "full of pock-holes." The same mark of identity is occasionally mentioned in the advertisements beyond the hundred tabulated, but not more frequently than before, the usual term in the later period being "pock-broken." This proportion of pock-marked persons among the London populace, sixteen in the hundred, or about twelve in the hundred excluding negroes, does not err on the side of under-statement, if it errs at all. Some such small ratio is what we might have expected in the antecedent probabilities, arising out of the varying degrees of severity of smallpox and the various textures of the human skin. Pitting after smallpox has always been a special risk of a certain texture of the skin, namely, a sufficient thickness of the vascular layer to afford the pock a deep base. Such complexions are common enough even in our own latitudes; and those are the faces that have always borne the most obvious traces of smallpox. It was some of the confluent cases, or rather, of such of them as recovered, that became pock-marked: the babe that became a changeling was not likely to survive. Adults retained the marks more than children, so that there must always have been a good many pock-marked faces in a population where the incidence of the disease was largely upon grown persons, as in the 17th century and in our own time. When smallpox was something of a novelty at the end of the Elizabethan period, a poet addressed a pathetic lyric to his mistress's pock-marked face. A medical writer of the same period reproduces the old Arabian prescription against pitting, to open the pocks on the face with a golden pin, and adds: "I have heard of some, which, having not used anythinge at all, but suffering them to drie up and fall of themselves, without picking or scratching,

have done very well, and not any pits remained after it[1]."
Whitaker, in 1661, dismisses the risk of pitting very briefly,
remarking that the means of prevention was "commonly the complement of every experienced nurse[2]." Morton, in his sixty-six
clinical cases and in his commentary, makes but slight reference
to pitting. In his 14th case, a severe one, "no scars remained";
in his general remarks he treats pitting as a bugbear: "women
set the fairness of their faces above life itself," which may mean,
as in Beaumont and Fletcher's comedy, that they would chill
themselves at all risks by the cooling regimen so they might drive
the pocks in[3].

The Epidemiology continued to the end of the 17th century.

What little remains to be said of smallpox in England to
the end of the seventeenth century may be introduced by the
following table of the deaths in London.

Smallpox Deaths in London 1661 to 1700.

Year	Total deaths	Smallpox deaths	Year	Total deaths	Smallpox deaths
1661	16,665	1246	1681	23,951	2982
1662	13,664	768	1682	20,691	1408
1663	12,741	411	1683	20,587	2096
1664	15,453	1233	1684	23,202	1560
1665	97,306	655	1685	23,222	2496
1666	12,738	38	1686	22,609	1062
1667	15,842	1196	1687	21,460	1551
1668	17,278	1987	1688	22,921	1318
1669	19,432	951	1689	23,502	1389
1670	20,198	1465	1690	21,461	778
1671	15,729	696	1691	22,691	1241
1672	18,230	1116	1692	20,874	1592
1673	17,504	853	1693	20,959	1164
1674	21,201	2507	1694	24,100	1683
1675	17,244	997	1695	19,047	784
1676	18,732	359	1696	18,638	196
1677	19,067	1678	1697	20,972	634
1678	20,678	1798	1698	20,183	1813
1679	21,730	1967	1699	20,795	890
1680	21,053	689	1700	19,443	1031

[1] Kellwaye, u. s., 1593.
[2] Dr Richard Holland in 1730 (*A Short View of the Smallpox*, p. 75), says: "A
lady of distinction told me that she and her three sisters had their faces saved in a bad
smallpox by wearing light silk masks during the distemper."
[3] As I do not intend to come back to the subject of pockmarked faces, I shall add
here that I have found nothing in medical writings of the 18th century, nor in its fiction
or memoirs, to show that pockpitting was more than an occasional blemish of the
countenance. At that time most had smallpox in infancy or childhood, when the
chances of permanent marking would be less. The disappearance of pockpitted faces

Sydenham's remarks throw some light on the smallpox of the several years. While the epidemic of 1667–68 was of a regular and mild type, that of 1670–72, which has fewer deaths in the bills, was of the type of black smallpox complicated with flux. The year 1674 has the highest figures yet reached; the type of the disease was confluent, and so severe that it "almost equalled the plague"; while the smallpox of the year 1681, with a still higher total, was "confluent of the worst kind."

It is not easy to make out what the differences of "type" described by Sydenham depended on; but it may be hazarded that those who fell into smallpox in an otherwise unhealthy season would die in larger numbers, being weakened by antecedent disease, such as measles or epidemic diarrhoea, influenza or typhus fever. An epidemic of measles in the first six months of 1674 was most probably the reason of the great fatality of smallpox in the second half of that year (see the chapter on Measles). The high figures of smallpox mortality in 1681 followed two hot summers, unhealthy with infantile diarrhoea, and coincided with a third season unhealthy in the same way. The deaths by smallpox in the last week of August, 1681, reached the very high figure of 168, the next highest cause of death that week, and the highest the week after, being "griping in the guts," or infantile diarrhoea. The smallpox of 1685 was more uniformly distributed over the months of the year, which was one of malignant typhus, the worst week for fever having 114 deaths (ending 29 Sept.), and the worst week for smallpox 99 deaths (ending 18 Aug.).

The deaths by smallpox in the London bills are the only 17th century figures of the disease. According to later experience, a high mortality in London in a certain year meant an epidemic general in England in that or the following year; and the same appears to have held good for the period following the

was discovered long ago. The report of the National Vaccine Board for 1822 says: "We confidently appeal to all who frequent theatres and crowded assemblies to admit that they do not discover in the rising generation any longer that disfigurement of the human face which was obvious everywhere some years since." The members of this board were probably seniors who remembered the 18th century; and it is quite true that the first quarter of the 19th century was singularly free from smallpox in England except in the epidemic of 1817–19. But the above passage became stereotyped in the reports: exactly the same phrase, appealing to what they all remembered "some years since," was used in the report for 1825, a year which had more smallpox in London than any since the 18th century, and again in the report for 1837, the first year of an epidemic which caused forty thousand deaths in England and Wales. These stereotyped reminiscences are apt to be as lasting a blemish as the pockholes themselves.

Restoration. In the parish register of Taunton, a weaving town, the smallpox deaths are many in 1658 ("all the year," which was one of agues and influenza), in 1670, 1677, and 1684 ("very mortal," the year being noted for a very hot summer and for fevers and dysenteries[1]). The highest total of deaths in London to the end of the 17th century fell in 1681, which is known to have been a year of very fatal smallpox at Norwich[2] and at Halifax. Thoresby's friend Heywood lost three children by it at the latter town in the epidemic of 1681, which does not appear to have visited Leeds. In 1689 Thoresby himself lost his two children at Leeds within a few days. In 1699 the epidemic returned, and he again lost two of the four children that had been born to him in the interval[3]. Similar calamities befell country houses, of which the following from the correspondence of a titled family in Cumberland is an instance:

"17th April, 1688,—Captaine Kirkby came hither, and told me that Mrs Skelton, my god-daughter, of Braithwaite, dyed the last week, and her two children, of the smallpockes[4]."

Rumours of "smallpox and other infectious disease" at Cambridge in the summer of 1674[5], and at Bath in the summer of 1675[6], threatened to interfere with the studies of the one place and the gaieties of the other.

Smallpox in London in 1694: the death of the Queen.

The epidemic of smallpox in London in 1694 was made memorable by the death of the queen. On 22 November Evelyn notes, "a very sickly time, especially the smallpox, of which divers considerable persons died"; on 29 December:

[1] Collinson, *Hist. of Somerset*, III. 226, citing Aubrey's *Miscellanies*, 33.
[2] Blomefield, *Hist. of Norfolk*, III. 417.
[3] Thoresby, *Ducatus Leodiensis*, ed. Whitaker. App. p. 151.
[4] *Cal. Le Fleming MSS.* p. 408 (*Hist. MSS. Com.*). There are also many references to smallpox from 1676 onwards in the letters of the Duke of Rutland at Belvoir, lately calendared for the Historical MSS. Commission.
[5] In the *London Gazette* of 11–14 May, 1674, the Vice-Chancellor and two doctors of medicine of the University of Cambridge contradicted by advertisement a report that smallpox and other infections were prevalent in the university.
[6] Marquis of Worcester to the Marchioness, [London] 8 June, 1675 (Beaufort MSS. *Hist. MSS. Commis.* XII. App. 9, p. 85): "They will have it heere that the smallpox and purple feaver is at the Bath, and the Dutchesse of Portsmouth puts off her journey upon it. The king askt me about it as soon as I came to towne. Pray enquire, and lett me know the truth." The *London Gazette* of 17–21 June and 28 June–1 July, 1775, had advertisements "that it hath been certified under the hands of several persons of quality" that Bath and the country adjacent was wholly free of the plague or any other contagious distempers whatsoever.

"the smallpox increased exceedingly, and was very mortal," the queen having died of it the day before. Queen Mary came of a stock to which smallpox had been peculiarly fatal, a brother and sister of her father, James II., having died of it at Whitehall in 1660. Some of the particulars of her illness and death come from bishop Burnet[1], who saw her in the first days of the attack and was about the Court until the end of it; the authentic medical details are by Dr Walter Harris, one of the physicians in attendance, who published them, by leave of his superiors, in order to meet the censures passed on the doctors "by learned men at a great distance[2]."

The symptoms of illness on the first day did not prevent the queen from going abroad; but, as she was still out of sorts at bedtime, she took a large dose of Venice treacle, a powerful diaphoretic which her former physician, the famous physiologist Dr Lower, had recommended her to take as often as she found herself inclined to a fever[3]. Finding no sweat to appear as usual, she took next morning a double quantity of it, but again without inducing the usual effect of perspiration. Up to that time she had not asked advice of the physicians. To this severe dosing with one of the most powerful alexipharmac or heating medicines, the malignant type of the ensuing smallpox was mainly ascribed by Harris, who was a follower of Sydenham and a partizan of the cooling regimen. On the third day from the initial symptoms the eruption appeared, with a very troublesome cough; the eruption came out in such a manner that the physicians were very doubtful whether it would prove to be smallpox or measles. On the fourth day the smallpox showed itself in the face and the rest of the body "under its proper and distinct form." But on the sixth day, in the morning, the variolous pustules were changed all over her breast into the large red spots "of the measles"; and the erysipelas, or rose, swelled her whole face, the former pustules giving place to it. That evening many livid round petechiae appeared on the forehead above the eyebrows, and on the temples, which Harris says he had foretold in the morning. One physician said these were not petechiae, but sphacelated spots; but next morning a surgeon proved by his lancet that they contained blood. During the night following the sixth day, Dr Harris sat up with the patient, and observed that she had great difficulty of breathing, followed soon after by a copious spitting of blood. On the seventh day the spitting of blood was succeeded by blood in the urine. On the eighth day the pustules on the limbs, which had kept the normal variolous character longest, lost their fulness, and changed into round spots of deep red or scarlet colour, smooth and level with the skin, like the stigmata of the plague. Harris observed about the region of the heart one large pustule filled with matter, having a broad scarlet circle round it like a burning coal, under which a great deal of extravasated blood was found when the body was examined after death. Towards the end, the queen slumbered sometimes, but said she was not refreshed thereby. At last she lay silent for some hours; and some words that came from her shewed, says Burnet, that her thoughts had begun to break. She died on the 28th of December, at one in the morning, in the ninth day of her illness.

[1] Burnet, *History of his own Time*, IV. 240.
[2] Walter Harris, M.D., *De morbis acutis infantum*. Ed. of 1720, p. 161.
[3] John Cury, M.D., *An Essay on Ordinary Fever*. Lond. 1743, p. 40.